At the Core of Mental Health

At the Core of Mental Health

Key issues for practitioners, managers and mental health trainers

Edited by Di Bailey

At the Core of Mental Health

Key issues for practitioners, managers and mental health trainers

Edited by Di Bailey

Published by:
Pavilion Publishing (Brighton) Ltd
The Ironworks
Cheapside
Brighton
East Sussex
BN1 4GD

Tel: 01273 623222
Fax: 01273 625526
Email: pavpub@pavilion.co.uk
Web: www.pavpub.com

First published 2000.

A Catalogue record for this book is available from the British Library.

ISBN 1 84196 049 7

Pavilion is committed to providing high quality, good value, current training materials and conferences, and bringing new ideas to all those involved in health and social care. Founded by health and social care professionals, Pavilion has maintained its strong links with key agencies in the field, giving us a unique opportunity to help people develop the skills they need through our publications, conferences and training.

Pavilion editor: Jo Hathaway with Julia Brennan
Cover and page design: Greg Levitt
Layout: Vanessa Good
Printing by: Ashford Press (Southampton)

Contents

Part Three

Part Four

Foreword

For many years now, it has been clear that more joint, shared and multidisciplinary approaches are needed across the mental health field, both in the management and delivery of services and in the training and education of workers. Many people, and indeed organisations, agree to this in principle. Yet it is the putting of this principle into practice that is the hard task. Organisational and professional barriers are often large and difficult to overcome. Sometimes it can feel like you have made a start and are beginning to break down the barriers with increased co-operation and sharing. Then, you can reach a sticky period and everyone retreats back behind their organisational and professional barriers – back to square one, so to speak.

So it is encouraging to read this book, aimed at mental health workers of all professions and persuasions and not at any one specific group.

The publication is a core text, which provides knowledge and understanding to underpin core competencies – competencies for all mental health workers.

It is great to have all this knowledge and understanding in one place, and it will save teachers/learners a great deal of effort and time.

The value-base for this book is equally important. Valuing the contribution of people who use services, as well as families and carers, should clearly be the basis of all contemporary mental health services. Valuing diversity is another important theme in this publication, and is clearly based on an understanding of discrimination and oppression within services as well as within the wider context of people's day-to-day lives. It is no surprise to find these values as Birmingham University has a fine record of being at the forefront in these important underpinning aspects of mental health work and services.

Birmingham University's postgraduate programme for staff within community mental health services is known to be one of the best in the UK and builds on their work at qualifying level in training for mental health. This book reflects the high quality of that programme. If we genuinely want to modernise mental health services, we must finally escape from the shadow of the large psychiatric hospitals, which were mainly built in the 19th Century. Now we have reached the 21st Century, we can use policies like the National Service Framework for Mental Health to help to build a more competent and skilled mental health workforce. Indeed, a workforce that is also able to communicate and speak a common language, and preferably a language that service users can understand.

This book provides knowledge and understanding for this workforce, and is a clear step in the right direction.

Thurstine Basset

Associate Consultant, Institute for Applied Health and Social Policy, King's College, London and External Examiner, Diploma in Mental Health Studies, University of Brighton

About the contributors

Annie Mitchell is a lecturer and clinical tutor on the Doctorate in Clinical and Community Psychology at the University of Exeter and was previously Lecturer in Complementary Healthcare for several years. She has worked as a researcher and as a clinical psychologist with various client groups, children with disabilities, adult mental health and people with chronic pain.

Peter Ferns is an independent training consultant with a wide experience of working in social services, health, probation services and voluntary sector organisations. He has undertaken practical research projects in the public sector and has engaged in service evaluation and development. He also undertakes leadership training and teamworking in the commercial sector. For several years he has been involved in the development of culturally appropriate community-based services.

Dr David Rothery is a consultant child and adolescent psychiatrist who has been working in the specialist adolescent service at Parkview Clinic in Birmingham for the past 15 years. He also has many years of experience in teaching other professionals in relation to the use of both The Children's Act legislation and The Mental Health Act legislation with children and adolescents.

Professor David Kingdon has been a professor of mental health care delivery at the University of Southampton since September 1998. He previously worked as Medical Director in Nottingham, Senior Medical Officer at the Department of Health and as Adult Psychiatrist in Bassetlaw, Nottinghamshire. He is Chairman of the Committee of Experts in 'Human Rights and Psychiatry' Council of Europe, Strasbourg and was a member of the NHSE National Service Framework External Reference Group.

Ann Davis is Professor of Social Work in the Department of Social Policy and Social Work at the University of Birmingham. She trained as a psychiatric social worker and has worked in hospital, residential and community settings. She has published and researched in the areas of poverty and mental health, and users' experiences of mental health services. She is a professional advisor for the National Schizophrenia Fellowship. She is a member of the TOPPS mental health training group for England.

Aidan Houlders has been a senior forensic social worker at the Reaside Medium Secure Unit in Birmingham since 1989. He has worked in a variety of settings including hospital and community-based social work teams and also as a social worker attached to General Practice. He also has experience of working with a range of client groups including young offenders, children and family work and as an approved social worker under the *1983 Mental Health Act*. Aidan acts as a practice teacher and is Chair of the Midlands, Northern England and Wales Forensic Social Workers Group. He was a member of the steering group for establishing the competencies for the Advanced Award in Forensic Social Work.

Dr. Mike Radford is a community consultant psychiatrist in a multi-ethnic inner city area of Birmingham where he works collaboratively to promote a recovery-oriented community mental health service. He is also Clinical Director for the South Birmingham Mental Health (NHS) Trust. Mike's commitment to community psychiatry and user involvement stems from his clinical and research experience in community development projects in Birmingham and northern Rhodesia and his work in therapeutic communities. He has worked as

At the Core of Mental Health © Pavilion 2000

a consultant child and adult psychiatrist in Bermuda where he was also medical director and advisor to the Minister of Health and Social Services. He has worked in the Bethlem and Maudsley Hospital and as a resarch fellow at the Institute of Psychiatry at London University.

Di Bailey is the Programme Director for the Postgraduate Multidisciplinary Programme in Community Mental Health at the University of Birmingham. She has many years experience in mental health, working with people with severe and enduring mental illness spanning the voluntary and statutory sectors and including working in the forensic setting. Di also has 12 years' training experience in a variety of settings. She has research and consultancy experience particularly in relation to mental health in primary care, multidisciplinary working, service delivery and implementing and managing change effectively.

Bryony Moore has worked as a clinical psychologist in the West Midlands since 1983, for the last 12 years within the Regional Forensic Mental Health Service, based at Reaside Clinic in Birmingham. Her other field of practice is in the provision of specialist clinical psychology opinion to the courts and related agencies.

Elizabeth Armstrong is Executive Director of the Depression Care Training Centre and a founder member and Director of PriMHE, Primary Care Mental Health Education. She is a general nurse and health visitor, a former theatre sister in Princess Mary's Royal Air Force Nursing Service and an experienced community nurse, primary care facilitator and trainer.

Carole Fernandez currently works as the Post Qualifying Co-ordinator for Cambridgeshire Social Services. She has 17 years' social work practice experience, 11 of which she spent as social worker for the West Midlands regional psychiatric adolescent unit (Parkview clinic, Birmingham).

Dr Graham Stokes is Consultant Clinical Psychologist at Premier Health NHS Trust, Staffordshire, with responsibility for psychology services to older adults. He is also Consultant Director of Mental Health at BUPA care, an honorary teaching fellow at Coventry University, and honorary lecturer in the Department of Social Policy and Social Work, as well as honorary tutor in the Department of Psychology University of Birmingham.

Zaffer Iqbal is Clinical Research Fellow at Birmingham University, although he spends most of his time in West Yorkshire where he is leading the research-led development of an early intervention service.

Max Birchwood is Director of the Early Intervention Service, Birmingham and Professor of Clinical Psychology at the University of Birmingham. Together with colleagues, he has pioneered the early intervention concept and established the first dedicated service in the UK. He has been closely involved in the development and implementation of psychosocial interventions for people with psychosis, including cognitive therapy for psychotic symptoms, early signs monitoring and family intervention. He is Patron to the National Schizophrenia Fellowship.

Marian Barnes is Reader and Director of Social Research in the Department of Social Policy and Social Work. She is a member of the national Health Action Zones evaluation team, focusing in particular on community involvement and inter-agency partnerships, and is leading a team undertaking research on public participation and social exclusion in the ESRC Democracy and Participation programme. She has worked with user and carer groups and with voluntary agencies seeking to develop greater citizen participation. As well as her university based work, she is a member of the Advisory Committee of WISH – Women in Special Hospitals and Secure Units, and acts as an Independent Chair of a social services complaints review panel.

Acknowledgements

Editing a collected work is rarely easy, and I am thankful that *At the Core of Mental Health* is at last complete!

This would not have been possible without the support of all the contributors and the administrative skills of Dee Partridge at the University of Birmingham, together with Chris Parker at Pavilion, who supported my initial suggestion that this book should be written.

I would also like to acknowledge all the service users and mental health workers who have inspired some of the theory and practice that is explored in the following chapters. Finally, can I thank all those readers who have come to this book looking for inspiration in their practice; I hope you find it here.

Di Bailey
Editor

Introduction

Anyone in the field of education and training will appreciate that when planning a training programme, setting the objectives which describe what the trainee will have achieved as a result of that training are an integral part of the overall training process. These objectives need to be considered in terms of the knowledge, skill and attitudes required of the individuals in order to do their job effectively on a day-to-day basis. Ideally, they should link to the strategic development objectives of the organisation employing the individuals.

Because of the increasing complexity of mental health practice in the community, as opposed to institutional settings, employers of mental health practitioners are keen to recruit people who can 'do the job' and make a difference to the care and treatment of people using such services. Not surprisingly, employers have looked to training programmes both at qualifying and at post-qualifying levels to provide the workforce with the skills, knowledge and attitudes they are seeking. As a result there has been a shift in emphasis towards training activities that are focused upon the skill-based element of learning. Participants are increasingly being asked to demonstrate what they can *do* as a consequence of the training.

An example of this shift in focus in relation to mental health can be seen by the changes that were made in 1993 to the framework for training approved social workers (CCETSW, 1993) with the result that in order to become approved, social workers needed to demonstrate 38 competencies in relation to mental health practice. Whilst a more recent revision of these competencies has reduced them in number (CCETSW, 2000) the approach essentially remains the same.

A similar emphasis on competencies is also evident in attempts that have been made to define the skills of mental health workers more generally, irrespective of discipline (Sainsbury Centre for Mental Health, 1997 and 2000; Institute of Health and Care Development, 1998). With the emergence of the National Service Framework in Mental Health (1999) the need to agree the core set of competencies required of practitioners to implement the framework has been identified and is being worked on currently.

The competence frameworks identified above are paralleled in the academic education and training arena by the identification of learning outcomes associated with mental health training programmes such as the postgraduate, multidisciplinary programme for staff working in the community mental health field which my colleagues and I have devised at the University of Birmingham.

Alongside this shift in emphasis to skills-based learning has been a recognition that more participative methods are required in the training room, such that participants are able to practise what is being 'preached' to them, at least in some limited way, before being required to transfer the learning and apply it in the work setting. Gone are the days when 'talk and chalk' lectures were the desired method for disseminating information. This has been replaced by the notion that learning through participant interaction is the way forward. This is coupled with a recognition, certainly at post-qualifying level, that learners bring with them a range of expertise. They should be encouraged to build upon this foundation and share experiences rather than be subject to an 'expert' at the front of the room, often sharing 'pearls of wisdom' that are outdated and far removed from the context of contemporary practice.

However, whilst this focus on action may be reassuring to employers, purchasers of services and practitioners to some extent (as, after all, they have to do the job), it is not supported by the knowledge we have about the way adults learn. Whilst adult learning needs to involve some learning by doing, it also must address needs to reflect upon the learning, practice or repeat the skills being taught, and facilitate transfer of the learning to the real world of the work setting. Several authors have proposed a cyclical process for effective learning. The one shown below is an amalgamation of the stages proposed by Honey and Mumford (1992) and those outlined by Kolb (1974) in his original work on problem-solving which Honey and Mumford adapted. The cycle illustrates that whilst some people have a preferred style of learning, effective learning can only be achieved if all elements of the process are accommodated.

There is no prescribed pattern for the learning process and the sequence of stages followed will depend upon the preference of the

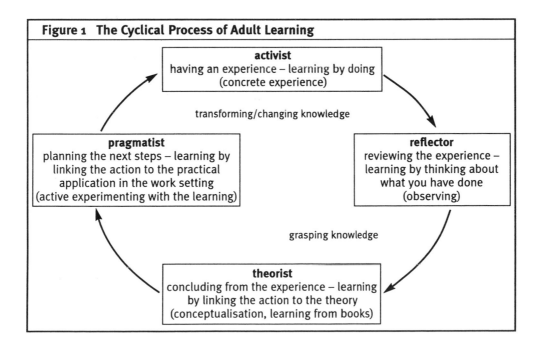

Figure 1 The Cyclical Process of Adult Learning

activist
having an experience – learning by doing
(concrete experience)

transforming/changing knowledge

reflector
reviewing the experience –
learning by thinking about
what you have done
(observing)

grasping knowledge

theorist
concluding from the experience – learning
by linking the action to the theory
(conceptualisation, learning from books)

pragmatist
planning the next steps – learning by
linking the action to the practical
application in the work setting
(active experimenting with the learning)

learner. However, it can be deduced from **Figure 1** that practitioners working in the mental health field who prefer to learn by doing, or by the practical applications of their learning, will probably most favour the competence approach to training. This leaves those who prefer to have a theoretical frame of reference to work from in a potentially disadvantaged position, if too much emphasis is placed upon competence frameworks.

No doubt those involved in education and training will also wish to debate the point as to whether a practitioner can be completely competent if they do not have the underlying knowledge base on which to build their practice. The answer of course is that they can't. Indeed, CCETSW have acknowledged the difficulty of encapsulating a knowledge base within the writing of practice-based competencies, and have listed the underpinning knowledge areas required of ASWs separately in their new guidance to programmes (CCETSW, 2000).

The Sainsbury Centre (1997) referred to 'knowledge and understanding' in a number of their core competencies (17 out of a total of 27) and the Programme in Community Mental Health at Birmingham, whilst focused on outcomes, recognises that some of these outcomes must be underpinned by a sufficient knowledge base if they are to be properly demonstrated. For example, practitioners cannot plan and implement cognitive behavioural therapy (CBT) interventions, or risk and relapse management plans without knowing something about what CBT entails and what areas a risk and relapse management plan should address.

For these reasons it was decided to produce a core text that would support practitioners on a number of mental health training programmes spanning the qualifying and post-qualifying levels. Whilst the underpinning knowledge in respect of the legal framework surrounding mental health practice is provided in the all-inclusive *Mental Health Act Manual* (6th Edition) (Jones, 2000), there is a lack of texts which cover the range of topics needed to inform the knowledge base in areas other than the law. It is thus envisaged that practitioners will use this textbook as a starting point from which to build their knowledge base as their practice becomes more advanced. The aim of this text is therefore to provide up-to-date coverage on some of the key issues being debated at the core of modern day mental health practice. It will hopefully replace the need for training providers to have to seek out numerous different handouts from several different sources to support the mental health training they are delivering.

For ease of access the book is organised into four parts, each reflecting a specific theme in relation to modern mental health care. However it must be made clear from the outset that the ordering of these sections and their constituent chapters in no way reflects a hierarchy of importance of the topics covered. The book is organised in this way to assist with the accessibility of material such that readers can easily locate relevant sections when studying related topic areas on training programmes.

Part One deals with signs and symptoms of presenting mental distress, concentrating mainly on depression, schizophrenia and affective psychosis. These topics were chosen as probably the most common types of disorders that people in the mental health field are working with. Signs and symptoms are then discussed more specifically in relation to two groups of young people and older adults, who tend to fall outside adult services but whom practitioners are also likely to come into contact with in the course of their day-to-day practice.

Part Two looks at service configuration spanning the primary and secondary care interface and the overlap with services for specific groups, particularly mentally disordered offenders and people with both mental health and substance misuse needs.

Part Three explores specific techniques for practice including care planning and keyworking, risk assessment, and early intervention alternatives to more mainstream approaches by including a chapter on social psychiatry and complementary therapies.

Finally, **Part Four** takes a look at anti-discriminatory issues in relation to women, Black people and service users themselves in an attempt to provide a balance of perspectives with an exploration of what users themselves want to see on offer from mental health services.

It is worth stating that the chapters are written from very different perspectives and in very different ways. Some, such as the chapters on depression and risk assessment, are very practical, almost step-by-step guides about how to assess and intervene. In contrast, the chapters on young people and older adults use case material to highlight the points being raised. This diversity of contributions is intentional for several reasons. Firstly, all the contributors come from different disciplines and backgrounds and as such provide a contribution to a core text which reflects multidisciplinary working as the core business in effective mental health care delivery. Secondly, having outlined the different needs of adult learners, it would be futile to try and provide chapters all written in the same style.

It is intended that the core text as a whole will appeal to the diverse population of all adult learners by offering a range and style of contributions to reflect their individual style and approach practice.

Finally, the editor and contributors wish to make a clear statement to the readers that as a group of professionals we value diversity in its widest sense and are keen to develop services and contributions to mental health practice which reflect this. This is a statement about our own 'value base'. We are committed to the development of user-centred practice which is anti-discriminatory and anti-oppressive. We are also committed to contributing to the knowledge, skills and attitudes required of practitioners if they too are to practise in this way.

Whilst it is not expected that this one text will provide all the answers in terms of contemporary thinking in the field of mental health, it is a drawing together of research, frameworks and models of practice which should underpin mental health training and should be used by practitioners and trainers alike to ensure that programmes are underpinned by a sound knowledge base on which to build.

At the Core of Mental Health © Pavilion 2000

References

CCETSW (1993) *Requirements and Guidance for the Training of Social Workers to be Considered for Approval in England and Wales Under the Mental Health Act 1983.* Paper 19.19, revised edition London: CCETSW.

CCETSW (2000) *Assuring Quality for Mental Health Social Work: Requirements for the Training of Approved Social Workers in England, Wales and Northern Ireland and of Mental Health Officers in Scotland.* London: CCETSW.

Honey, P. & Mumford, A. (1992) *Manual of Learning Styles.* Maidenhead: Honey.

Institute of Health and Care Development (1998) *Core Competencies for Mental Health Workers:* A project commissioned by the NHS Executive North West Regional Office Bristol. London: Institute of Health and Care Development.

Kolb, D. A. (1974) *Experiential Learning.* New Jersey: Prentice Hall.

Jones, R. (1996) *The Mental Health Act Manual* (6th Edition). London: Sweet and Maxwell.

NHS (1999) *Mental Health National Service Frameworks: Modern Standards and Service Model.* London: DoH.

Sainsbury Centre for Mental Health (1997) *Pulling Together: the future roles and meaning of mental health staff.* London: Mind.

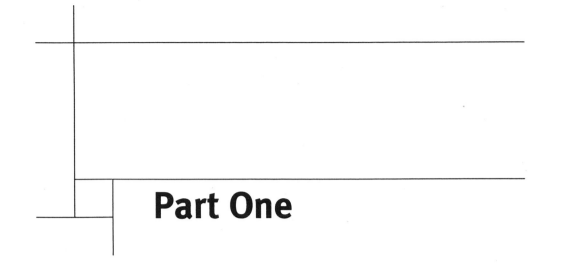

Part One

Chapter 1

Depression: signs and symptoms, assessment and intervention

Martin Davies

What is Depression?

The word 'depression' has different meanings to different people, with a range of interpretations extending between normal low mood and a life-threatening disorder. Depression is clinically different from the 'blues' and involves chemical changes. It is an illness that has both psychological and physical symptoms with a high morbidity rate. It is as common as asthma and more common than diabetes, heart disease and any cancer.

Depression is the 'common cold' of mental illness, affecting one in twenty adults at any one time (Paykel & Priest, 1992). Its prevalence in the general population is approximately 5% (6.4% in women and 3.2% in men). Anxiety is a common feature, with a mixed depression-anxiety state being more common than the separate disorders.

Primary care services are in the front line of all mental illnesses, accounting for up to 40% of GPs' consultations. Research shows that up to 50% of depression cases is missed in general practice (Tylee &

Freeling, 1989). Specialist psychiatric services will encounter only a small percentage of this large group (less than 10%) as depression is more usually recognised and managed within the primary care setting (see **Chapter 5**).

Perhaps one of the simplest ways to illustrate the incidence of depression is to consider an average general practitioner's caseload of 2000 people. Amongst this population there will be approximately 100 people with minor symptoms, 200 people with moderate depression symptoms, and 100 people with major depressive illnesses. An established link exists between the presentation of depressive symptoms and suicidal behaviour. Currently there is one suicide every two hours in the United Kingdom, and two thirds of the victims will have a depressive illness (Department of Health, 1992). If recognised early, depression can be successfully treated using drug and non-drug options. Recognising risk factors and using good consultation skills can help this early recognition, thus intervening at a point that may in fact prevent the illness from developing further.

In summary, depression, though common, is treatable and often preventable.

Depression can be described in terms of a *'continuum'* (Paykel & Priest, 1992):

Normal low mood	Normal low mood + loss of functioning	Abnormal low mood + loss of functioning

Severity ⟶

As one moves along this continuum, functioning decreases, whilst the severity of the symptoms increase. The ability to cope with the changes in mood decrease as the chemical changes that take place in depression become more profound. This continuum can be divided into three categories of depression, dependant on the severity – **mild**, **moderate**, and **severe**.

The **range of symptoms** often includes low mood, poor concentration, sleep and appetite disturbance. There are often co-existing symptoms of anxiety. These symptoms can become evident through a loss of *libido*, feelings of worthlessness and suicidal ideas, worries over health, and negative thinking.

Major depression is identified by the World Health Organisation (WHO) International Classification of Diseases (ICD-10, 1992) as depressed mood and loss of interest and pleasure plus four or more of the following:

- feelings of worthlessness or guilt

- impaired concentration

- loss of energy and fatigue

- thoughts of suicide

- loss or increase of appetite and weight

- insomnia or hypersomnia

- retardation or agitation.

These signs must be in evidence for a duration of at least two weeks.

A diagnosis of depression can be secondary to organic factors which include endocrine disorders, brain disorders, drugs, blood disorders, infections, drug withdrawal, kidney disease and some malignancies. It is important, as part of the assessment process to fully investigate any possible organic causes.

Causes of depression

The causes of depression are multi-factorial. External factors such as life events and circumstances may influence internal factors, such as self-esteem and the ability to cope, and vice versa. Depression does appear to run in some families, but this may be more due to learning than to genetic factors. There appears to be some evidence that certain types of depression, such as manic depression, may be affected by a genetic predisposition. Children who suffer the loss of a parent in early life appear to be more predisposed to depressive illness than those who continue to have a parent throughout their childhood and adolescent years. Other factors such as self-esteem, problem-solving abilities, social and spiritual wellbeing, and personality all play their part in an individual's emotional and psychological health.

The factors which can contribute to the presentation of depression can be grouped under four headings:

- **life events** eg relationship problems, bereavement, financial difficulties, loss

- **lack of social support** eg not having someone to talk to, to share worries

- **chronic illness** eg back pain, arthritis, diabetes, asthma, heart disease, cancer

- **predisposing factors** eg a family history of depression and/or anxiety, and/or personality disorders. The use of alcohol and illicit drugs can also induce depressive symptoms.

Traditionally, definitions relating to depression have used terms such as 'endogenous/reactive' and 'psychotic/neurotic'. They have been replaced with the terms mild, moderate and major, referred to earlier. Whatever the reason for the illness, it should still be treated appropriately. Simply because an individual has a 'reason' for their depression (eg suffering a bereavement), this should not mean that it is not treated. Older definitions may have contributed to inappropriate or inadequate treatment of what is a very disabling illness. Modern drug treatments, talking treatments and self-help approaches all have their place in the prevention and treatment of depression.

Why is it missed?

Research has shown that there are essentially three reasons why depression is missed (Freeling & Paykel, 1985):

1 **patient** reasons – something the patient does that inhibits the detection of depression

2 **clinician** reasons – something that the clinician does to inhibit detection

3 **consultation** reasons – something that happens within the dynamics of the consultation.

These can be because the individual presenting:

■ does not mention any psychological symptoms

■ somatises their emotional pain into something physical

■ does not disclose, due to embarrassment and the stigma of having a mental health problem

■ harbours misbeliefs about the clinician's role and time

■ has no insight or understanding of the illness

■ has experienced depression over a long period of time

■ covers up any signs by smiling and being dismissive

■ focuses on a physical problem.

The clinician can miss depression as a result of:

■ lack of time for the consultation

■ lack of skills and confidence in detection

■ not asking any psychological type questions

■ their own suffering, misery or worries

■ not recognising 'at risk' factors

■ having few resources or options

- showing signs of being in a hurry

- being preoccupied with physical/organic factors

- showing little empathy

- poor listening skills

- making little in the way of eye contact.

A consultation will render detection difficult if the discussion involves:

- no mention of anything psychological

- the environment created is not conducive to a sensitive discussion.

Recognising depression

Recognising depression requires the use of particular skills and sensitive questioning. Skills required are the ability to listen, to use silences effectively, to show empathy, and to pick up non-verbal cues. When asking questions, it can be easier to ask 'closed' questions – those that have only a 'yes' or 'no' answer, but this will not help towards gaining the information that is required. Sensitive and 'open' questions are essential in recognising an early difficulty. An example of such an approach can be as follows:

Practitioners should use screening questions:

'How bad is it?'

'How long have you felt like this?'

'Have you lost interest in things?'

'Are you more tired than usual?'

If the person replies 'yes' to any of these, the practitioner should ask:

'Have you lost confidence in yourself?'

'Do you feel guilty about things?'

'Do you find it difficult to concentrate?'

'How are you sleeping?'

'Have you lost appetite/weight?'

'Do you feel life is not worth living?'

(Armstrong & Lloyd, 1994)

Screening tools can be helpful to detect the more detailed nature of the presenting problem.

Screening tools are used in physical health assessments such as asthma, where one such tool is the peak flow meter. This can help identify when people are falling below the 'normal' lung function expectation. This helps the practitioner, alongside a full assessment, to identify a possible clinical condition before it becomes problematic or unmanageable. In depression, there are many such tools in the form of screening questionnaires, that are well researched and validated. Examples of these are:

- the HAD scale (Hospital Anxiety and Depression scale)
- the GHQ (General Health Questionnaire)
- the Beck Depression Inventory (France & Robson, 1986)
- the GDS (Geriatric Depression Scale)
- the EPDS (Edinburgh Postnatal Depression Scale).

When a diagnosis or assessment is unclear or disputed, such screening tools become extremely valuable. The person presenting completes the questionnaire within the consultation, which will only take a few minutes, and a score is calculated by the practitioner. The score will help clarify whether there is evidence of illness or reasons for further assessment. These questionnaires are suitable for use in general practice, and by other healthcare workers such as psychologists, psychiatric nurses, social workers, psychiatrists and counsellors. Their value is in the measurement of outcomes which can be helpful in evaluating 'recovery'.

The **advantages** include:

- saving time by addressing many issues at once and in a 'safe' manner

- clarifying on initial assessment

- validating an assessment

- helping the person to acknowledge the illness

- allowing the person an 'easy' method of expressing themselves

- demonstrating to the person that the practitioner is interested in their distress

- showing the person that this is a common illness, by using a standardised form

- standardising a common language between practitioners which improves communication

- by repeating the questionnaire at intervals, practitioners and the individuals themselves can monitor the course of the illness

- by repeating its use, it can be seen whether an intervention is working or not.

Assessment

There are specific points that must be addressed when assessing depression. These are:

- severity

- duration

- biological symptoms

- social support

- suicidal thinking

- view of self and the world.

Having a series of specific questions for each of these broad headings allows a structured approach to be adopted. Using the screening tools mentioned above to accompany such an assessment can be a useful addition. It must be pointed out that such an assessment may require several sessions to carry out, and that the practitioner must accept an assessment of this nature may need to be staged and time should be allocated accordingly. It is therefore important to ask the individual to return at a time that will allow this to be completed. It must also be noted that asking one question may generate the answers to several others. Looking at the assessment in more detail, it can be broken down into individual questions:

Assessment of:	Possible questions:
severity	– how bad is it?
	– have you felt like this before?
	– on a scale of 0 to 10 how do you feel just now? (screening questionnaire can help determine severity)
duration	– how long have you felt like this?
	– have you been feeling like this constantly for...?

biological symptoms	– how are you sleeping?
	– how are you eating?
	– how is your concentration?
	– do you feel tired most of the time?
	– have you lost interest in things?
	– have you lost any weight?
	– have you lost interest in sex?
	– are you worrying about your health more than usual?
	– are you feeling anxious and tense much of the time?
social support	– is there someone you can talk to?
	– is there a person you feel you can turn to?
	– do you have a good friend or member
	– of your family to help?
	– do you still see your friends as much as usual?

Assessment of suicide risk

It is important to assess the thoughts/ideas, intentions and plans that a person may harbour in respect of self-injurious behaviour (Hawton, 1987).

These questions need to be asked in a sensitive way and it is important to act upon the inter-personal cues displayed by the individual being assessed.

Potential questions may include:

'Do you ever feel like harming yourself?'

'Do you feel that life isn't worth living?'

'Do you feel that you sometimes can't go on?'

'Are these thoughts with you all the time?'

If the person answers 'yes' to any of these, then:

'Have you thought about how you might harm yourself?'

'Have you thought of how you might carry this out?'

If 'yes':

'Have you thought of when you might do this – a plan?'

'Have you already tried this out at some point?'

End by checking with the person:

'What reason/s do you have for not acting on your thoughts?'

It is worth being aware of the risk factors for self-injurious behaviour which include:

- isolation
- recent bereavement
- unemployment
- psychiatric illness
- past suicide attempt
- physical illness.

It is also important to explore the individual's view of themselves. This can be done by asking:

'Is there anything that you are looking forward to?'

'Looking back on your life, how would you summarise it?'

'Was there a time that you felt good about yourself?'

In order to conduct an assessment successfully, the following skills are required:

- empathy
- listening skills

- noticing non-verbal behaviours

- using the patient's language and answers

- summarising

- allowing good use of silence

- not showing signs of hurry

- clarifying points

- good use of eye contact

- avoiding jargon and theory

- direct questions – using questions that require more than a 'yes/no' response.

Treatment/intervention

Treatment and intervention strategies will depend upon the severity of the illness and the functioning of the individual and should combine various approaches. Seldom does one single approach to treatment work in the long term. If medication is indicated, it should also be accompanied by either a talking therapy or self-help. Medication is for symptoms only, talking (or self-help) is for easing the distress often caused by the symptoms. In accordance with good practice any intervention must be *negotiated* between the practitioner and the individual, otherwise compliance may be poor. There is a considerable difference between the approaches adopted for mild depression and those of severe depression. Looking at a model of care it can be seen that as the illness progresses, the level of care changes:

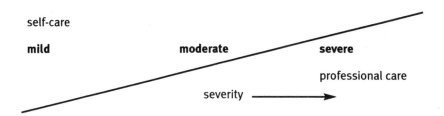

At the Core of Mental Health © Pavilion 2000

From this model (Davies & Smart 1994) it can be seen that the interventions required during a 'mild' depressive illness should focus primarily on self-help and not drug treatment. While at the other end of the spectrum, in 'severe' depression, professional intervention is essential usually by the use of anti-depressant medication. There is no indication for the use of anti-depressants in mild depression. Medication should be reserved for moderate and severe presentations.

Drug treatments

The first real breakthrough in anti-depressant therapy came in the late fifties with the discovery of the **Mono Amine Oxidase Inhibitors (MAOIs)**. These were quickly superseded by the **Tricyclic anti-depressants (TCAs)** which led the field for the next 30 years. More recently, the newer **Selective Serotonin Reuptake Inhibitors (SSRIs)** have been added to the options available for clinicians. An even more modern class of medication has also now entered the frame with the availability of the Modified Tricyclics, having similar properties of the older TCAs but with the advantages of the SSRIs in terms of the side-effect profile.

The MAOIs are very rarely used nowadays, mainly due to their toxicity. When taking MAOIs they also interact with certain foods and cause very severe complications. If a person is taking a MAOI, there are important dietary restrictions to be aware of. These should be checked in detail with the psychiatrist who is responsible for prescribing the medication. An example of a MAOI is Nardil (Phenelzine).

The tricyclics include:

- Prothieden (Dothiepin)
- Amitriptylene (Lentizol)
- Surmontil (Trimiprimine)
- Imiprimine (Tofranil)
- Anafranil (Comiprimine)

Typical side-effects of the tricyclics include:

- dry mouth

- sedation

- blurred vision

- gastric upset

- nausea

- shaking

- constipation

- weight gain

- sexual problems

- confusion.

Dosage should start at around 50 – 75mg, building up in stages to a minimum of 150mg/day. **Lower doses are ineffective.**
Contra-indications to the use of these drugs include:

- recent myocardial infarction

- heart block

- mania

- pregnancy.

The SSRIs include:

- Prozac (Fluoxetine)

- Seroxat (Paroxetine)

- Lustral (Sertraline)

- Faverin (Fluoxamine).

Typical side-effects can include:

- headache
- nausea
- anxiety
- gastric problems
- sexual problems
- sweating.

Dosage is usually one 20mg tablet/day, increasing to 30 or 40mg if necessary.

Contra-indications may include:

- renal or hepatic failure
- mania
- cardiovascular disease
- epilepsy
- pregnancy.

Examples of the Modified Tricyclics include:

- Lofepramine
- Venlafaxine.

The advantages and disadvantages of the two main anti-depressant groups are summarised in the table below:

Table 1 Types of anti-depressant: advantages and disadvantages		
Group	**advantages**	**disadvantages**
tricyclic	• aids sleeplessness • anxiolytic • cheap • familiar	• toxic in overdose • dose requires being built up • high side-effect profile
SSRI	• single dose – no building up • non-sedating • not as toxic in overdose	• expensive • may have severe side-effects • long-term use is unknown

General

Anti-depressants take between ten days and three weeks to begin to have an effect. Both the tricyclic and SSRIs are as effective as each other, and some consultants will consider the tricyclics as the first line of treatment unless indicated otherwise. It is the individual's needs that must be considered first, rather than the choice of drug. **Anti-depressants need to be prescribed for between four and six months after the patient has improved, and treatment should continue for up to two years if necessary.**

There is a high level of relapse if treatment is either stopped early or if there is under-dosing of the medication (most common with TCAs). It is therefore important that the individual is encouraged to comply with their medication. This can be achieved by giving accurate information about side-effects, the length of treatment necessary and regular reviews conducted. The **key message** here is **information**. This approach still causes some difficulties as some practitioners are reluctant to give people the information they require, feeling that by giving details of side-effects and pointing out the length of treatment, this will encourage the person to 'adopt' the side-effects. It is also a problem for many practitioners to provide information in a form that is 'person-centred', tending to either jargonise or use confusing language. Relying on the information provided in the prescription pack does not seem adequate, again because it tends to be highly technical. Below are some examples of the kind of information people need in relation to anti-depressants.

- Anti-depressants are not addictive.

- This medication will take between ten days and three weeks to start working.

- It must be taken exactly as prescribed by your doctor.

- All medication has side-effects, but if these become a problem, talk to your doctor.

- Most of the side-effects will pass with time, and will not cause you any physical harm, though some may remain (eg dry mouth).

■ If you are having difficulty with persistent side-effects see your doctor.

■ Do not stop taking your medication without speaking to your doctor first.

■ Even when you start to feel better, you must keep taking your tablets as prescribed.

■ Stopping anti-depressants does not cause any withdrawal effects.

■ Remember that tablets will not solve the problem, they only help the symptoms.

■ You may require other help (eg counselling or self-help) to prevent any relapse.

If an individual is not responding to a specific anti-depressant, it is better to prescribe a different group of anti-depressant, rather than switching to another within the same category. For example, if a tricyclic is not having the desired effect, it would be better to switch to an SSRI, rather than to try another TCA. There is no real evidence that 'mixing' treatments (using a TCA *and* an SSRI) has any benefit.

Talking treatments

In addition to anti-depressants, interventions that involve talking about the mental distress in a structured way may also be advocated for people with mild to moderate depression. This may be the preferred approach as an alternative to drug therapy, or as an attempt to reduce the distress before medication is tried.

Talking treatments are rarely offered in isolation from other interventions for people who are experiencing moderate to severe depressive symptoms. This is because talking to someone about mental health difficulties is effortful in itself and people with significant depressive symptoms may lack the motivation to be able to engage in such interventions initially until their symptoms have improved.

Talking therapies do not always mean in depth 'counselling' but basic counselling skills can be adopted to engage and develop a relationship between the individual and the practitioner. Research has shown that when individuals are helped to simply *acknowledge* that they may have a depressive illness, the outcome is immediately improved (Paykel & Priest, 1992). This acknowledgement is therefore not only desirable, but essential. Part of any intervention therefore must be to assist this process. Sensitive listening and good use of communication skills is a basic necessity to begin the process of engagement.

Counselling

This may be on offer from within the primary care team and it is now more common for GP surgeries to have a counsellor attached to the practice. Counselling comes in many forms and approaches, and increasingly general practice is demanding that shorter and more direct approaches be employed such as solution-focused therapy. Counselling has always had difficulty in providing firm evidence of positive outcomes, and this continues to be the case. There is no doubt that most people seem to be positive about their counselling encounter, but little measureable evidence is yet available to confirm the clinical value.

Cognitive Behavioural Therapy (CBT)

There is much evidence to show the effectiveness of this approach with people with depression. Usually, interventions are carried out by a trained mental health practitioner and a number of courses are available nationally where this intervention is the main focus of the training. CBT aims to identify the distorted thought processes and underlying negative beliefs of the individual. These are then systematically challenged and replaced with more factual and positive thoughts, thus increasing the feelings of wellbeing and pleasure. It deals with the distress caused by the symptoms as opposed to the symptoms themselves. Sometimes, behavioural techniques are used alongside a cognitive approach, thus influencing what the individual does about the distress as well as what they think and feel. **Stress and anxiety management programmes** often use cognitive behavioural techniques. Cognitive behavioural interventions are particularly useful for people who perhaps cannot directly influence what is happening in their world, but can be helped to react to their circumstances more positively by thinking about them in a different way (Beck *et al*, 1979).

Problem-solving

Recently there has been reliable evidence indicating that this approach can be highly effective for mild to moderate depression. The basis of problem-solving is to help the individual work through a series of practical and constructive steps relating to their difficulties. Unlike cognitive approaches, this technique is intended for people who have problems where there *are* solutions and options, but the person is not sure of what they are or how to act on them. Problem-solving encourages the person themself to work through the following steps:

- **listing** all their problems or difficulties

- **prioritising** these difficulties

- **choosing** which **difficulty** to tackle first

- listing *all* the **possible options/solutions** for this problem – from the silly to the serious

- working out the **pros and cons** of each of these options in full

- **choosing** which **option/solution** to work at

- designing an action plan and what **steps** need to be taken to achieve the solution, and then breaking them into small practical steps

- planning **when to carry out the steps** identified

- **evaluating** how the problem-solving approach went and if it was unsuccessful, tracing back the steps to re-plan, or start again

- if the approach was successful, moving on to the next chosen problem and repeating the strategy.

Self-help

It must be the aim of all interventions to help the individual back to a position of self-care. Not everyone is equipped with a range of coping methods to rely on, and even these may fail should the circumstances be so traumatic or unbearable. It is therefore important to encourage the person to build up and practise a range of methods that can be used in the future. **Self-help involves:**

Patient information

Giving the individual information such as leaflets, books, audio tapes, video tapes, and self-help packs. This should occur on every occasion, as it is the cornerstone of all interventions, and yet is the least used. There is now a wide range of excellent sources of information available in many different forms. These include written material, audio and video tapes which are often multi-lingual. Information may also be of value to carers, family members and friends.

Self-monitoring

Encouraging individuals to take a daily note of their mood and tension levels is an easy method of encouraging them to take some responsibility for their recovery and ongoing self-management. This form of self-monitoring, using mood charts and self-scoring diaries, can help both the individual and the practitioner to monitor the progress and pattern of the depression over a period of time.

Support

It is important to ascertain whether there is a source of support within the individual's network. This can be a highly desirable component of intervention and should be encouraged. It is useful to check if there is a close friend, confidant, advocate or family member to accompany the individual for some sessions.

Homework

Homework can take many forms, but it is essentially something that should be encouraged as part of the intervention. It may involve simply practising relaxation techniques or challenging negative thoughts. It should be pointed out that new coping strategies will only be effective if practised. It must also be mentioned that with all practice comes failure – failure is actually a necessity for us to learn, rather than perceiving it as something which is just 'bad'. Giving patients 'permission' to fail is always a useful step, but encouraging them to learn from each setback is important. Homework should always be realistic and achievable.

Self-awareness

Self-esteem is one of the most common building blocks to coping, and low self-esteem one of the commonest signs of depression. Perhaps the person's self-esteem was never as healthy as it should have been or perhaps it has been shaken up by recent events or difficulties. A healthy self-esteem is an essential part of recovery. Information, as mentioned earlier, is a good start to this approach. It may require a more focused approach through an assertiveness or self-help group. Checking out what the local psychology service has to offer may prove useful also.

Follow-up

Anyone who is prescribed anti-depressants or who is involved in talking-type interventions should initially have regular reviews. These reviews can be carried out by the person's GP, but could be conducted by other members of the primary or secondary care team such as the practice nurse or health visitor and community psychiatrist. Certainly in the beginning, the person should be seen within two to three weeks and at similar intervals for the next three follow-up consultations. Review periods should be much shorter if there is felt to be a suicide risk. One must remember that the greatest risk of suicide is when the person starts to improve after the first few weeks of treatment. If there is any suspicion of possible self-injurious behaviour or harm to others, specialist advice should be sought, or the person should be referred to the specialist mental health services immediately. Where a depressive episode is severe, reviews are likely to be undertaken by, or in conjunction with, a practitioner from the community mental health team.

The re-use of the depression screening questionnaires referred to earlier can be a valuable part of the review process. Planning a prevention strategy can be tackled towards the end of the intervention programme and should encompass coping methods and problem-solving strategies.

Consulting a specialist

Referral to a psychiatric specialist may also be necessary if there is any doubt about the diagnosis or treatment, or a high level of risk to self or others has been identified. Liaison with local mental health specialists differs between geographical areas and there are examples of both good and poor practices across the UK. Good communication across the primary/secondary care interface is essential and, generally, secondary care colleagues are only too happy to be contacted by telephone for advice. Encouraging primary care teams to invite their local community psychiatric nurse (CPN) or psychiatrist to one of their team meetings can also be extremely beneficial in improving communication. Although mental health teams are geared to dealing with severe and enduring mental health problems, they will usually be able to offer valuable advice on milder forms of mental disorders.

Guidelines

Using shared guidelines has proved useful in improving the care of individuals in many areas of physical health. There are now various guidelines available on depression which can be shared across the primary and secondary interface to provide practitioners with a common language and structure that can significantly improve the recognition and management of depressed patients. An example of such guidelines is shown in **Table 2** below.

Table 2 Depression – Shared Care Guidelines	
How severe is it?	**What to do about it?**
Mild	1 acknowledge and see again
	2 give suitable information/literature/advice on sleep, exercise, diet, relaxation, problem-solving/audio information tape
	3 assess social difficulties/give details about helping agencies or resources
	4 consider counselling
	5 treat any underlying physical health problems
Moderate	6 undertake steps 1 to 5 as above
	7 prescribe suitable anti-depressants and arrange to monitor
	8 offer/refer for counselling or cognitive behavioural intervention
	9 do carers/family require support? If so, refer to local mental health service
Severe	10 carry out all steps as above, but see more frequently
	11 refer to specialist mental health team
	12 consider request for specific intervention and support for carers/family members

Adapted from: Armstrong & Lloyd (1994)

Resources

Keeping a list of local and national resources at hand can save a lot of time and energy. Some mental health trusts have produced local resource directories. Giving an individual a contact telephone number of a helpline for accessing information empowers the person and offers hope as well as additional support from people who understand exactly what they are feeling.

Table 3   Some national agencies (self-help organisations, information resources)

Organisation	Address	Telephone number
Depression Alliance	PO Box 1022￼London SE1 7GR	020 7721 7672
Samaritans	10 The Grove￼Slough SL1 1QP	01753 532713
Relate	Herbert Gray College￼Little Church Street￼Rugby CV1 3AP	01788 573241
Phobic Action	Hornbeam House￼Manor Rd￼Essex IG8 8PR	020 8559 2551
British Association￼of Counselling	1 Regent Place￼Rugby CV21 2PJ	01788 550899
Asian Family Counselling	74 The Avenue￼London W13 8LB	020 8997 5749
Association for Postnatal Illness	25 Jeral Place￼Fulham￼London SW6 1BE	020 7386 0868
Black Mental Health Centre	277 Chapeltown Road￼Leeds LS7 3HA	0113 237 4229
Centre for Stress Management	156 Westcombe Hill￼London SE3 7DH	020 8293 4114

Table 4   Sources of literature (leaflets, booklets and audio tapes)

Organisation	Address	Telephone number
The Royal College￼of Psychiatrists	17 Belgrave Square￼London￼SW19 8PG	020 7235 2351
Mind	Granta House￼15–19 Broadway￼Stratford￼London￼E15 4BQ	020 8519 2122
Wendy Lloyd Audio￼Productions	PO Box 1￼The Wirral￼Merseyside￼L47 7DD	

Useful reading for people experiencing depression include:

Pitt, B. (1994) *Down with Gloom.* Gaskell/Royal College of Psychiatrists.

Hauck, P. (1973) *Depression.* London: Sheldon Press.

Milligan, S. & Anthony, C. (1993) *Depression and How to Survive It.* London: Ebury Press.

Useful reading for practitioners include:

Wright, A. (1993) *Depression: Recognition & Management in General Practice.* London: Royal College of General Practitioners.

Summary

In summary, depressive symptoms may span a continuum from low mood through to loss of functioning, and culminate at the severe end with abnormal low mood and loss of functioning. Treatments range from anti-depressant medication to talking therapies coupled with approaches to self-help. Of key importance to the process of recovery is the prescribing of appropriate levels of medication and accessible information to the individual and their family on its effects and side-effects. Information on resources and national organisations and support networks can also be useful. The assessment of someone who is depressed should be holistic and cover areas of social difficulties in addition to signs and symptoms. Only by offering a co-ordinated response on all fronts is the approach to the depressed individual likely to be effective.

References

Armstrong, E. A. & Lloyd, K. (1997) *Management of Depression in Primary Care.* Card produced for the Defeat Depression Campaign. London: Royal College of Psychiatrists.

Beck, A. T., Rush, A. J. & Shaw, B.F. *et al* (1979) *Cognitive Therapy of Depression: A treatment manual.* Guildford: New York.

Beck, A. T., Steer, R. A. & Garbin, M. G. (1998) Psychometric Properties of the Beck Depression Inventory. *Clinical Psychiatric Review* 8 77–100.

Cox, J. L. & Holden, J. (1994) *Perinatal Psychiatry: Use and misuse of the Edinburgh Postnatal Depression Scale.* London: Gaskell.

Davies, M. (1996) Educational Programme on Depression in Primary Care.

Davies, M. & Smart, D. (1994) *Northamptonshire Defeat Depression – a team approach.* Northamptonshire Health Authority.

Department of Health (1992) *Health of the Nation: Suicide prevention – the challenge confronted.* London: DoH.

France, R. & Robertson, (1986) Behaviour Therapy in Primary Care: A practical guide. *The Beck Depression Inventory.* Kent: Charles Press.

France, R. & Robertson, M. (1997) *Behaviour Therapy in Primary Care: A Practical Guide.* Kent: Croom Helm.

Freeling, P., Rao, B. M., Paykel, E. S., Sireling, L. I. & Burton, R. H. (1985) Unrecognised depression in general practice. *British Medical Journal Research* **290** 1880–1883.

Golner, R. (1990) *Brief Therapy Practice.* London: Shireland Mews.

GRIPP (Getting Research into Practice and Purchasing) (1996) *Project Guidelines for the Recognition and Management of Depression in Primary Care.* Northamptonshire Health Authority.

Hawton. K. (1987) Assessment of suicide risk. *British Journal of Psychiatry* **150** 145–53.

Katona, C., Freeling, P., Hinchcliffe, K., Blanchard, M. & Wright, A. (1995) Recognition and management of depression in late life in general practice: consensus statement. Geriatric Depression Scale. *Primary Care Psychiatry* **1** 107–113.

Mynors-Wallace, L. M., Gath, D. H. & Lloyd Thomas, A. R. *et al* (1995) Randomised clinical trial comparing problem-solving treatment with amitripltyline and placebo for major depression in primary care. *British Medical Journal* **310** 441–5.

Paykel E. S. (1989) The Background: Extent and Nature of the Disorder. In: K. Herbst & E. S. Paykel (Eds) *Depression: An integrative approach.* Oxford: Heinemann.

Paykel, E. S. & Priest, R. G. (1992) Recognition and management of depression in general practice: consensus statement. *British Medical Journal* **305** 1198–202.

Tylee, A. T. & Freeling, P. (1989) The Recognition, Diagnosis and Acknowledgement of Depressive Disorder by General Practitioners. In: K. Herbst & E. S. Paykel (Eds) *Depression: An Integrative Approach.* Oxford: Heinemann.

World Health Organisation (1992) *ICD – 10 Classification of Mental and Behavioural Disorders: Clinical descriptions and diagnostic guidelines.* Geneva: WHO.

Other useful references

Sireling, L. I., Freeling, P., Paykel, E. S. *et al* (1985) Depression in general practice: clinical features and comparison with outpatients. *British Journal of Psychiatry* **147** 119–25.

Sireling, L. I, Paykel, E. S., Freeling. P. *et al* (1985) Depression in general practice: case thresholds and diagnosis. *British Journal of Psychiatry* **147** 113–19.

Blacker, C. V. R., Clare, A. W. (1988) The prevalence and treatment of depression in general practice. *Psychopharmacology* **95** S14–17.

Goldberg, D. P., Jenkins, L. Millar, T. *et al* (1993) The ability of trainee general practitioners to identify psychological distress among their patients. *Psychiatric Medicine* **23** 185–93.

Truax, C. B. & Cakhuff, R. R. (1967) *Toward Effective Counselling and Psychotherapy: Training and practice.* Chicago: Aldine Atherton.

Balwin, D. S. & Priest, R. G. (1995) The Defeat Depression Campaign. *Primary Care Psychiatry* **1** 71–6.

Secretary of State for Health (1993) *Key Area Handbook: Mental illness.* London: Department of Health.

Secretary of State for Health (1993) *The Health of the Nation: A Strategy for Health in England.* London: HMSO.

Davies, M. (1996) *Educational Programme on Depression in Primary Care.* Mental Health Facilitator, Northamptonshire Health Authority. Unpublished.

Chapter 2

Schizophrenia and Mood (Affective) Disorder

Professor David Kingdon

Discussion of the presentation of schizophrenia and mood (affective) disorder has frequently led to disputes between psychiatrists, social workers, psychologists and users of services. Social and biological perspectives often referred to as the medical and social models of mental ill health, have seemed to be diametrically opposed. However, this is not the case and current training initiatives encourage mental health workers to accept the importance of a biosocial model recognising that severe mental illness may often have social determinants as well as biological.

Research has shown that life events and circumstances experienced by the individual are influential in relapse, especially in relation to the family environment. There is increasing evidence to clarify the role that biological factors may play. An example is that groups of people with schizophrenia and other mental disorders have larger ventricles – the internal spaces in the brain. However, despite these developments, diagnosis remains problematic as the training of psychiatrists and mental health nurses has been based on the work of Karl Jaspers and others. These individuals have stressed the 'unintelligibility' of delusions and hallucinations which has led to generations of trained professionals who have been encouraged to make mental state assessments of what people say and do to achieve a diagnosis but ignore the content of the delusions and hallucinations experienced. In practice, because professionals have been trained to take a full personal history, this has led to situations where personal events of self-evident significance are elicited but their relationship to both schizophrenia and affective disorders have been denied.

Approached from a social perspective, this has seemed even more contradictory. Medication has been important but not sufficient for many people, who may not be prepared to take it because their beliefs about the origin of whatever their problems are. The evidence that delusions and hallucinations are 'unintelligible' has now been challenged (see **Chapter 10** by Iqbal and Birchwood). This chapter is written in the hope that these contemporary perspectives may lead to a rapprochement in the future, such that psychological, social and pharmacological approaches are valued.

The chapter will begin with an exploration of the signs and symptoms of severe mental health problems before returning to the debate surrounding diagnosis.

Symptoms and Signs

Severe mental health problems such as schizophrenia and affective disorders are characterised by positive and/or negative symptoms and/or thought disorder. They are referred to by mental health professionals as 'psychotic' disorders.

The term **'positive symptoms'** is used to describe delusions and hallucinations. **'Negative symptoms'** refer to the loss of personal abilities and feelings whilst **'thought disorder'** encompasses distortions in thoughts that make communication difficult.

Symptoms of depression and anxiety are also common in this group of disorders. Many other mental health problems can also occur, although not as commonly, eg obsessive-compulsive and eating disorders, and social phobia. The signs and symptoms are deliberately described together in the following sections but will be differentiated into separate categories under the section **Diagnosis or Labelling** (page 47).

Lack of insight denotes psychotic states but this can be variable in intensity, timing and its effects on actions (David, 1990). **People who discuss psychotic experiences may vary in the strengths of their beliefs or in how they act in relationship to them, for example, they may deny they are ill but readily accept medication or hospitalisation.**

Early Signs

The first signs of the development of severe mental illness may long precede a person seeking or being brought to the attention of mental health services. Alternatively, signs and symptoms can arise and climax within days. In the former, the early signs may be fluctuations in mood, mild eccentricity, confusion, slightly odd behaviour, increasing isolation, and deterioration in concentration and educational performance. In the latter, it may be the quite sudden development of bizarre ideas or hallucinations.

There is some evidence that suggests that early intervention improves the outcome for a person and so early identification and management is important (see **Chapter 10**). It can certainly reduce the distress and negative effects of psychotic episodes on job prospects, friendships, family relationships and self-esteem. There are currently some major European and Australian studies exploring the area of early intervention in relation to schizophrenia.

The person may develop a **'delusion mood'** – something strange and mystifying seems to be happening around them. They may become uneasy and suspicious. This may be due to the abuse of hallucinogenic drugs, although drug use is not essential to the onset of psychotic disorder. Sometimes, people present with schizophrenia after very little use of such drugs. During the 'psychotic experience' lights and colours may become brighter whilst events and observations may begin to take on meanings that seem of unusual importance. When people discuss the beliefs experienced as part of the psychotic state they are usually uncommon and not shared by others.

Positive Symptoms

Hallucinations

Hallucinations can be **visual** – as visions, auditory – or **somatic** – as smells or feelings of being touched, often sexually.

They are described as **false perceptions**. What the person feels, hears, sees or smells seems to be caused by something external and seems absolutely real. This is, however, a misinterpretation of such phenomena – either thoughts in their own mind or sometimes, bodily sensations. Most commonly these thoughts are heard as 'voices' speaking either directly to the person themselves or around them. They can be derogatory, abusive, violent, sexual or neutral in content, but sometimes positive and comforting. They can sound like muffled whispers or as someone speaking or shouting aloud. Sometimes it sounds to people that their thoughts are being echoed back to them, or that a running commentary is going on about what they are doing, or that they are being discussed by the originators of the voices.

People will frequently discuss their hallucinatory experiences openly but sometimes conceal them for a number of reasons. The content may seem too unpleasant to say to someone else; the voices may tell them not to trust anyone or tell anyone about them, and the voices may threaten them if they do so; or they may fear being hospitalised or having their medication increased. People may sometimes appear to be responding as if someone were talking to them, either by speaking aloud or by gesture and movement. Whilst this can mean that they are hallucinating, it can also be a response to distressing or confusing thoughts; for example, when angry with a partner or authorities, an internal conversation may be developed which the patient recognises as their thoughts rather than as a voice. Asking if thoughts or voices are troubling a person can sometimes elicit this.

It can be possible to confuse voices with **misinterpretations of sounds and delusions of reference** (see below). Some individuals report they have both these phenomena and hallucinations occurring sequentially.

Delusions

Delusions have been described as irrational beliefs which are not amenable to reason and which are out of keeping with the person's cultural background. However, recent work demonstrating the effectiveness of the application of structured reasoning techniques is leading to a revision of this description (see **Chapter 10**).

This means that **delusions appear irrational without an understanding of their origin**. Tracing the development of the beliefs with the individual often makes them more understandable, although the beliefs themselves are still inaccurate. By nature, delusional beliefs appear bizarre and incorrect. Assessment needs to embrace the degree of bizarreness in the cultural context of beliefs held. The strength of conviction attached to the belief determines whether it is appropriate to describe them as delusions, overvalued ideas or simply idiosyncratic beliefs.

The themes of delusions are frequently guilt, paranoia or grandeur. They can also be of bodily change or nihilistic. The beliefs of guilt may be quite out of context with the person's situation, though so strongly held they are thus delusional. Examples may include ideas that someone or some group is persecuting them, following them or interfering with them. They may believe themselves to be a special person, such as Christ, or to have special powers which can influence the course of the Universe. They may feel they have done something special which they are not given credit for, such as having invented the compact disc for example. Often these themes inter-relate, such that paranoia follows grandiose beliefs, as the individual is being persecuted for their special powers. They may believe that other people know what they are thinking, or even that they are putting thoughts into or taking them out of their mind. This is known as **thought interference** which feels like an extraordinary invasion of one's privacy. Sometimes people can develop the belief that others control what they think, or do, or feel. This is known as **passivity phenomena** or, more simply, 'made thoughts, feelings or actions'.

Delusions can develop over time or sometimes occur quite abruptly, in response to something happening such as hearing words in a song which are taken to have specific meaning, for example, that 'I am the chosen one'. This is known as **delusional perception.**

Delusions tend to refer to the person themselves although sometimes include important others in their lives. **Delusions of reference** are said to occur when things said by others, in the same room or street, or on the television, radio or in music, are taken personally when the individual is not actually being referred to. The misinterpretations are usually critical to the formulation of a diagnosis.

Accompanying and often intermingled with delusional ideas are concerns about philosophical questions or scientific belief. For example, the person may be preoccupied with the theories of the development of schizophrenia or science fiction. These ideas may be derived from conventional scientific and philosophical discussion but go far beyond, stretching evidence and logical discussion to lengths that would normally be unacceptable to most people and certainly to scientists or philosophers.

Thought interference

Thoughts may seem to stop dead (**'thought block'**). Alternatively, individuals may deny that these thoughts are occurring at all. They may say that someone is taking their thoughts from them. (This is known as **'thought withdrawal'**). Speech may be slow, repetitive, stereotyped or absent (**poverty of content of speech**). Sometimes people develop the belief that their thoughts are being broadcast to others so that they know what that person is thinking (**'thought broadcasting'**). This seems to occur especially where thoughts are embarrassing to the individual, such as those with a sexual or violent content. Similarly, individuals may believe that other people are putting thoughts into their mind. (This is known as **'thought insertion'**.)

Passivity

If people describe their actions being controlled by others – 'the voice made me break my next door neighbour's door down', for example – this is described as **passivity phenomenon** or in simple terms **a 'made' action**. This is distinct from a person attempting to excuse him or herself from an action that they shouldn't have committed. In 'made' actions people genuinely believe they have no power over their behaviour. Similarly they may describe feelings or thoughts that they are convinced are controlled by others (**'made' thoughts and feelings**).

Behavioural problems

As a consequence of the bizarre experiences described above, it is not surprising that abnormal behaviour is observed as part of the severe and enduring mental health problem. People can act in an eccentric way in response to their delusional ideas or hallucinations. Disinhibited behaviour may be a response to a grandiose belief that, for instance, because they are God, they are entitled to behave as they wish, or because they are convinced of someone's love for them, they can act as if that person were their spouse. Self-caring behaviour may be affected and people may become neglectful of their appearance or personal hygiene.

People may also describe certain **movement abnormalities** such as posturing or waxy flexibility. This is where a person remains in a fixed position when moved into it by another.

Stereotypy is the name given to describe repetitive stereotyped movements. **Catatonia** presents as overwhelming excitement or, the opposite, stupor; these are similar to mania and depressive symptoms of retardation – gross slowing. These movement abnormalities are now described as being seen much less frequently. It has been suggested that they may have been symptoms of institutionalisation rather than schizophrenia and affective disorder, as they seem to be much less common in modern, community-based services. However, over-activity does occur commonly in mania, and sometimes in schizophrenia. This behaviour is known as **negativism** as demonstrated when people act in direct opposition to requests.

There has been much controversy about whether **aggression** is more common in someone with severe mental illness. Aggression and irritability seem to be more likely to occur in someone with schizophrenia than in the general population, although serious offences are very uncommon. Where these do occur, they are associated with acute psychosis where individuals react in response to paranoid beliefs or hallucinations which command, and are believed to have the power to make them commit an aggressive act. The use of illicit drugs and excess alcohol are also major risk factors. Early intervention and readily accessible services available on a 24 hour, 7 days a week basis are important in reducing the likelihood of these happening.

Negative symptoms

Negative symptoms include **poor motivation** and **a lack of drive** to do anything, including speaking, and even it seems, thinking. The person may spend long periods in relative isolation from others, for example, spending most of the day in bed and then getting up at night, seeming to say and do little of consequence. The lack of volition is associated with poor adherence to treatment, increased severity of illness and frequent admissions to hospital. Individuals can develop **anhedonia** – the inability to enjoy anything, which is perhaps less intense but merges into depression. They may appear depressed or elated, sometimes flat or with **'incongruous affect'**. The effect appears incongruous because the mood expressed doesn't match the circumstances or things being said – laughing whilst discussing a fatal accident, for example.

These symptoms are thought likely to be biological in origin. They may sometimes be understandable in their context. For example, seeking isolation and turning night into day can be a coping strategy used by individuals to reduce stimulation and thus also reduce the positive symptoms. Laughing or giggling at distressing events can be a nervous reaction. It can be difficult to distinguish negative symptoms from depression, and both may be present. Anti-psychotic medication may also cause similar symptoms because of sedation and Parkinsonian side-effects, such as stiffness, rigidity and reduction in facial expression.

Thought disorder

Thought disorder presents as speech that seems muddled or disconnected to the extreme of seeming quite unintelligible. The association between the words and the sentence seem difficult to understand (**'loosening of associations'**). Sometimes a remote connection can be seen, called **'knight's move' thinking** or **'clang associations'** where the connection seems to be based in similar sounds. It can be circumstantial or a 'word salad' seeming completely disconnected. Metaphor or punning may occur; words may be used in an idiosyncratic way or new words invented. Some evidence is emerging that such thought disorder in schizophrenia may have meaningful themes within it. Indeed, sense can be made of it by careful enquiry of the individual and understanding of their background (Harrow & Prosen, 1998). Diagnosis of thought disorder can be a particular problem where cultural, language or dialect differences exist. Speech can sometimes become rapid and pressured, which contributes to the lack of clarity.

Mood changes

As described by Martin Davies in **Chapter 1**, the core features of depression are low mood, loss of interest, energy and enjoyment, pessimism, guilt and low self-esteem. Concentration and attention are reduced which interferes with the person's memory. Sleep is frequently disturbed with problems getting off to sleep and/or waking early or repetitively through the night. Appetite can be reduced or increased with corresponding weight changes. Ideas of self-harm or suicide are frequent.

Anxiety often accompanies depression or may exist on its own. There are a wide variety of symptoms that can occur and be frightening in their own right, such as breathlessness, numbness, tingling, abdominal discomfort and giddiness. They can be misunderstood as early signs of a serious physical illness, like cancer or Aids, or, delusionally, as being signs of interference from outside agencies. Anger and irritability can also occur in response to circumstances as with anxiety or depression. This can fuel paranoia and depressive symptoms. Conversely, elation may occur, sometimes as a response to the development of grandiose beliefs. Reduction in sleep may be linked to the elated mood and often to plans being worked out.

Diagnosis or labelling?

The need to provide a diagnosis based on the signs and symptoms of the mental health problem presented often results in a debate between medical and social models of mental disorder. It can be construed that the process of diagnosis seems to reduce an individual to a disease entity. However, most individuals and their families seek a name – a label or diagnosis – for what is happening to them so that they can find out more about their mental health problem and what they can do to improve matters. Rightly, they see the name as simply referring to their mental health problem, not themselves as a person, ie they do not want to be dismissed as *a* 'schizophrenic'.

Stigmatisation, however, remains a major problem and unfortunately, schizophrenia and other forms of mental illness, are associated inappropriately with frequent violence and inevitable deterioration.

Kraeplin made the distinction between dementia praecox and affective disorder in 1896 and Bleuler (1911) renamed the former 'the group of schizophrenias'. There are some problems with this classification as the distinction between schizophrenia and affective disorders is not absolute. There is even a category, **schizo-affective disorder**, that is designed to include individuals who present with characteristics of both disorders, highlighting the continuum that exists. There is also evidence that the symptoms used in their description – delusions and hallucinations – are continuous with 'normal' beliefs and imagination (Strauss, 1969).

The problems encompassed by these disorders are broad and diverse although many attempts have been made to reclassify them in a way that is clinically appropriate. Differentiation of symptoms into 'positive', 'negative' and 'thought disorder' has been broadly accepted, although regrouping of people displaying signs and symptoms into different, more specific sub-groups has not. However, criteria developed over the past 20 to 30 years are now used much more reliably to determine whether someone has schizophrenia or affective disorder. Their use has gained international recognition in the *International Classification of Diseases*, 10th revision (WHO, 1992) and the *American Classification, Diagnostic and Statistical Manual*, 4th revision.

There is, therefore, considerable overlap between affective disorder, schizophrenia and other disorders and it seems likely that they exist on a continuum with schizo-affective disorder, so called, occupying the middle area. There is some evidence that schizo-affective disorder is more like schizophrenia than affective disorder in terms of its outlook or prognosis. The presence of affective symptoms – detected through prominent changes in mood – seems to correlate with a generally better outcome.

The diagnosis of schizophrenia is made where certain symptoms occur. The list of symptoms chosen (known as **'first rank symptoms'**) is based on a description by Schneider in 1959 (see *a*) to *d*) in **Table 1**, below). This has been supplemented by other symptoms *e*) to *i*) in the International Classification of Diseases, 10th Revision). For a diagnosis to be made, one of symptoms listed as *a*) to *d*) and two of those listed as *e*) to *i*) must be present for a period of a month or more. These criteria have been used to produce international agreement on diagnosis. They seem to be reliable in use across countries, so that, at least in research studies, a person with a diagnosis of schizophrenia in Nigeria, for example, would receive the same diagnosis as they would in the UK.

Table 1 Symptoms of special importance for diagnosis of schizophrenia	
'First rank symptoms'	**Other symptoms**
a) broadcasting, insertion, withdrawal or echoing of thoughts	e) persistent delusions of other kinds that are culturally inappropriate or completely impossible, such as:
b) passivity symptoms: delusions of control or influence	• religious or political identity
c) delusional perception (a delusion arising from a normal perception)	• superhuman powers and abilities
d) auditory hallucinations ('voices')	• persistent hallucinations of any type when accompanied by:
■ giving running commentary	– fleeting or half-formed delusions without clear affective ('mood') content
■ discussing the person among themselves	– persistent over-valued ideas
■ coming from some part of the body	– occurrence for weeks or months on end.
	f) breaks or interpolations in the train of thought leading to incoherence or irrelevant speech, or neologisms ('new words')
	g) catatonic behaviour
	h) 'negative symptoms'
	i) significant and consistent change in overall quality of some aspects of personal behaviour

A diagnosis of schizophrenia takes prominence over diagnoses of affective or neurotic disorders such as depression or anxiety. This can seem confusing, as psychiatrists will insist that someone has schizophrenia when they, their carers and others may see the most important symptoms being depression and/or anxiety. The reason given for this by psychiatrists is that treatment of the schizophrenic symptoms is most important, as other symptoms often improve as a result. The prognosis for the individual is dependent on the diagnosis of schizophrenia. This approach is partially, but not wholly, accurate as treatment of depression and anxiety in their own right by drugs or psychosocial measures may be necessary.

If the 'schizophrenic symptoms' have a clear physical cause such as delirium from a chest infection or drug abuse, a diagnosis of schizophrenia is not made. This can also be problematic because some individuals abuse hallucinogenic drugs in the early stages of a schizophrenic illness and it can be difficult to determine the root of the problem. A situation can arise where individuals initially present with schizophrenic symptoms and have clearly been abusing drugs. This can progress to where the person claims to have stopped such abuse, or is using substances intermittently, and yet still has the same symptoms of the mental health problem.

The triangle in **Figure 1,** below demonstrates this hierarchy used in diagnosis but it is important to bear in mind the reservations mentioned above.

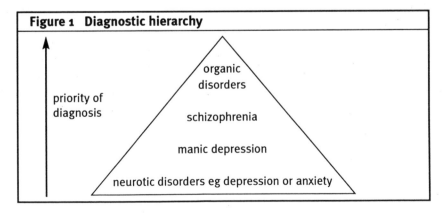

Figure 1   Diagnostic hierarchy

priority of diagnosis

organic disorders

schizophrenia

manic depression

neurotic disorders eg depression or anxiety

People who are given a diagnosis of schizophrenia can vary considerably in the symptoms that they experience. Bleuler (*ibid*), who first used the term, described 'the group of schizophrenias' and most psychiatrists agree that, indeed, it is a number of different conditions that are being described. However, finding ways of describing them better is problematic. Attempts based on the analysis of clusters of symptoms have not been particularly helpful. Classically, **groupings were based on clinical impression: paranoid; hebephrenic** (young with predominantly positive symptoms); **catatonic** (either stuporose or very excited) and **simple** (predominantly negative symptoms). Work is currently progressing which is looking at other possible groupings.

A diagnosis of affective disorder is made when significant depression or mania occurs. The term **'manic depressive'** has often been misused to mean someone with rapid mood swings, such that they suddenly become angry then calm again. Where emotional changes are fleeting, they are not usually of diagnostic significance but where these are pervasive they are more likely to be. This type of disorder may be described as **bipolar affective disorder** where episodes of depression and mania have occurred, or **unipolar** where only one type of episode has occurred. **Hypomania** is a term used, according to ICD 10, to mean a state of less pronounced over-activity or disruption of everyday activities than mania and without the presence of hallucinations or delusions. **Depression is classified** (as described in **Chapter 1**) **according to whether it is mild, moderate or severe in intensity**. However, as with any continuum, the point at which mild depression becomes moderate or moderate depression becomes severe is **a matter of clinical judgement**. It is also important to recognise that in bipolar illness, periods of normality occur between episodes. Nonetheless, persistent depressive states can also occur.

What causes schizophrenia and affective disorder?

The causes of schizophrenia and affective disorders are multi-factorial. It is almost certainly an interaction between individual vulnerabilities and stressful circumstances that leads to such illnesses becoming manifest, rather than any one biological or social cause in isolation. In both conditions, genetics appear to play a part. In schizophrenia, identical (monozygotic) twins are much more likely to both have the illness (50%) than non-identical (dizygotic) twins (15%) as shown in a number of studies. As the environment is likely to have similar effects on both types of twins, the fact that the genetic constitution is identical in monozygotes but differs in dizygotes, would seem to be the reason why they are both more likely to have the illness. However, even where the environment is different – such as where twins have been reared separately – identical twins are still much more likely to both have the illness. Where both parents have schizophrenia, 50% of children born to them are also likely to have the disorder. Despite these statistics, 50% of children and of identical twins do not become ill, indicating that other factors in addition to genetics are necessary.

A similar genetic predisposition has been shown for affective disorders. Some individuals seem to have vulnerability factors such as a family history, and genetic factors seem to be relevant in some. Personality also seems important such that people with certain personality characteristics which can be described as **schizoid** (cold and aloof) or paranoid, seem more likely to develop schizophrenia.

For a number of years now, it has been recognised that when brain scans of groups of people with schizophrenia (and also some other mental illnesses) are compared with 'normal' controls, there appear to be some abnormalities. In particular, as mentioned earlier, in the areas where fluid circulates inside the brain, the ventricles are relatively larger. Also the volume of the creases in the outer part of the brain – the sulci – are decreased. The volume reduction is in areas associated with language development.

Position Emission Tomography (PET) of the brain allows functioning to be assessed. These scans have been used whilst individuals perform psychological tests, to assess different types of brain functioning. Reduced performance has been found in assessments of flexibility in problem-solving, especially involving strategy planning and verbal fluency. Decreased blood flow and activity in the frontal area of the brain has been shown whilst doing these tests and this is also associated with the negative symptoms of schizophrenia. Conversely, auditory hallucinations show increased blood flow in the area of the speech centre. This supports the hypothesis that such hallucinations are **'inner speech'** which individuals misinterpret.

The introduction of chlorpromazine and other drugs which are effective in reducing the positive symptoms of schizophrenia has suggested that their mechanism of action might reveal clues to an underlying abnormality. These drugs have been shown to universally affect a chemical called **dopamine**, which is a neurotransmitter. It is released by some nerve cells in the brain and stimulates others to react. Dopamine is broken down into noradrenaline and subsequently adrenaline, which is, of course, a chemical involved in anxiety. Some other drugs, which cause symptoms like those occurring in schizophrenia – such as the amphetamines – act on the nerve receptors stimulated by dopamine. This seemed to confirm the importance of dopamine in the disorder. However, other drugs, such as LSD, which has hallucinogenic properties, act on another neurotransmitter, serotonin. This suggests that other, or a combination of, neurotransmitter abnormalities are relevant. Specific abnormalities of the nerve cells in the brain or the chemicals involved have not been demonstrated conclusively.

For depression, anti-depressant drugs act to increase levels of dopmaine and serotonin. This suggests that these compounds are important in some way in the development of affective disorders.

A suggestion that schizophrenia is caused by complications during birth has been put forward but is also unproven. Similarly, viral theories have been proposed, such as influenza at the time of the fifth month of pregnancy. This again has not been conclusively confirmed. There do however seem to be definite signs of abnormality emerging in childhood in some people who later develop schizophrenia. Comparative evidence from the National Childbirth Study (Jones *et al*, 1993) and video recordings revealed factors that were more likely to be seen in children who later develop schizophrenia. These were:

- milestones of motor development reached late, particularly walking

- more speech problems, up to age 15

- low educational test scores, at ages 8, 11, and 15 years

- preference for solitary play, at ages 4 and 6

- individuals rated themselves as less socially competent at 13 years

- teachers rated the children more anxious in social situations at 15 years old

- a health visitor's rating of the mother as having below average mothering skills and understanding of her child at age 4.

The evidence that life events and circumstances are of importance has come for a variety of studies (eg Bebbington *et al*, 1993). These have shown an increased incidence of events in the periods before illness onset and during relapse. Some of these events are directly related to the illness itself. For example, a reduction in concentration and drive can lead to losing a job. However, other events which seem quite independent also appear to increase in frequency. It is certainly the case that many individuals and their families attribute the illness, at least in part, to significant events in their lives.

How common are schizophrenia and affective disorders?

The National Psychiatric Morbidity Survey completed by the Office of Populations, Censuses and Surveys (OCPS, 1996) revealed an overall rate of 0.4% of the population with functional psychosis at any time in private households. The prevalence of functional psychoses varied from city to countryside areas. In cities, it was 0.5%; in semi-rural areas, 0.3% and in rural areas, 0.2%.

Three hundred and fifty people with functional psychoses were also contacted through community mental health teams (CMHTs) using randomised methods. A further 1200 people living in residential establishments, including hospitals for people with mental health problems were also interviewed. Important results from the survey are given in **Tables 2** and **3** (below and overleaf). They show the degree of disadvantage suffered by the group and the amount and type of services currently made use of. The relatively low use of services, medication and counselling conditions causing considerable distress and disability is notable.

Table 2 Adults with functional psychoses living in private households	
Equal male to female:	**About half were receiving some form of treatment:**
■ 50% married or cohabiting	■ a third were receiving therapy or counselling
■ twice as likely to be unemployed or economically inactive	■ about a third were on drugs used in psychosis and related conditions
■ living in rented accommodation	■ 20% on anti-cholinergics (drugs for side-effects of anti-psychotic medication)
■ living alone	■ 10% on anti-depressants
■ divorced or separated	■ 3% on hypnotics (for sleeping problems)
	■ 82% received some service in 12 months prior to interview
Two thirds also had significant neurotic symptoms (predominantly depression and anxiety)	■ two thirds had seen a general practitioner for a 'mental or emotional problem'
	■ half had been seen in an outpatient clinic
	■ a quarter had had a hospital inpatient stay
	■ 11% had had a home visit from a psychiatrist or psychiatric nurse

Table 3 Adults with functional psychosis in residential establishments for people with mental health problems	
70% have schizophrenic disorders	**Residents with schizophrenia** ■ three quarters were men ■ 98% in hospital and 90% in residential accommodation were given anti-psychotic medication ■ non-compliance with medication was twice as likely if: – aged 16-34 compared to 55-64 – having 'A' level or other higher qualification compared to no qualification – living in unsupervised compared to supervised accommodation
8% have affective disorders	**Residents with affective disorders** ■ a quarter were divorced ■ 8 in 10 were on anti-psychotic medication including anti-manic medication ■ 3 in 10 were on anti-depressants

The onset of schizophrenia usually occurs before the age of 30 but there is another peak in the 40s and it can even come on later in life, including after retirement age. Men develop schizophrenia, on average, 5 years before women, making their average age of onset between 15 and 25, with females between 25 and 35. Over a lifetime, nearly 1% of the population develop schizophrenia, and slightly more, 1–1.5% develop bipolar affective disorder.

There has been some uncertainty about whether the incidence of schizophrenia is lower in higher social classes. Evidence supports that there is certainly a drift downwards before and after the illness occurs. There is also an 8% excess of people who develop schizophrenia who are born in the winter months. This is from January to April for people living in the Northern Hemisphere, and July to September for those in the South. No conclusive explanation has been given for these findings.

The International Pilot Study of Schizophrenia concluded that there was a similar incidence of schizophrenia across the wide range of different countries they investigated but there are some individual groups with higher incidence. In the UK, the incidence in second-generation African Caribbean men is markedly raised but there is much controversy as to why this should be so. The diagnostic instruments used and the way they are used seem to be similar to the way they are used in other populations and so diagnosis does not seem to be in error. It is believed that environmental factors are the most likely causes of the raised incidence and these would include stressful life experiences arising from racism.

Interventions and treatments

Intervention in schizophrenia and affective disorders needs to occur early. It should be as effective as possible whether it involves measures to improve social circumstances or symptoms. Treatments need to be aimed at meeting needs rather than just reducing symptoms. For example, some people are only minimally distressed by their voices, and strenuous efforts to get rid of them simply leads to impairment in other areas of their lives through over-sedation or other side-effects. Social interventions are discussed elsewhere in this book and so not mentioned further here. Psychological interventions are being shown to be effective, especially where based on cognitive behavioural principles (see **Chapter 10**).

Medication does seem to be of value and numerous studies have shown that it reduces relapse in the period after an episode of schizophrenia or affective disorder. After a first episode, many individuals and their doctors will agree to discontinue medication although there is evidence that it is protective for the first couple of years. After repeated episodes, long term maintenance is indicated using an anti-psychotic drug in schizophrenia or a mood stabiliser in affective disorder. Exactly how these drugs work is unclear. Perhaps they offer the individual a 'buffer' from the effects of stress, and they certainly assist with sleep and improving mood. People's adherence to medication regimes is not good according to some studies, suggesting that two thirds fail to take medication properly. However, there is some evidence that cognitive behavioural intervention can improve compliance with a medication regime (Kemp *et al*, 1996).

Commonly used anti-psychotic drugs include chlorpromazine, haloperidol, thiorodazine, trifluoperazine and sulpiride. These all have trade names such as 'Largactil', 'Stelazine' etc and are usually given by depot injection weekly to monthly, which assists in adherence to treatment regimes. Side-effects are common and can include tremor, stiffness, involuntary movements and sedation. A number of drugs have recently been introduced which have different and generally fewer side-effects. These include clozapine which requires regular blood monitoring and other newer drugs such as respiridone, seroquel, sertindole and olanzapine.

Mood stabilisers include the standard 'tricyclic' anti-depressants, such as imipramine and amitryptiline, and the newer SSRIs (see **Chapter 1**). Drugs such as lithium carbonate and carbamazepine, if taken long term, reduce the likelihood of depressive or manic relapse. Electro Convulsive Therapy (ECT) still has a place when someone is severely depressed or manic, as both conditions can be life-threatening if they persist. There are also well conducted research studies showing that ECT can be effective especially where delusions are present.

What about the future?

The outcome or prognosis for an individual depends on their presentation, response to treatment and the quality of aftercare. Outcomes surprisingly seem to be better in developing countries compared to the 'developed world' with 45% compared to 25% clinically recovered after five years.

Affective disorders have a significant effect on people's lives and relapse is quite common. Suicide in particular is a serious risk, and is estimated at 15%. It is also a significant risk in schizophrenia. Ten per cent of people with schizophrenia die from suicide early on in the course of their illness. This is possibly related to insight developing and feelings of hopelessness about the future. Young males with repeat admissions as a result of multiple delusions and hallucinations are at risk but the risk does appear to remain throughout the course of the illness. Physical illness is also a significant problem with death rates which are two to three times higher than in the general population. This is partly due to habits which contribute to poor health, for example 90% of individuals with persistent schizophrenia smoke and their diet is frequently poor.

Despite these statistics there are some positive indicators. Early intervention appears to lead to a better prognosis. Studies in Vermont and Nottingham have provided quite positive results in people with functional psychosis even where they have been institutionalised for many years.

Summary

In summary, the symptoms of schizophrenia and affective psychosis can be classified into positive, negative and thought disorder. There is a significant degree of overlap of symptoms between the different disorders. Causation is multifunctional with social, biological and environmental variables playing a part.

Treatment should be aimed at meeting needs rather than reducing symptoms and should embrace social and psychological approaches rather than medication *per se*. Early intervention seems to play a role in promoting a better prognosis. It is important to regard any label or diagnosis as referring to the mental health problem not the individual themselves as this can lead to professionals dismissing the individual as a person in their own right.

References

American Psychiatric Association (1994) *Diagnostic & Statistical Manual of Mental Disorders* (4th Edn). Washington D.C.: APA.

Bebbington, P., Wilkins, S., Jones, P. *et al* (1993) Life events and psychosis. Initial results from the Camberwell Collaborative Psychosis Study. *British Journal of Psychiatry* **162** 72–79.

Blueler, M. (1911) *Dementia Praecox or the Group of Schizophrenias* (trans. J. J. Zinkin, 1950). New York: International Universities Press.

David, A. S. (1990) Insight and psychosis. *British Journal of Psychiatry* **156** 798–808.

Harrow, M. & Prosen, M. (1978) Intermingling and disordered logic as influences on schizophrenic 'thought disorders'. *Archives of General Psychiatry* **35** 1213–1218.

Jones, P., Rodgers, B., Murray, R. & Marmot, M. (1993) Child development risk factors for adult schizophrenia in the British 1946 birth cohort. *Lancet* **344** 1398–1402.

Kendler, K. S. & Robinette, C. D. (1983) Schizophrenia in the National Academy of Science. National Research Council Twin Registry. *American Journal of Psychiatry* **140** 1551–63.

Kingdon, D. G. & Turkington, D. (1998) Cognitive Behaviour Therapy: Styles, Groups and Outcomes. In: T. Wykes, N. Tarrier and S. Lewis (Eds) *Outcome and Innovation in the Psychological Treatment of Schizophrenia.* Chichester: John Wiley.

Kemp, R. Hayward, P., Applewhaite, G., Everitt, B. & David, A. (1996) Compliance therapy in psychotic patients: a randomised controlled study. *British Medical Journal* **312** 345–349.

Kraeplin, E. (1896) Psychiatrie. (5th Edn.) Leipzig: Barth.

Leff, J., Satorius, A., Jablensky, A. *et al* (1992) The International Pilot Study of Schizophrenia: five year follow-up findings. *Psychological Medicine* **22** 131–45.

Liddle, P & Barnes, T. R. E. (1990) Syndromes of chronic schizophrenia. *British Journal of Psychiatry* **157** 558–561.

Meltzer, H., Gill, B., Petticrew, M. & Hinds, K. (1995) *OPCS Surveys of Psychiatric Morbidity in Great Britain. Report 1.* London: HMSO

Office of Populations, Censuses and Surveys (1996) *The National Psychiatric Morbidity Survey.* London: OCPS.

Schneider, X. (1959) Clinical Psychopathology (trans. M. Hamilton). New York: Grune and Stratton.

Strauss, J. S. (1969) Hallucinations and delusions as points of continua function. *Archives of General Psychiatry* **21** 581–586.

World Health Organisation (1992) *The ICD-10 Classification of Mental and Behavioural Disorders: Clinical descriptions and diagnostic guidelines.* Geneva: WHO.

Chapter 3

Mental Health Problems in Young People

Carol Fernandez & David Rothery

Introduction

At any one time, between 10% and 20% of young people up to the age of 16 have emotional or behavioural difficulties severe enough to need help in overcoming them (Department of Health, 1994). The causes of these problems are often related to stress and aversive life experiences. It is not true to say, as is sometimes asserted, that adolescents generally tend to grow out of these difficulties.

Young people who are or have been sexually or physically abused are particularly at risk of developing emotional or behavioural difficulties. However, being subjected to peer bullying, being poorly or inconsistently parented, emotionally abused or losing important adult figures can often give rise to problems too. In addition to this, young people who are unable to cope with managing the adolescent maturational tasks associated with growing up, with the increased independence and responsibility that this entails, are also prone to developing difficulties. These maturational tasks include the development of emotional, social and work identities as well as separation from their family of origin or other caretaking situation.

Unhappiness, anxiety, social phobia, risk-taking behaviour, conduct problems, delinquency, self-harming behaviour and more specific attempts at suicide can all be indications of young people running into problems (NHS Health Advisory Service, 1995).

Adolescents can also develop specific psychiatric disorders. These include:

- depressive illness
- specific phobias such as school phobia
- obsessive compulsive disorders
- eating disorders (anorexia and bulimia nervosa)
- manic depression
- schizophrenia.

Disabilities or disorders, such as learning disabilities/difficulties, autism and attention deficit hyperactivity disorder (ADHD), which have been present from an early age, can give rise to increased and in some cases different types of problems during the adolescent period. Young people with temperamental difficulties are also more at risk of developing problems. However, there are no psychiatric disorders which are unique to adolescence.

Differentiating between what may be called reactions to development and environmental stressors and the development of a specific psychiatric illness can on occasions be very difficult. It must also be borne in mind that there is a degree of overlap in that development and environmental stressors can precipitate psychiatric disorder, and psychiatric disorder always has implications for an adolescent's development and how they might respond to the environment (Rutter *et al*, 1994).

Emotional problems

At some time in their adolescence nearly all young people have periods when they feel frightened, sad or upset about things. Indeed, up to half of all young people have felt so low in mood that they have cried and wanted to get away from everything and everybody, and up to a fifth have felt that life was not worth living at some time.

When these feelings do not go away quickly and start to affect school work or relationships with family and friends, then a mental health problem can be said to have developed. Emotional disorders are often not recognised by adults, even those close to the teenager. Withdrawal from usual activities, worry about appearance and unusual behaviour can all be indicators of emotional difficulties in a teenager. This does not necessarily mean however that the teenager has developed a psychiatric disorder such as a depressive illness.

Treatment may entail offering a range of interventions which might include general supportive psychotherapy and advice, suggestions for changing the young person's environment, eg their school, as well as more formal psychotherapy such as cognitive-behavioural and family therapy (Graham & Hughes, 1995).

Self-harm and suicide

Deliberate self-harm peaks in late adolescence and research shows that it is more commonly carried out by females than males. The opposite is true for completed suicide where males outnumber females. Self-harm is usually an impulsive act. Common motives include wanting to get out of an intolerable situation, making other people feel sorry and wanting to draw attention to personal distress. The teenager is rarely found to be suffering from a specific psychiatric disorder and serious suicidal intent is often low. However, care must be taken to identify those adolescents who are at increased risk of further self-harm, as suicide, although uncommon, is the third commonest cause of death in adolescence. Adolescents most at risk are those alienated from society in general, with long-standing low mood and drug or alcohol abuse. Multiple losses or changes, such as the breakup of a close relationship, or problems at school may precipitate the attempt. Suicide of a relative or close friend or a media figure may also be important. Ten per cent of adolescents who attempt suicide repeat the act within a year. When suicidal behaviour is associated with being male, there are several factors which have been identified as indicating an increased risk of the young person succeeding in killing themselves. These include previous attempts at suicide, persistent depression, isolation and alienation from family and social support, a suicide plan and note and a family history of depression or suicide.

Self-injurious behaviour such as cutting, biting, burning or inserting objects such as needles into parts of the body tends to occur in adolescent girls who have problems in their personality development. This is often associated with low self-esteem and poor relationships. Self-injurious behaviour is also associated with eating disorders. Commonly it seems to be used by the teenager as a means of releasing intolerable tension. After the self-mutilation the young person generally feels detached and calm before experiencing shame and guilt associated with the act.

In the management of a young person who has self-harmed, the first task is to keep them safe while an assessment of their mental state is carried out. Typically the issue which needs to be addressed first is whether or not the young person is suffering from a mental illness. Often there is no mental illness. It is more usually the case that there are relationship problems with parents or carers, friends, or problems at school which have precipitated the self-harm episode. It is usually these problems that need to be addressed (NHS Health Advisory Service, 1994).

The key factors in addressing these issues include providing the young person with a stable environment and providing psychotherapy. Both these interventions will allow the young person to express their distress in a more appropriate way and to help them develop more appropriate coping strategies. In addition to this, it is helpful to involve other significant adults such as parents or carers to listen to the young person.

It is not unusual for those who harm themselves to provoke considerable anxiety for both carers and professionals who come into contact with them. As emphasised above, the most important task is to ensure that the young person is safe from further acts of self-harm, thus consideration may need to be given to the use of a statutory order to ensure their safety. It can be difficult to decide if involving the *Mental Health Act* is warranted on the grounds that the young person may be suffering from a mental illness. It is therefore important that any mental health assessment is conducted jointly between a social worker, and a child and adolescent psychiatrist. Assessment usually concludes that the young person is not suffering from a mental illness as defined by the *Act* and that action under childcare legislation should be considered if removal to a safe place is required. This will involve an assessment of the ability of the young person's parents or carers to deliver a 'reasonable' level of childcare (*Children Act 1989*). There might also be grounds to invoke the *Children Act* if the young person is beyond the control of their parent or carer.

Sometimes, for those young people who need safe accommodation as a result of self-harm, the most appropriate resource is local authority secure accommodation. This will involve using Section 25 of the *Children Act 1989*. However, as an alternative, some young people may be suitably accommodated in a children's home or in a teenage foster placement.

Problems with behaviour

A young person with behavioural problems from a health point of view is often said to be suffering from a **conduct disorder**. A significant conduct disorder is characterised by persistent and significant anti-social, destructive and aggressive behaviour. In order to fulfil the criteria for the diagnosis to be made, a teenager needs have more than transient behavioural problems. Conduct disorders can be associated with severe emotional problems. It is separate from, but overlaps with **delinquency** which includes behaviours such as theft, assault and serious vandalism. Delinquency is often associated with alienation from parents and identification with a delinquent peer group (NHS Health advisory Service, 1995).

Young people with conduct disorders are more usually referred to in social service contexts as those who are 'beyond control'. The most useful way to intervene with these young people is to aim interventions at both changing their behaviour and at helping them to look at improving their handling of interpersonal relationships. A combination of individual psychotherapy and behavioural intervention, sometimes including anger management techniques, is often helpful. In addition, family work or a combination of individual work with the young person, along with separate work with parents or carers, can help (Rutter, *et al, ibid*).

Eating problems

Problems with eating, body weight and shape seem to be increasing within the teenage population. The two main eating disorders are **anorexia nervosa** and **bulimia nervosa**. Anorexia nervosa may present very insidiously with weight loss very advanced before parents notice anything amiss. It is a disorder where females account for between 90% and 95% of cases. The central symptoms of this disorder are weight loss, ammenorrhoea (cessation of menstruation) and preoccupation with body weight together with the pursuit of continued weight loss. This can be a life-threatening condition with anything up to 15% of sufferers dying either from malnutrition or, more commonly, suicide. On occasions professionals need to resort to using the *Mental Health Act* in order to ensure that a sick teenager receives appropriate treatment.

In the treatment of anorexia nervosa the first and most important task is to enable the young person to gain weight. It is often the case that if a person's weight is very low they are unable to usefully engage in individual psychotherapeutic work. Our own experience at the adolescent unit in Birmingham is that a combination of individual, group and family work can help a young person consider the issues which have contributed to the development of their illness. Russell and his colleagues (1987) have demonstrated that family work aimed at restructuring the family behaviour is helpful in dealing with anorexia in younger individuals. In older adolescents it is often the case that the young person themselves will eventually take responsibility for eating. However, family work can still be useful in these situations as the illness itself can cause considerable problems and tensions within family relationships.

Bulimia nervosa tends to be a disorder of older adolescents. The main symptoms consist of a cycle of binge eating followed by vomiting, and sometimes purging by the use of laxatives. In the main it is a chronic secretive disorder as the teenager is often extremely ashamed of their behaviour. Unlike someone suffering from anorexia nervosa the teenager is usually of normal weight or in some cases overweight. On occasions, young people suffering from this disorder can became seriously depressed with the possibility of suicide attempts being made.

It is not usually helpful to admit young people with bulimia nervosa to hospital. Individual therapy using a cognitive behavioural approach is usually the best way to help them to change their abnormal eating patterns. It is also important to look with them at the emotional difficulties that so often precede the bulimia. Treatment with fluoxetine, a new generation anti-depressant, has also been shown to be helpful in this condition (Rutter, *et al, ibid*).

Substance abuse

Adolescents are growing up in a world where alcohol, drug use and abuse are increasing. This, combined with peer group pressures, easy access, and glamorisation in the media means that experimentation with drugs and alcohol is occurring at an earlier age. Drug and alcohol abuse can cause medical problems such as overdosage and infection with HIV or hepatitis, as well as psychiatric problems such as depression, attempts at suicide, and drug-induced psychoses. The latter can be caused by using LSD and amphetamines. Drugs can also precipitate a psychotic illness in a teenager who is vulnerable to developing such an illness. Alcohol misuse and abuse by teenagers causes more problems than other drugs.

A teenager who is abusing substances may present with serious, sudden changes in behaviour. However, most young people who try drugs never get beyond the experimentation phase and hence do not develop problems.

In terms of treatment approaches it is important to try and engage the young person in the treatment process. Generally this is best done on an outpatient basis. There needs to be a range of treatment options available including individual, group and family treatments. Unfortunately, there is a dearth of suitable treatment resources for adolescents with substance abuse problems. This is particularly true of suitable residential units (Rutter, *et al, ibid*).

Specific psychiatric illness

Anxiety states, phobias and obsessive compulsive disorders can affect teenagers. However, serious mental illnesses, such as severe depression, manic depression and schizophrenia, though rare in young adolescents, become more common in older teenagers and in the early twenties.

Depression

A low mood in an adolescent does not mean that the person is necessarily suffering from clinical depression. Unhappiness is very common at one time or another during this period of development. However, low mood that is totally unresponsive to external events, and which is associated with irritability and loss of enjoyment in previously pleasurable activities, does suggest a depressive illness. Biological symptoms such as weight loss and sleep disturbance may not be prominent symptoms in teenagers but do occur. It can be difficult distinguishing true depressive illness from a reaction to developmental issues or external events. However, this distinction is important as research suggests that depressive illness in teenagers is both under-recognised and under-treated. Treatment of depressive disorder in teenagers involves support and discussion of any particular difficulties in the young person's life. Anti-depressant medication can be very useful despite evidence that it is less successful in teenagers than adults.

Anxiety disorders

These disorders often arise out of fears commonly held at this age stage. Examples include a fear of global catastrophe and concern about personal appearance and gender issues. However, more adult type disorders may occur, such as a panic disorder and agoraphobia. They may present with fear of certain aspects of school (such as assemblies or undressing for sports), fear of personal failure or anxiety about personal appearance. Physical symptoms such as abdominal pain and headache are common. Anxiety-based disorders can produce quite bizarre behaviour in teenagers such as total social withdrawal, refusal to communicate with anybody at all or reversal of the normal day/night rhythm such that the young person is active at night but asleep during the day. Treatment involves understanding the young person's anxiety in the context of their life. It is important that they have access to support and a listening ear as well as more specific treatments such as relaxation therapy and behavioural interventions. In general, treatment with medication is rarely used as it can lead to problems with dependence.

Obsessional disorders

This disorder in young people presents with very much the same symptoms as in adults. The features of an obsessional disorder are **obsessional thoughts** and **compulsive acts**. Obsessional thoughts are ideas, images or impulses that recurrently enter into consciousness in a stereotyped fashion. These are distressing and the sufferer often tries unsuccessfully to resist them. They are, however, recognised as the person's own thoughts. Compulsive acts are stereotyped behaviours that are repeated again and again. In extreme cases in teenagers it can sometimes be difficult to distinguish an obsessional disorder from a psychotic illness. Indeed, the onset of a schizophrenic illness can sometimes present with obsessional symptoms. Treatment involves various behavioural approaches such as modelling, response prevention and thought-stopping. Two anti-depressant drugs, clomipramine and fluoxetine, appear to have an anti-obsessional effect and are on occasions useful as an additional treatment, along with behaviour therapy.

Schizophrenia

Schizophrenia is rare in early adolescence and only becomes more common in the late teenage years and the early twenties. Classical symptoms of schizophrenia, such as clear auditory hallucinations and delusions, are less common in adolescents as compared with adults.

The onset of the illness can be vague, characterised by gradual social withdrawal and marked social and educational difficulties. Symptoms may also be intermittent. The mental state may include vagueness of thought and confusion, with suspicion, intermittent fear and distress. Symptoms such as delusions, auditory hallucinations and paranoid ideas may also occur. It can be very difficult to differentiate between schizophrenia and mania in adolescence and it is not uncommon for the diagnosis to change during subsequent episodes of illness.

Assessment

Essentially, the assessment and treatment of young people with psychotic disorders is no different from the assessment and treatment of adults with such presenting problems. Occasionally it will become necessary to consider detention under the *1983 Mental Health Act*. If the person is assessed as having a psychiatric illness, and is of sufficient age and maturity to make their own decisions regarding treatment, and yet is refusing such treatment, then use of the *Mental Health Act* should be considered. If the young person is not of sufficient age and understanding to make their own decisions regarding treatment, then the responsibility for this decision lies with whoever has parental responsibility (Section 2 of the *Children Act 1989*). If the person with this responsibility is considered not to be acting reasonably then social services will need to consider the use of childcare legislation to mandate assessment and treatment. However, it should be remembered that children retain the right to refuse examination and treatment, and this right can only be overturned by recourse to the Court (*Children Act 1989* – Section 8 Specific Issues Order or Section 100 Wardship).

As presented by the Government guidance, it should be national practice that young people under 16 years of age who have been detained under the *Mental Health Act* are made subject to the Care Programme Approach (Department of Health and Welsh Office HC (90)23/LASSL(90)11).

Use of the *Mental Health Act* with adolescents

In order to illustrate the issues which have been described so far, four case examples are outlined and discussed below and opposite.

Case study 1   Susan

Susan is a white 15-year-old girl and has been seen as an outpatient by a child psychiatrist. Her initial presenting problem was of feeling unhappy and wanting to die. The psychiatrist has been seeing her for six months, has prescribed anti-depressants and has also provided psychotherapy. After a session she discloses that she was sexually abused by her father some years ago. Additionally she does not have a good relationship with her mother and mother's boyfriend. Today at the appointment Susan says she has cut herself and if she has to go home she will do so again. The psychiatrist requests an approved social worker to assess Susan to establish whether compulsory admission to a psychiatric hospital is a viable and appropriate option.

Case study 2   Halima

Sixteen-year-old **Halima** is a Pakistani Muslim girl, with mild learning disabilities. She lives with her parents and two younger siblings. She has been suffering from a psychotic illness for the last 18 months and has been treated as an outpatient by both a child psychiatrist and a psychiatrist in the field of learning disability. Halima has not been in school for two years and has been referred to the regional adolescent inpatient services because her illness has deteriorated. Halima is reported to still be hearing voices and responding verbally to them by swearing at them to go away. She is also refusing to take medication or to eat and drink. She is not sleeping and has been verbally and physically aggressive to her parents. Halima is seen by an adolescent psychiatrist and an approved social worker (ASW). She agrees she has problems but does not want to go into hospital. Her parents had originally requested hospital admission but are now saying they will persevere with her at home.

Case study 3 Justin

Justin is 13 years old and lives with his mother, and stepfather, who has legally adopted him. He has had no contact with his biological father who left his mother when she was pregnant. Recently, Justin had an argument with his stepfather and swallowed some bleach. This is the second time he has done so in six months. In Casualty at the district general hospital he tells the child psychiatrist that he hates his stepfather. He thinks his mother loves his half-brother more than she loves him and wishes he were dead. He also says he does not want to go home. On further questioning it appears Justin has been unhappy for some months. He is agreeable to going into an adolescent unit for assessment. His mother tells the psychiatrist that Justin swallowed the bleach out of anger because his stepfather had reprimanded him for hitting his 6-year-old half-brother. She says that usually Justin and his stepfather get on very well. She also thinks bumping into his biological father last week may have upset Justin. She thinks he should be back at home and is sure that things will 'sort themselves out'. She thinks the bleach-swallowing episode should be ignored.

Case study 4 Michael

A 15-year-old boy called **Michael** has been in local authority accommodation since the age of 4 and is subject to a Care Order. He does not know his biological mother who left him with his father when he was 1 year old. His father died when he was ten. Originally in foster care, Michael was moved to a children's home at the age of eleven. Michael has since been in two other homes. Michael took an overdose of tablets some twelve months ago. As a result he was assessed by a psychiatrist who offered outpatient appointments which Michael failed to attend. Things had seemed to settle down until the last two weeks when he took two further overdoses of twenty five paracetamol tablets. Following the last overdose Michael was seen in the Accident and Emergency department. Staff would like to admit him for a further assessment. Michael refuses to go into hospital. He says he took the overdoses because of bullying from peers at school and in the children's home. He says he just wants to go into foster care. His social worker is concerned he might take another overdose.

Key questions and issues to be considered with all four examples include:

- ■ Is this a mental health problem?

- ■ Is the young person giving consent to assessment/treatment?

- ■ Is the young person deemed able to give consent (Devereux, Jones & Dickenson, 1993)?

- ■ If the young person is not deemed able to give consent, who has parental responsibility and is therefore in a position to give consent?

- ■ Is the person with parental responsibility acting 'reasonably' – within the meaning of the term in the *Children Act 1989* (Section 31)?

The legal position

The question of whether the problem is a mental health one or not is a matter of both clinical and ASW judgement and ideally the decision should be reached jointly. The *Children Act* states clearly that *'the child may, if he is of sufficient understanding to make an informed decision, refuse to submit to the examination or other assessment'*.

Similarly the *Mental Health Act Code of Practice 1993*, (Para 30.7(a)) notes that:

> *'If a child has "sufficient understanding and intelligence" he can take decisions about his own medical treatment in the same way as an adult'.*

The decision as to whether a young person has sufficient understanding to give valid consent is one of clinical judgement. However, Paragraph 15.10 of the *Mental Health Code of Practice* (*ibid*) places a responsibility on the clinician to ensure that the treatment has been explained to the young person in a way he or she can understand. Importance is placed upon the use of 'interpreting services' in certain situations – especially those where the person's and nearest relative's first language is not English or those who have a hearing disability.

A young person's biological mother automatically has parental responsibility. If the parents were married at any time, the father too will automatically have parental responsibility. If the parents are not married, the father may have parental responsibility only if he acquires it through the Court. Additionally, other adults may also obtain parental responsibility through the Courts. If another adult acquires parental responsibility it does not mean that those who already have it lose it. Therefore, consultation with the adults involved in the care and welfare of the young person may need to go beyond interviews with one or both biological parents.

Specific issues to be considered in relation to each example are as follows:

In **Case study 1** it may be that despite the anti-depressant medication and the psychotherapeutic treatment **Susan** has become increasingly depressed and is at risk of serious further self-harm. One way to establish this would be to ascertain the degree of cutting and the events surrounding the act, together with her reasons for wanting to further harm herself. If the cutting is severe and if the psychiatrist's assessment is that she is at risk of further serious self-harm because of a depressive illness then it may be appropriate to consider the need for her to be admitted to hospital. However, it may be that Susan's act of self-harm was precipitated by unhappiness or anger about her home situation or following some emotional distress precipitated through the psychotherapeutic work she was engaged in. This would not in itself be a reason to consider admission to psychiatric hospital. Alternatively, it may be more appropriate to consider how able her mother is to provide emotionally stable care for her or how able she is to assist with the impact the feelings are having on Susan. If the assessment is that Susan's mother is not sufficiently able to provide a safe, emotionally stable and caring environment it may be appropriate to consider Susan moving somewhere else, to relatives, friends or to accommodation provided by the local social services department. If the intent to harm were serious (or if there were a history of previous self-harm) it may be more appropriate to conclude that for the time being Susan's mother is not able to provide a sufficiently safe environment for her and that a placement in a secure setting should be more appropriate. It may well be necessary to consider using Section 25 of the *1989 Children Act* (*Secure Accommodation*).

With regard to **Case study 2**, the answer to the question of 'Is this a mental health problem' would most probably be 'yes'. However, it would still be important to assess whether admission to hospital would be '*in all the circumstances of the case the most appropriate way of providing the care and medical treatment of which the patient stands in need*' (Section 13.2 *Mental Health Act 1983*). In **Halima's** case, does she need admission? Can she be deemed to be able to consent to treatment? How much does her learning disability, or indeed her current mental ill health, mean that she does not have the capacity to give valid consent? Can she continue to be treated at home?

Anti-discriminatory issues to be considered would include avoiding the assumption that because Halima has a learning disability she does not have the capacity to consent to treatment, and avoiding the racist assumption that Halima's Asian family will be able to care for her better than hospital staff – thus denying her the right to treatment and her nearest relative's right for her to be admitted in the interests of their protection.

In **Case study 3** it may well be that at 13, **Justin** is not deemed to have sufficient understanding and intelligence to give his own consent to treatment. However, note that the person with parental responsibility seems to be saying there is no problem, whereas Justin's comments suggest he may be in need of further assessment of his mental state. In this case it may well be appropriate to consider use of the *Children Act* on the grounds that Justin's mother is not giving care which '*it would be reasonable to expect a parent to give to him*' (Section 31.2b (I) *Children Act*

1989). In this case, an Emergency Protection Order, with a direction concerning medical examination (assessment), would be appropriate.

In **Case study 4, Michael** is already on a Care Order, thus it would be important to decide if there is sufficient information to suggest he may be suffering from a mental illness. If there is sufficient information, should there be consideration of the use of Section 2 of the *Mental Health Act*? Alternatively, use of Wardship (*1989 Children Act* Section 100) could be considered, as the inherent jurisdiction of the High Court could be used to direct assessment.

When considering the use of the *Mental Health Act 1983* in relation to work with young people it is vital to refer to Section 30 of the *Code of Practice*. This section in the revised code makes some areas clearer than before.

In practice, problems arise more often when a young person refuses assessment or treatment. Case law examples would suggest that a young person can be deemed competent to give consent to treatment but not competent to refuse consent.

We have alluded already to anti-discriminatory practice in this area; it should be remembered that in all work with young people it is important not to abuse our power as adults but to make decisions on their behalf if they are not capable of doing so themselves.

Resources

Most district health authorities have district child psychiatric services – usually staffed by a multidisciplinary team of psychiatrists, psychologists, community psychiatric nurses, and social workers. These services will have links with their local inpatient facilities and all should be aware of the procedures for referral to them.

The majority of adolescents are treated as outpatients. Inpatient units for adolescents are limited in number although there is one in most regions. However, the criteria for admission can be somewhat idiosyncratic to each unit. In general they are under considerable pressure to respond adequately to the demands placed on them. Few, if any, are able to accept emergency admissions. This means that those young people who need emergency admission, often in a severe crisis, have to go elsewhere on a temporary basis, such as an adult psychiatric hospital. This is by no means the most helpful solution for young people in mental health crises. The Health Advisory Service (1986) has advised of the importance of young people to be nursed in an appropriate adolescent environment. Secure psychiatric units for adolescents are even scarcer as there are only two NHS facilities in the country.

Summary

Young people can present with signs and symptoms of mental distress as a consequence of the difficulties and dilemmas involved in growing up. Others do display signs and symptoms of specific psychiatric illnesses and, as such, require treatment. This usually involves a combination of medication and psychotherapy, which should involve both the individual and family members or significant adults.

The legislative framework for intervening with young people in times of crisis can involve either the *Mental Health Act 1983* or the *Children Act 1989*. Practitioners should conduct assessments jointly and ensure that the most appropriate legislation is used and takes account of the power imbalance that can exist between adult professionals and young people in their care.

References

The Children Act (1989) London: HMSO.

Department of Health and Welsh Office (1993) *Code of Practice Mental Health Act 1983*. London: HMSO.

Department of Health and Welsh Office (1994) *Health of the Nation. Mental Illness: Can children and young people have mental health problems?* London: The Stationery Office.

Department of Health and Welsh Office HC(90)23/Lassl(90)11. *The Care Programme Approach for people with a mental illness referred to the specialist psychiatric services*. London: The Stationery Office.

Devereux, J. A., Jones, D. P. H. & Dickenson, D. L. (1993) Can children withhold consent to treatment? *British Medical Journal* **306** 1459–1461.

Graham, P. & Hughes, C. (1995) *So Young So Sad So Listen*. London: Gaskell/West London Health Promotion Agency.

Mental Health Act (1983) London: HMSO.

NHS Health Advisory Service (1986) *Bridges Over Troubled Waters: A report on services for disturbed adolescents*. London: HMSO.

NHS Health Advisory Service (1994) *Suicide Prevention: The challenge confronted*. London: HMSO.

NHS Health Advisory Service (1995) *Child and Adolescent Mental Health Services: Together we stand*. London: HMSO.

Russell, G., Szmuckler, G., Dare, C. & Eisler, I. (1987) An evaluation of family therapy in anorexia nervosa and bulimia nervosa. *Archives of General Psychiatry* **44** 1047–1056.

Rutter, M., Taylor, E. & Hersov, L. (Eds) (1994) *Child and Adolescent Psychiatry: Modern approaches* (3rd edition). Oxford: Blackwell.

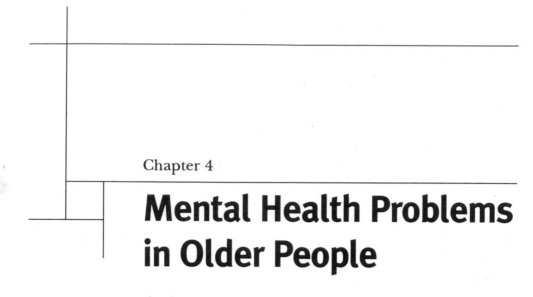

Chapter 4

Mental Health Problems in Older People

Graham Stokes

Introduction

The range of mental disorder to be found in later life is as broad and varied as that observed at any age. As such, a robust mental health assessment must not be limited in scope to the two most common disorders of old age, namely dementia and depression. Yet these are the archetypal referrals for assessment, even though many elderly people suffering from these conditions are not known to health services (Macdonald, 1985; O'Connor *et al*, 1988).

Despite their prevalence, neither dementia nor depression is an inevitable accompaniment of ageing. They are not the unavoidable outcome of an ageing biology, nor are they the inescapable response to adversity. They are, instead, exceptional aberrations requiring, not passive acceptance, but assessment, diagnosis and therapeutic intervention.

At the Core of Mental Health © Pavilion 2000

Dementia – a clinical syndrome

The Royal College of Physicians (1981) defines dementia as:

'... the global impairment of higher cortical functions, including memory, the capacity to solve the problems of day-to-day living, the performance of learned perceptuomotor skills, the correct use of social skills and the control of emotional reactions, in the absence of gross clouding of consciousness [ie drowsiness and a lack of alertness in the person]. The condition is often irreversible and progressive'.

Having described what dementia is, it is also necessary to know what it is not. Although we speak of diagnosing dementia (from the Latin 'demens', which means 'being out of one's mind'), it is not a disease in its own right. It is an umbrella term employed to denote the existence of a neuro-psychological syndrome. As such, dementia represents a clinical description without any supposition to an underlying aetiology (Wade & Hachinski, 1987).

'There are many specific disorders or diseases which can give rise to this grouping of symptoms.'
(Jorm, 1987)

These include Alzheimer's disease, multi-infarct dementia, Pick's disease, dementia with Lewy bodies, Creuzfeldt-Jakob disease and chronic alcohol abuse, which are themselves *'all referred to as dementia'* (Jorm, *ibid*).

For example:

'Dementia is a group of progressive diseases...' (Murphy, 1986)

'Dementia is a set of diseases of the brain ...' (Marshall, 1998)

'Dementia is a disease...' (Moniz-Cook, 1998)

Jorm (1987) questions why we persist with the descriptive term of 'dementia' which is non-specific as to causation, rather than focusing on the specific pathological conditions which give rise to it? The answer is that, when used judiciously, 'dementia' can be a useful concept in practice as the possible causes of dementia are often hard to tell apart, especially in the early stages. It can be seen, therefore as a **'compromise diagnosis'** when faced with brain pathology for which there are no ante-mortem markers. It acknowledges both a set of characteristic signs and symptoms and excludes a number of alternative diagnoses.

Figure 1 (below) illustrates how the term 'dementia' is used as both a descriptor of intellectual and behavioural dysfunction, and as an explanation for that dysfunctional performance.

Figure 1 'Dementia' – both a descriptor of, and explanation for dysfunctional cognition and behaviour	
Clinical Syndrome Progressive and irreversible: ■ memory impairment ■ disorientation and (confusion)* ■ intellectual deficits ■ language impairment ■ perceptual impairment ■ social incompetence ■ ADL** dependency ■ (challenging behaviour) ***	**'Dementia' as a description**
Presumptive Pathology ■ Alzheimer's disease ■ Lewy body dementia ■ Multi-infarct dementia ■ Fronto-temporal dementia	**Dementia as a compromise diagnosis**
* not always observed ** activities of daily living *** not always observed; when present, may possess remedial potential	

It is essential however to appreciate that the presence of cognitive deficits and behavioural incompetence cannot automatically be assumed to be evidence of dementia. The case of **Mrs W** (below) illustrates the multi-factoral nature of cognitive impairment in old age and how the term 'dementia' is often used injudiciously.

Case study	**Mrs W**
Client	Mrs W, aged 81 years
Diagnosis	Dementia of the Alzheimer Type
Demographics	Widowed for 5 years. Lived alone

History

■ Over a two year period noticed to be absent-minded, at times muddled and 'cantankerous'.

■ Admitted to a residential home six months ago as considered to be at risk.

■ Since entry to the home she has been observed to be subdued, withdrawn and increasingly disoriented.

■ Visited by a psychiatrist who asked such questions as day, date, town, country and the name of the Prime Minister and residential home. She was assessed using the Mini-Mental State Examination (MMSE). The MMSE has a series of questions – like 'spell WORLD backwards'; recall 3 objects; copy a design – that test a range of cognitive functions.

■ Poor performance on the MMSE led to both an assumption of severe cognitive impairment and a diagnosis of dementia.

Reformulation

■ At the time of her interview and assessment Mrs W had been confined to bed for the previous six days with a chest infection.

■ Mrs W had been registered blind since 1981, and had worn a hearing aid since 1987.

Opinion   Ill health and profound sensory disadvantage severely compromised Mrs W's ability to comprehend her world, and significantly interfered with her capacity to respond to questions and perform tasks. A 'diagnosis' of dementia was both ill-founded and prejudicial.

The case of **Mrs W** illustrates that a reliable diagnosis of dementia can only follow accurate assessment of performance and the exclusion of physical morbidity, psychological disorder and sensory impairment that may also be responsible for cognitive decline and dependency in later life. Alternative explanations include delirium, caused, for example, by chest infection, urinary tract infection, constipation and toxic states, which include the effects of prescribed medication (Pitt, 1987). Reversible dementia can result from brain tumour, vitamin B12 deficiency, hypothyroidism and subdural haematoma (Byrne, 1987). Other explanations can include benign senescent forgetfulness (Kral, 1962; 1978); and severe depression (Jorm, *ibid*), but not '*being old*' (Stokes, 1992). A 'diagnosis' of '*What do you expect at their age?*' is both wrong and demeaning.

Dementia – prevalence

Recent prevalence studies estimate that there are 636,000 people in the United Kingdom with dementia (Alzheimer's Disease Society, 1995). Yet as there are no reliable ante-mortem markers for the causes of dementia, epidemiological studies rely on 'cases' of dementia based upon clinical symptoms alone (Jagger & Lindesay, 1993). This immediately raises the question, '*What are researchers measuring*'? For example, the previously mentioned Mini-Mental State Examination (Folstein *et al,* 1975) is a widely used screening instrument for the detection of cognitive impairment. Yet Jagger and Lindesay (*ibid*) report the number of studies that have demonstrated that poor education, extreme age, manual social class, visual impairment and even manual dexterity, can give rise to poor performance and cause people to be mis-classified as cases of 'dementia'. Caution is therefore required. As illustrated in the case of **Mrs W**, the MMSE, as well as other brief screening measures, such as the Clifton Assessment Procedures for the Elderly (Pattie & Gilleard, 1979), do not allow a diagnosis of dementia to be made. Despite a general belief that they possess '*diagnostic value*' (Pattie, 1988), these instruments are no more than measures of cognitive functioning and useful indicators of whether further investigations are necessary.

Acknowledging the methodological weaknesses inherent in epidemiological studies, Jagger and Lindesay (1993) consider that the 'norm' in present studies appears to be an overall rate of moderate and severe dementia (both points on a continuum of impairment rendering a person incapable of independent self-care) in those aged 65 years and over, of between four and seven per cent. There are, however no prevalence studies of dementia in Third World countries as longevity is less common in developing countries. Henderson (1986) reports that *'dementia... is extremely rare'* for those adults who enter old age; it is possible they constitute a survival elite who may be resistant to the onset of dementia.

Although prevalence estimates differ across studies, research always confirms the steep rise of dementia prevalence with age (eg Jorm *et al*, 1987; Hofman *et al*, 1991). Just over 1% of people in their late sixties has dementia, while about a third of those over ninety years of age are similarly affected. It is estimated that around 17,000 younger people in the United Kingdom have **'early onset dementia'** (EOD), a term used to describe a syndrome which first begins before the arbitrary cut-off age of 65 years of age.

There are no major differences in prevalence of dementia between men and women, but as women are more likely to live into advanced old age (for example, 75% of adults over 85 are women) there are far more women with dementia than there are men.

The causes of dementia

For most of this century, dementia in late life (**'senile dementia'**) was considered to be an extreme variant of normal age-related changes. Intellectual deterioration was considered to be an almost inevitable consequence of ageing, and as such, attracted little interest from either practitioners or researchers. The commonest cause was felt to be cerebral arteriosclerosis – hardening of the arteries. The brain was thought to be starved of its blood supply because of diseased arteries, which resulted in a progressive dementia. However, knowledge was disfigured by myth and distorted by disinterest. Today, dementia is acknowledged as a major public health challenge. **We now possess a better understanding of the clinical presentation, risk factors and pathogenesis of the four main disorders that result in dementia:**

1 Alzheimer's disease (AD)

2 Multi-infarct dementia (MID)

3 Dementia with Lewy bodies (DLB)

4 Fronto-temporal dementia (FTD).

It is appreciated that the role of arteriosclerosis as a cause of dementia was greatly overestimated (eg Blessed *et al*, 1968; Tomlinson *et al*, 1970).

Alzheimer's Disease (AD)

Alzheimer's disease or senile dementia?

Alzheimer's disease is an acquired neurological disease of the cerebral cortex. It is progressive, irreversible and pursues an insidious unremitting course over a number of years. Following its description by Alois Alzheimer at the beginning of the century, it was regarded as a rare disorder afflicting people in middle age. As a consequence, until recent times, it was described as a '**pre-senile dementia**'. A distinction was made between AD and senile dementia, the latter having an onset at or after 65 years of age. While the characteristic pre-senile picture of intellectual and behavioural deterioration represented an abnormal and tragic deviation from normal ageing in mid-life, senile dementia was considered to be a distinct and separate entity characterised by a sense of inevitability.

Several autopsy studies during the 1960s and 1970s, however, showed that the majority of elderly people with 'senile dementia' had the characteristic neuro-pathological features of AD. In addition, the

At the Core of Mental Health © Pavilion 2000

clinical picture of senile dementia is, in the main, clinically indistinguishable from AD. In essence, AD and senile dementia differ primarily through an arbitrary age cut-off point. As with other diseases, younger people may be more rapidly and severely affected, but there is little evidence to support the *continued* use of the age distinction. With the current tendency to refer to *all* cases as AD, regardless of age at onset, AD has been transformed from a rare dementia affecting middle-aged people, to the most common dementing illness.

Risk factors

Epidemiological studies have identified very few risk factors so far. Aside from age – which is the most important risk factor for AD – no other risk factors have been adequately established.

■ Family history

Despite methodological difficulties, reliable data suggest that first degree relatives (eg siblings, children) of AD victims do have a greater risk of developing the disease. Probably the most rigorous genetic study of AD is that of Heston (1981). He found that the risk to relatives varies greatly depending on the age that AD began. Genetic factors appear to decrease in significance with later age of onset in the index case.

■ Head trauma

Both early-onset and late-onset cases of AD are more likely to have experienced a serious head injury at some point in their lives. A single severe blow resulting in loss of consciousness can predispose someone to AD in later life. In most cases, this accident occurs several decades before the onset of dementia. Mortimer *et al* (1985) found the average time elapsing between the head injury and the signs of dementia was 35 years.

■ Down's Syndrome

As people with Down's Syndrome grow older, an above average incidence of Alzheimer's disease has been noted. Fifty years ago, post-mortem studies revealed that between 90 and 100% of people with Down's Syndrome over the age of 35 had the characteristic cellular changes of Alzheimer's disease (Thase, 1982). It appears, however that many will not develop signs of dementia when alive (Oliver & Holland, 1986). A review of the link between Down's Syndrome and Alzheimer's disease is provided by Barr and Campbell (1995).

■ **Environmental toxins**

AD could be due to some toxic agent that affects the brain, which reacts by producing plaques and tangles. The most discussed possibility is aluminium. AD sufferers have been shown to have high levels of aluminium in their brains. Although aluminium is a common substance, in geographical areas where the aluminium content in the water supply is high, it is suggested there is a higher prevalence of AD. The case, however, remains unproven.

Clinical picture

The course of cognitive, behavioural and emotional change varies from person to person. However, while there is no common pathway, a stage model describing broad characteristics is generally accepted. A typical early AD dementia may not however be easy to differentiate from benign age-related changes.

The 'forgetfulness phase' (minimal dementia)

Evidence of memory impairment is a necessary condition for the diagnosis of AD, and in the great majority of cases it is present at the earliest stage. At this point the most prominent feature is an impairment of storage, wherein memory for recent events is affected, and there is a tendency to forget where objects have been placed and what was intended next. Disorientation in time frequently occurs. Names of places and people that were once familiar may also be poorly recalled. Overall, the memory disorder is usually apparent as a mild, exaggerated forgetfulness.

Fatigue and poor concentration may be observed. The learning of new information is deficient. Abstract thinking shows signs of patchy impairment. The structure of conversational speech (eg phrase length, grammar) is relatively normal in the early stages of AD, but the speech content tends to be abnormal. There is an over-reliance on stock phrases and mild word-finding difficulties (known as anomia).

Aside from cognitive impairment, there are changes in mood and adaptive behaviour. The new or unexpected is feared or disliked. The person appears egocentric as they seek sanctuary in established routines. At this early stage, activities of daily living in familiar surroundings are usually unimpaired, but when in new situations a shifting pattern of incompetence is revealed. Impairments become apparent more quickly if the person leads an active, varied life than if they have a routine lifestyle.

There may be emotional changes such as anxiety and irritability. While depression is often fleeting and variable, Alexopolous *et al* (1988) estimated that up to 50% of people with dementia may also suffer from depression. For others, mood disturbance and anxiety are conspicuously absent.

In the early stages of AD, most people display some form of insight into their impairments, although awareness is often less apparent in late-onset dementia. However, insight may be distorted by memory dysfunction, cultural expectation and psychological defence mechanisms. Reactions to the distressing changes may not simply manifest as appropriate concern, but instead result in the onset of additional psychopathology that may obscure the advancing cognitive decline. Denial may be used as a defence against the emotional trauma of losing one's intellectual capacity. The dementing person may also appear 'paranoid' as they attempt to avoid the frightening implications of a deteriorating memory:

> *'Making accusations against others to explain why items cannot be found or why an arrangement was*

*forgotten can provide external sources of blame for
internally caused errors.'*
(Stokes, 1990)

The 'confusional phase' (mild-moderate dementia)

This stage is characterised by progressively failing memory,
increasingly poor attention-span and a generalised decline in
intellectual performance. Learning becomes increasingly impaired.
Disorientation in place can result in the person getting lost in
unfamiliar surroundings. Forgetting internally produced plans and
objectives is, in many ways, responsible for the discontinuity and lack
of purpose that characterises the dementia. Behaviour is seen to be
increasingly random and disorganised. As retrieval of familiar
information from memory is affected, the person may acquire a
reality different from our own. To us they have become confused.

All aspects of language become more impaired, although structural
features show slowest deterioration. Berrios (1987) notes that the
interacting effects of memory loss, cognitive degeneration and
perceptual dysfunction lead to a peculiar disintegration of spoken,
written and read language in dementia. Defects in comprehension
become evident.

Judgement and the capacity for abstract thought are significantly
deteriorated. Apraxia and agnosia evolve. Apraxia is the impairment
of the ability to carry out purposeful movements even though motor
skills and comprehension of the action to be carried out are intact.
Agnosia is a disorder of recognition resulting in an inability to
identify an object by sight alone. As Holden (1990) writes:

> *'...(it) is not only an inability to name or demonstrate
> the use of an object without touching it, but also a lack
> of recognition of the object's meaning or character'.*

Case illustrations of the neuro-psychological changes that may form
part of a person's dementia are to be found in Sacks (1985).

Complex tasks are slovenly and inaccurately performed. Mistakes are not acknowledged or corrected. Skills necessary for social independence are the first to be markedly eroded, although during this stage, basic self-care skills are also compromised. Behaviour is considered to be increasingly 'risky'. There is a withdrawal from demanding situations. Mood is characterised by emotional flattening. Indifference, apathy and a loss of interest in events in general is to be expected. Emotional indifference should not be taken as incontrovertible evidence that distress is absent, for a traumatic victim response is to present as indifferent and accepting.

Confabulation (giving an imaginary account of activities and actions) conceals failures of memory. The environment may be seen as threatening as demands exceed limited competence. Heightened sensations of fear and foreboding may result in disruptive behaviour such as wandering, aggression and calling out. There is a deconstruction of habit and action leaving behind apparently bizarre and meaningless conduct. While there is little empirical investigation of challenging behaviour, clinical impressions indicate that, in part, such disruptive actions are the consequence of an inability to articulate significant psychological needs (Stokes, 1996; in press).

The dementia phase (moderate-severe dementia)

This can be defined as beginning at the point at which remaining intellectual and self-care abilities would no longer sustain survival if the person were left on their own. Profound difficulties in fundamental activities of daily living are the hallmarks of this phase. There is gross destruction of all intellectual capacities. Memory worsens to such an extent that personal history is eroded. At this stage, recognition of oneself and close relatives is lost. All aspects of language are severely impoverished and ultimately lost. Sufferers lose the urge or ability to practise intimate self-care skills and so need assistance in dressing, toileting and eating.

The dementing person is unaware of their experiences and surroundings. The personality is now submerged by the disease. There is a progressive physical wasting as the person declines to a state of passive, incoherent dependency. General motor abilities overtly decline. Ultimately, physical feebleness will mean they require help with walking. Life may continue for one or more years in an almost vegetative state. At this point the person is unable to control their bodily functions and is either chair- or bed-bound. Attention is not focused on stimuli, and the person appears to stare blankly and is invariably unresponsive.

Without longitudinal data, the temporal gradient in AD cannot be truly identified. However, clinical data based on cross-sectional methodology give general support to this stage approach. Progress through each of these stages is gradual and unique. A person may spend several months, if not years, in each phase, displaying characteristics and actions that indicate who they once were and who they remain. Stokes and Holden (1990) note that while remorseless deterioration is inevitable, a number of 'islands' of relatively intact ability may be found until late in the process. What functions are preserved and for how long will depend on the personal characteristics and history of the dementing person, as well as the encouragement received from supporters.

Multi-infarct dementia (MID)

With a few exceptions, the consensus is that late-onset AD is a considerably more common disorder than MID. Kay and Bergmann (1980) suggest that men are more prone to MID in 'young-old' age (65–74 years), whereas women mainly suffer from AD in 'old-old' age (75 or over). There is no reliable distinction between AD and MID yet possible in field settings, and until reliable and valid criteria are established for the diagnosis of presumed cause, prevalence rates derived from epidemiological studies must be treated with caution.

Cerebral pathology

Despite accounting for a significant proportion of late-life dementia, MID has not been subject to anywhere near the same volume of research as AD. MID is a vascular dementia, and thus the old concept of cerebral arteriosclerosis was not completely wrong. Although restriction of the blood supply to the brain does not cause dementia, narrowing of the arteries has been found to make people more prone to stroke. In a stroke, or infarct, there is a blockage of an artery supplying blood to a region of the brain. After several strokes, sufficient brain tissue may be destroyed to result in dementia. Hachinski *et al* (1974) labelled this form of dementia, multi-infarct dementia. At post-mortem the brain may present with a 'moth-eaten' appearance as the surface is marked by many infarcts.

Strokes do not always lead to dementia. Most often they produce quite specific deficits, the nature of which depends on the region of the brain affected. A person may even suffer several strokes without showing signs of dementia, despite evidence of marked physical disability. In contrast, a person can suffer from severe MID with only minor physical handicap. Pitt (1982) offers the explanation that in MID the cerebral infarcts mainly affect the smaller vessels nearer the brain's surface, and thus mainly spare the tracts lying deeper in the brain which govern movement.

Risk factors

■ **Ageing**

As with AD, the prevalence of MID rises sharply with age.

■ **Family history**

Parents and siblings of people with MID have a greater risk of developing the dementia themselves, although there is no data on whether the children of parents with MID are at greater risk.

■ **High blood pressure**

As has already been noted, not all stroke victims develop dementia. A comparison between stroke victims with and without dementia revealed that high blood pressure was the main difference between them. Ladurner *et al* (1982) found that while 68% of stroke patients with dementia had high blood pressure, only 23% without dementia had raised blood pressure.

■ **Stroke is much more common in Japan**

This frequency is possibly related to high salt levels in the Japanese diet. Salt raises blood pressure, and as high blood pressure predisposes to stroke, this could be why MID is the most common cause of dementia in that country.

■ **Life habits**

Smoking and alcohol use are possibly related to MID. As a consequence it is possible that lifestyle changes may lead to a decline in its incidence. In fact there is good evidence from several countries that the incidence of stroke is declining and so it is almost certain the MID is on the decline as well.

Clinical picture

MID is a fluctuating and remitting dementia characterised by an abrupt onset. It is generally observed in the seventh and eighth decades of life, although it may occur as early as the mid-40s.

The course is typically that of a series of small strokes or 'strokelets' which vary in frequency, intensity and location from individual to individual. They cause episodes of confusion and loss of specific cognitive function, sometimes associated with minor neurological signs (eg slurring of speech, weakness down one side of the body). After the infarct there is usually limited clinical improvement until the next episode, which sometimes takes place in a matter of weeks or months, and sometimes not for more than a year. On occasions, the strokelet can be so small to be silent at the time of trauma, leaving the behavioural and cognitive consequences as testimony to the 'invisible' infarct.

Although vascular disease is extensive, the cortex is less uniformly affected than in AD. As a consequence the clinical picture is patchy, inconsistent and at times intriguing. Certain intellectual functions are significantly deteriorated, while others are unimpaired. Emotions are often labile and weeping may be induced easily. Not all emotionalism is shallow, however. There is a relative preservation of personality and insight, and as a consequence profound depression is more frequently encountered.

Eventually, after a succession of infarcts there is less and less recovery, until by a process of *'step wise'* deterioration, dementia as widespread as AD develops. However, many victims die before they reach the stage of advanced dementia, most often from a major stroke.

Dementia with Lewy bodies (DLB)

In 1912 Frederic Lewy described lesions found in the brains of people suffering from Parkinson's disease. Known as Lewy bodies, these are established pathological markers of this most common neuro-degenerative disease that results in progressive impairment of mobility in old age.

During the 1970s and 1980s an atypical dementia was identified at post-mortem that was found to have Lewy bodies present in areas of the brain not usually affected in Parkinson's disease, namely the cerebral cortex.

Earlier neuropathological studies (eg Tomlinson *et al*, 1970) had indicated that around 60% of older people with dementia suffered from AD, approximately 20% had MID, and a further 20% had a mixed diagnosis of AD and MID. More recently, however, several groups of workers have reported significantly different figures. Perry *et al* (1991), using post-mortem findings, found that AD was the most common cause of dementia (50%), but the next most common group was characterised by Lewy bodies in the neocortex (between 15 and 25). Perry *et al* (1990) described this pathology as 'senile dementia of the Lewy body type'. Other researchers have reported similar findings, but have used different terminology. Byrne *et al* (1989) suggested the term 'diffuse Lewy body disease (DLBD)', while McKeith *et al* (1996) refer to dementia with Lewy bodies (DLB).

Figure 2 (below) details proposed criteria for probable diagnosis (McKeith *et al*, 1992).

On cognitive testing the main feature differentiating people with DLB and those with AD is a marked fluctuation in memory and intellectual performance for which there is no underlying treatable cause. These fluctuations are eventually as marked within a day as between days. Psychiatric symptoms are common in DLB with around 80% of cases reporting visual hallucinations and paranoid delusions (McKeith *et al*, 1992). People also suffer from movement disorder (for example, stiffness, slowness, shuffling gait) and falls, often typical of mild Parkinsonism.

Figure 2   The holistic model of dementia

- Fluctuating cognitive impairment affecting both memory and higher cortical functions (such as language, visuospatial ability, praxis, reasoning). The fluctuation is pronounced, with both episodic confusion and lucid intervals.
- At least one of the following:
  - visual or auditory hallucinations, or both, which are usually accompanied by paranoid delusions
  - mild spontaneous extra-pyramidal features or neuroleptic sensitivity syndrome – an exaggerated adverse response to standard doses of neuroleptics
  - repeated unexplained falls or loss of consciousness.
- The illness progresses to an end stage of severe dementia.
- Exclusion of any underlying physical illness adequate to account for the fluctuating cognitive state.
- Exclusion of past history of confirmed stroke.

(Adapted from McKeith *et al*, 1992)

For mental health workers, the challenge to be faced is often at the time of pre-discharge from hospital. As the fluctuating profile of dementia is consistent with delirium, and as falls and unsteadiness often give rise to concerns over physical safety, hospital admission is frequently requested. On return to a lucid state, discharge is advised. Unfortunately, there may be a failure to appreciate that the progress of the dementia will be characterised by fluctuating clinical features. Hence, an assessed care package that meets the needs of a client at the time of discharge, may be ill-equipped to resource the client during their next episode of heightened dementia. Recourse to anti-psychotic medication at this point in order to manage behavioural disturbance and psychosis is contra-indicated, for a cardinal sign of DLB is a neuroleptic sensitivity syndrome. This is manifest in an extreme adverse reaction to standard doses of neuroleptic medication, often resulting in death. It is therefore imperative to assess for need not at the point of temporary recovery, but at the stage of greatest dependency and distress. For it is to this level of severity the person will return. The following case study illustrates the social worker's dilemma.

Case Study   **Mrs P**

Client   Mrs P, aged 79 years
Diagnosis   Dementia with Lewy bodies
Demographics   Widow, living alone. Caring daughter living nearby

History
- Fifteen month history of fluctuating memory impairment and confusion, visual hallucinations and depression. Episodes of lucid thought and conduct.

- Admission to hospital following an episode of marked dementia and a series of falls. On arrival, also observed to be hallucinating and manifesting signs of paranoia.

- Over a 10-day stay Mrs P demonstrates a marked recovery, although at times subject to disorientation and delusions.

- Despite reservations of the clinical team, the social worker is under immense pressure from both Mrs P and her daughter to enable a discharge back home. The responsible medical officer (RMO) favours a discharge, but is inclined to recommend a continuing care nursing home placement. Assessment of current need suggests a supported return home. The social worker acting as an advocate for the client and her family ensures a return home with domiciliary support arranged.

Outcome

Initially the care package meets the needs of Mrs P, but within weeks further episodic dementia and unpredictable falls result in physical injury and a crisis admission.

Fronto-Temporal Dementia (FTD)

Research studies have revealed a dementia that is associated with cellular pathology affecting the fronto-temporal lobes of the brain (Brun, 1987; Mann *et al*, 1993). The prevalence of FTD has been estimated at approximately ten per cent. As with AD, frontal dementia is observed as both an early and late-onset syndrome. Unlike AD, however, more cases of FTD occur in middle age. A family history of dementia occurs in almost half of cases. The length of illness is variable. In some people a rapid decline is noted over two or three years, whereas in others, only minimal change is observed over a decade (Neary *et al*, 1994).

FTD is a clinical syndrome related to atrophy of either the frontal or temporal lobes or both, which may in a minority of cases implicate cellular degeneration known as Pick's disease. Symptoms reflect the relative involvement of the frontal or temporal lobes. If temporal lobe atrophy predominates, a decline in language is more apparent; frontal pathology is associated with personality change.

The clinical features of FTD are characterised by a slow and insidious onset involving predominantly personality, emotion and judgement. The change in personal and social conduct is dramatic. There is a lack of initiative, indifference, inertia and neglect of responsibilities, leading to a breakdown in domestic and occupational performance. Emotions become shallow and empathy with others is lost. In contrast to this hypoactive-hypomanic profile, some become hyperactive and hypermanic. These people are restless, highly distractible, impulsive and overtly disinhibited. Their manner may appear fatuous and inappropriately jocular, and they may exhibit stereotyped behaviours such as repeated singing or recitation of a repertoire of phrases. Hypochondriasis can often lead to negative physical investigations. Obsessive compulsive behaviour is common. While patients tend to polarise in the early stages of the dementia, differences are eventually submerged as the person loses insight and degenerates into a state of total dependency.

Changes in eating habits are common early symptoms. Excessive and indiscriminate eating is superseded by selective food fads, usually involving favoured sweet foods. Sleep pattern alterations occur, with prolonged somnolence, especially in people who exhibit the clinical profile of apathy and inertia.

In the early stages of FTD, features of personality and behavioural change outweigh specific cognitive symptoms. This may invite a variety of psychiatric diagnoses. As the disease progresses there is a gradual yet subtle reduction in spontaneous conversation. Remarks are brief, concrete and unelaborated. They do not converse, but present others with statements. In impulsive, hyperactive patients a press of speech is sometimes observed. In the beginning, orientation in time and place is normal, and information about present and past biographical events is available. Hence, clinical amnesia is absent. Results obtained on simple screening batteries, such as the Mini-Mental State Examination, are invariably normal (Hodges, 1994). This belies a widely held misconception about dementia, namely that it primarily and essentially involves the impairment of memory and intelligence. Only with progression of the disease will people affected by FTD conform to the classical picture of generalised cognitive destruction.

Person first, dementia second – transforming our understanding

> *'My every molecule seems to scream out that I do, indeed exist, and that existence must be valued by someone! Without someone to walk this labyrinth by my side, without the touch of a fellow traveller who understands my need for self-worth, how can I endure the rest of this uncharted journey?'*
> (Diana Friel, 1993)

To assume a simple linear causal relationship between neuropathology and dementia fails to acknowledge that in dementia the origins of behaviour remain complex. Although the underlying pathology eventually determines a state of incoherent dependency, as the disease progresses psychological and environmental factors influence the rate and pattern of decline. These factors do not cause dementia, but they offer an explanation for the contrasting and variable signs observed in people suffering from the same presumptive pathology.

Kitwood (1989) reported that the relationship between the severity of dementia and the degree of neuro-pathological change established at post-mortem leaves *'some 80 per cent of the variance unexplored in moderate or severe dementia'*. Without doubt, the dementing illness is inextricably woven into the pattern of an individual's life history, personality, social relationships and environmental circumstances.

An assessment of the mental health needs of older people with dementia must include an appreciation of their inner world, a subjective realm that *'is often denied to people with dementia'* (Stokes, 1995). They acquire the status of a non-person, a *tabula rasa*, banished from the human milieu. All we see and hear is degraded to the state of symptoms. Yet we cannot allow the destruction of language, memory and reasoning to be an insurmountable barrier to understanding who people with dementia are and why they do what they do (Stokes, 1996). If we make contact with the person behind the barrier we are offered the opportunity to *'stand the prevailing opinion of dementia on its head and assert that much behaviour in dementia is not meaningless, but meaningful'* (Stokes, 1995).

Goudie and Stokes (1989) proposed that much behaviour in dementia defined by others as challenging can be understood within the framework of poorly communicated need. Stokes (1996; in press) describes the inconstant psychology of dementia and identifies the range of need and feeling to be acknowledged and assessed. This does not mean that actions can be readily associated with the inner world of need and motivation. Instead we observe behavioural ruin and chaos. For example, the experience of fear and the need for security in dementia may present as withdrawal, calling out, searching (*'wandering'*), violence or asking for parents, a behaviour described by Miesen (1993) as *'parent fixation'*. As was noted long ago by Hebb (1955), needs are *'an engine, not a steering wheel'*. This applies even more to the person with dementia.

Furthermore, a person with dementia acquires a concept of self, based not on what they do or who we *know* them to be, but on who they know themselves to be – knowledge that may be based on known features of their history; a time passed, but again restored to the here-and-now. The destruction of recall and awareness follows the principle of Ribot's Law. What was learned or experienced last, is lost first; that which was experienced first or most often survives the longest. It is not that they experience a chronologically determined unfolding of historical events, re-experiencing their lives as lived. Instead, their acting out of personal history encompasses overlearned ways of being and themes of emotional significance – a world not of belief, but of entrenched and enduring conviction (see Stokes, in press). This is their reality; an appreciation of self founded not on the objective features of a situation, but on subjective awareness. An awareness that in itself is transient, for dementing people live their lives in fragments. A fragmentation determined by the limits of their impoverished memory span. That is why so much of their conduct appears disjointed and without purpose.

Unfortunately, for those with dementia, attempts to understand, act out their reality and fulfil their needs may serve to obscure who they are rather than providing us with a gateway to their inner world of need and emotion. Despite the understandable protests of grieving carers that *'for all the intimate familiarity of that face and body ...I did not feel his presence beside me, only his absence'* (Morris, 1995), the person remains. A person who is increasingly unrecognisable, but an individual with needs and rights, to be acknowledged and validated.

The person-centred model of dementia replaces the reductionistic causal frame of the biomedical paradigm, based as it is *'on false logic and inadequate evidence'* (Kitwood, 1993). In similar vein, Kitwood (1990) has developed a Dialectical Model of Dementia. This model focuses on the social psychological milieu surrounding the person with dementia, and the effect interpersonal relationships have on the wellbeing of a dementing person. The progression of dementia depends primarily on the interplay between neurological impairment and social psychology. This interaction is defined as dialectical. Using a research methodology known as ethnogenic, Kitwood (1993) has described the key aspects of the social-psychological milieu which often bear down on those with dementia, undermining their sense of self and destroying personhood. This is termed the *'malignant social psychology of dementia'*, wherein genuine disability is exacerbated at the level of interpersonal interactions. Tragically for the person with dementia:

> *'the malignant social psychology is so much a part of the taken-for-granted world of later life that it generally passes unnoticed.'*
> (Kitwood, 1990)

Clearly, this paradigm has similarities to social models of disability wherein the attitudes of people towards a person perceived as different, actively disempowers the person with the disability and denies them a voice, thus exacerbating existing disabilities and attracting even more negative attitudes. Using a dialectical model we get an explanation for the observation of catastrophic decline following admission to institutional care and the phenomenon of transitory '*re* mentia' observed in supportive, person-centred care settings (Sixsmith *et al*, 1993), all of which are inadequately explained by the medical disease model.

These psychosocial models challenge the therapeutic nihilism that permeates dementia care and advocate a response to the individual

Figure 3

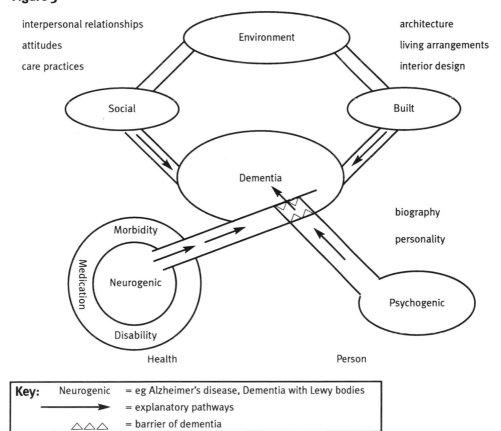

needs of dementing people. The behavioural and emotional aspects of dementia are not dismissed as artefacts of the process of neurodegeneration, but are interpreted as compromised reactions to what they experience and distorted expressions of who they subjectively are (see **Figure 3**, previous page).

Guidelines for assessment

A significant proportion of what is called dementia in old age is the consequence of, or related to ill-health, sensory losses, personal biography, communication of self, altered living arrangements and changing relationships. Cerebral pathology is not, and can never be, the sole explanation.

Assessment must therefore be holistic. It is also both descriptive and analytical, following a sequential methodology. First, information-gathering and observation yields a true and accurate description of a person's mood, cognitive abilities and performance. A meaningful account that cannot be achieved through the process of labelling (Stokes, 1996). This is the baseline from which we can determine the severity of impairment and monitor future change. As such, assessment is regarded as an ongoing, continuous process, not an end-product in itself.

The second stage determines 'why' a person has changed. Having established 'what' a person is like, we now seek the reasons. Understanding 'why' subjects the heuristic explanatory pathways of the model (**Figure 3**) to examination, and appreciates the balance between a number of interacting and dynamic factors. These variables include:

- physical state, including sensory impairment

- medication

- mental health

- personality and biography

- relationships

- care-giving practice

- living arrangements

- accommodation design.

Issues pertaining to who sees the person's behaviour as a problem, the frequency and severity of that problem, and the circumstances in which it occurs should also be addressed.

Effective assessment depends on good practice. This implicates not only the measures selected, but also good communication and interpersonal skills – and critically, the assessment location. Arguably, the most reliable and meaningful assessment of older people will be in their usual place of residence (RCN, 1997; Jolley & Arie, 1978; Murphy & McDonald, 1993). This is the situation in which the person feels comfortable, and is less likely to trigger atypical distress, disorientation and confusion. Given that environmental circumstances contribute to a person's behavioural profile, there is limited merit in moving a client to the unnatural environment of an assessment unit, where they will spend their time alongside others who they may perceive as frightening or threatening. Any assessment made in these circumstances is unlikely to yield a true appraisal of the client's mood and conduct, bearing in mind that the move in itself is also likely to disorientate. Assessment at home, which is where most people return, also allows a person's living conditions and family support to be assessed. We gain a greater appreciation of functional abilities when domestic appliances and spatial configuration are familiar. Finally, with supporters more readily at hand, whether they be family members, friends or neighbours, we learn more about the person and their difficulties.

Finally, the description of problems is transformed into the positive language of need (Stokes, 2000). The transformation of behavioural deficits into needs is achieved through the positive frameworking of problems. So the person is no longer wetting, bored or unable to dress, but *'needs to toilet successfully'*, *'needs to be occupied'* or *'needs to dress themselves'*. How we respond to these unfulfilled needs depends on the reason for their skill deficiencies.

But what about behavioural excesses? These are the challenging behaviours that others wish were not committed, such as verbal abuse, assault, destructive acts, screaming, shouting, wandering, smearing, repeated questioning and sexual indiscretions. What are the needs of people who commit these acts? How can these be positively frameworked to express needs? They cannot. So are we left simply with problems that require management and control? No, for what we need

Case Study	Mr B
Client	Mr B, aged 72 years
Diagnosis	Probable dementia of the Alzheimer Type
History	Retired postman who has suffered dementia for three years.
Circumstances	Lives with his unsupported wife.
Presenting problem	Referred to social services by GP as *'he wanders constantly around the home following, and searching for his wife. Mrs B cannot cope. Please assess and advise'*.
Formulation	The demonstrably exhausted Mrs B is unable to cope with her husband's wandering around the home. She gets little peace during the day and is frequently disturbed throughout the night. She has been told by a CPN that some people with dementia become agitated and constantly wander. This has, however, provided neither solution nor solace.

Action   Mr B attends a specialist day centre where he presents with disturbed behaviour. He assaults other clients, repeatedly shouts 'help' and demands to go home.

Explanation   Mr B's conduct is further evidence of his advancing dementia.

Revised formulation

■ At home, Mr B demonstrated a type of wandering described as *'trailing and tracking'* – clinging behaviour motivated by separation anxiety. When apart, Mr B cannot recall the whereabouts of the person who represents security and so he resolves his anxiety by seeking her presence.

■ The problem was 'wandering', yet his *need* is to be secure.

■ Mr B's conduct at the day centre reveals the extent of his fear and insecurity, and is evidence that the service response to the *problem* of his wandering failed to acknowledge his *need*.

to articulate in the form of a need, is the reason for the behaviour, an explanation that is only rarely expressed successfully in terms of neuropathology. The case example of **Mr B** illustrates how establishing the explanation enables a need to be identified.

The outcomes of a needs-based analysis are creative interventions that address individual need. Adherence to the medical model offers little in the form of need, and inevitably leads to a slavish commitment to the desirability and necessity of control. The identification and meeting of need, however, holds the prospect of behavioural improvement in dementia, despite the progressive neuropathology. (For a detailed exposition of need in dementia see Stokes, 1996; 2000 and Goudie & Stokes,1989.)

Depression

In this section we leave dementia and look at a quite different disorder, yet one that can give rise to a similar profile of symptoms – depression. While the principal symptom of depression is a marked change in mood, a British study of patients admitted to hospital with dementia found 8% were in fact suffering from depression (Marsden & Harrison, 1972), while a study in Australia established a similar rate of 5% (Smith & Kiloh, 1981). A further complication is that major depression is approximately 10 times more frequent among people with dementia than in the general population.

Prevalence

Depression is the most common emotional disorder affecting elderly people, yet too often it is regarded as an inevitable feature of old age rather than a potentially treatable condition (Coleman, 1986). The underpinning knowledge for this belief is enshrined in the question *'Are you looking forward to being 79?'* When for many that answer is '*no*', it is so easy to define 'depression' as simply a new word for 'old age' (Bucks, 1990).

You can live next door to an elderly woman who you rarely see from one week to the next. When you do, she clearly is diminished. She looks shabby and has clearly lost weight. She never smiles and hardly ever engages you in conversation as she walks slowly to the gate. After a few moments staring vacantly into space she will return to her increasingly dilapidated house and the front door will close behind her. Who is she? Just the 'old girl' next door who lost her husband a few years ago. Yet if she was 29 years old and presented in a manner indistinguishable to that described, we would know she was suffering and would not passively accept her diminished state. This is why depression in late life remains 'a silent epidemic' – a clinical phenomenon often unnoticed behind a barrier of social distance and isolation.

If we cannot interpret depression as an inevitable concomitant of old age, how prevalent is the condition? Unfortunately, depression in late life is a vague concept to grasp, with no consensus regarding typology, and so efforts to establish prevalence rates are somewhat unreliable. Investigations adopt different criteria for case definition, some including transient changes in mood, others focusing on the syndrome of major depression. Support for the view that it is possible to discriminate between symptoms of depression (for example, unhappiness, self-disdain) which may commonly occur in old age yet not interfere with functioning (Busse, 1985) and the presence of a coherent syndrome is widespread (eg Blazer, 1980; Zemore & Eames, 1979).

Blazer (1980) found that 25% of his sample showed symptoms, but only 3.7% satisfied the criteria for major depression. Lindesay *et al* (1989) found 4.3% having a severe depression and a further 13.5% having a mild to moderate degree of depression. Most studies find higher rates of depression in women (eg Copeland *et al*, 1987).

States of depression are clearly common in later life, but they are not more common in older people. Henderson (1989; 1990; 1994) suggests that rates of depression in elderly people are lower than in other age groups, when mental status and education are controlled, although older people might indeed have more depressive symptoms.

Depression – the clinical syndrome

Chapter 1 has explored the signs and symptoms most commonly associated with depression. However, for older adults there are some important differences.

- Tiredness, sleep disturbance and weight loss may be less prominent among older adults, while low mood is sometimes denied (Burns & Hallewell, 1995).

- Many older people may present with somatic rather than emotional complaints.

■ Vague physical symptoms, and hypochondriacal concerns may be clues to the diagnosis of depression.

Burns and Hallewell (1995) suggest that a loss or reduced ability to take pleasure from activities that are usually enjoyed is very common. Enquiring about favourite television programmes or visits from friends or family may elicit the necessary information.

Depressive thoughts, such as ideas of guilt, reduced self-esteem, worthlessness, hopelessness and pre-occupation with death and suicide, are commonly observed.

When sleep disturbance as evidenced by early waking is observed, consideration needs to be given to the time the elderly person is going to bed. If they are going to bed (or more accurately being put to bed) in the early evening, then the normal reduced sleep requirement in late life will result in the person waking in the early hours of the morning. Similarly, a sedentary lifestyle characterised by inactivity will result in daytime cat-napping, further reducing the need for sleep at night. Hence, early waking cannot automatically be seen as evidence of depression.

Agitation, as evidenced by wringing hands and restlessness, tears, and expressions of sadness and despair have obvious clinical significance. Decline in self-care – for example unwashed hair, unkempt appearance, stale body odour in a formerly smart person – is an indicative sign of depression.

The origins of depression in older adults

Whilst similar to the origins of depression outlined generally in **Chapter 1**, there are some important differences in respect of older adults.

Life experiences

Murphy (1982) compared elderly depressed adults with 'normal' people of the same age and found the former were more likely to have experienced major stressful life events, such as the death of, or serious illness in, someone close. They were more likely to have housing problems and relationship difficulties. Those who were most vulnerable were those who lacked a close, confiding relationship to act as a buffer at times of adversity.

Brown and Harris (1978) established that what may precede the onset of depression is an accumulation of mostly minor adverse life experiences. Stenback (1980) considers that depression is not necessarily the outcome of distressing loss, but the consequence of a loss of futurism. A limited forward time perspective may mean the person considers that it is not worthwhile to attempt to find replacements for losses experienced. Depression is common in residential homes (Ames *et al*, 1988) and may be the reason for their admission in the first place, but could also arise as a result of the experience of life in such settings.

Negative emotion is, however an expected response to loss, dissatisfaction and disappointment. It is only characteristic of an emotional disorder when it is out of proportion in terms of severity, duration, or both and impairs personal and social functioning.

Cultural factors

The prevailing negative attitudes, prejudice and stereotypes about old age in western industrial societies may lower self-esteem, invoke a sense of uselessness and produce a state of depressed mood.

Physical illness

Poor physical health is also related to depression. Kay *et al* (1964) found moderate or severe physical disability in 41% of their elderly sample with functional mental illness, compared with 16% among their 'normal' group. The impact of poor health on mood may be mediated by the inability to perform personally significant activities, and chronic pain.

Cerebral changes in depression

Although social circumstances appear to be significant risk factors, a biological basis of depression cannot be denied. Some older people experience no adverse circumstances prior to their depression, which may indicate a biological predisposition to depressive illness. This is often referred to as an 'endogenous' depression.

The question of how organic brain changes are related to the emergence of depression in later life is as yet unresolved. Contemporary work suggests that when depression occurs for the first time in later life, it is more likely to be associated with degenerative brain changes than if depression occurs earlier in life. Reding *et al* (1985) found that 57% of depressed elderly people developed dementia within three years of the depression being diagnosed. Whether the depression represents a reaction to the insidious onset of the dementia, or is related to the same biological changes as the presumptive dementing illness is open to question.

Heredity

Heredity is a factor, for there is a family history of major depression in 44% of those developing the disorder in old age (Pitt, 1982). However, it appears that heredity is of less significance in late-onset depression than in episodes of depressive disorder in early adult life.

Models of treatment and intervention for depression

These are covered in some detail in **Chapter 1.**

Prognosis of depression in older adults

Anumber of studies on the prognosis of depression in old age have been undertaken, and reflect the effectiveness of the usual treatment regime, which in most instances has been anti-depressant medication (Woods, 1996). Burvill (1993) found that over a timescale of a year, 42% of elderly patients remain depressed, make only a partial recovery, or recover, but then relapse within 12 months. As many as a third of older people with depression remain depressed three years later, with only around 20% sustaining a complete recovery (Livingston & Hinchcliffe, 1993). Similar findings have been reported by Murphy (1983) who found that only one third of depressed elderly people recovered and did not subsequently relapse. While there continues to be some debate regarding the interpretation of such figures (eg Baldwin, 1991), it is evident that a significant number of older people with depression are not restored to emotional health with the standard treatments available. As such, pessimism has long been typical of the attitude toward the treatment of depression in late life.

The reasons for this sense of therapeutic nihilism are complex. Woods and Britton (1985) believe some elderly people are simply 'written off'. Poor treatment responses are attributed to cumulative losses, poor physical health, anticipated decline in intellectual functioning as part of the 'normal' ageing process and 'rigidity' of old age which prevents elders from looking at problems from a psychological perspective and changing the way they think or behave.

There is, however, increasing evidence that psychological therapies can benefit older people (eg Gallagher & Thompson, 1983) if the content areas of therapy are 'modified to take physical and psychological issues relevant to the ageing process into account' (Goudie, 1990). Not only do Nemiroff and Colarusso (1985) consider that elderly people are good candidates for psychotherapy, Knight (1996) suggests that in some cases older adults may respond better than younger patients.

Elderly people do not traditionally respond well to therapeutic intervention because they typically present themselves (or are presented) for treatment when their depression has become chronic, at which time they are offered treatments which are not tailored to their specific needs. For example, while anti-depressant medication is useful with many older depressed people, in instances of reactive depression, where medication is the only therapeutic response, it is rarely of value. Plopper (1990) suggests that effective treatment requires a multifocal approach, including psychological therapy, family and social intervention and, when indicated, pharmacological treatment.

Suicide

Suicides are disproportionately common among older people, therefore suicidal ideas, no matter how trivial, should be openly addressed. While elderly people constitute around 16% of the UK population, approximately 25% of all suicides involve people 65 or over (Lindesay, 1986). As Woods (1996) reports, older adults *'are more likely than any other age group to die by committing suicide'*. On the other hand they are much less likely to attempt suicide unsuccessfully, or indulge in *'manipulative overdoses'* (Burns & Hallewell, 1995).

The majority of older adults who commit suicide are suffering from depression, most of whom will not have been receiving treatment (Barraclough, 1971). An elderly man living alone, with a history of social isolation and in poor physical health is a suicide risk. Lindesay (1991) identifies the loss of income and status following retirement as powerful risk factors for men. Chronic alcoholism especially heightens the risk (Addario, 1990). The disinhibiting effects of alcohol may facilitate the act, and its interaction with other drugs may potentiate their effects (Woods, 1996).

In an analysis of suicide notes, Kulawick and Decke (1973) found physical illness most frequently mentioned, especially for elderly women. The relationship between ill health and suicide is complex, however and is often mediated by pain (Cattell, 1988).

Although social isolation and loneliness are frequently cited as precipitants of suicidal behaviour (eg Cattell, 1990), Stenbeck (1980) found that suicidal intent was not associated with the frequency of social contact, but with the intimacy experienced in social relationships ('qualitative isolation').

Of contemporary relevance, hospital discharge and, conversely, the fear of hospitalisation or being placed in a nursing home have been identified as precipitants of suicide (Loebel *et al*, 1991). While it is of value to identify precipitants of suicide in older people, for these to translate into suicide intent, a psychological framework is required. It is widely recognised that hopelessness is implicated in linking depression and suicide attempts. Attitudes to suicide will also influence the likelihood that suicidal intent will progress to an attempt.

As suicide possesses a multi-factoral base, a model of risk and potential can be of assessment value (see **Figure 4**, overleaf).

At the time when a decision to commit suicide has been taken, there may be an apparent recovery of mood and the observation of adaptive behaviour. This 'spontaneous recovery' reflects the move away from a state of helplessness as the person regains control of their destiny, and the wish of many people who commit suicide to leave their lives in good order. We thus observe a 'tidying up' of life's affairs (for example, paying household bills, contacting friends and family) that conceals the darkness of their intent. 'Spontaneous recovery' in the absence of attitude change and in the presence of continuing hardship, allied to 'tidying up' should alert the practitioner to the potential of a suicide attempt.

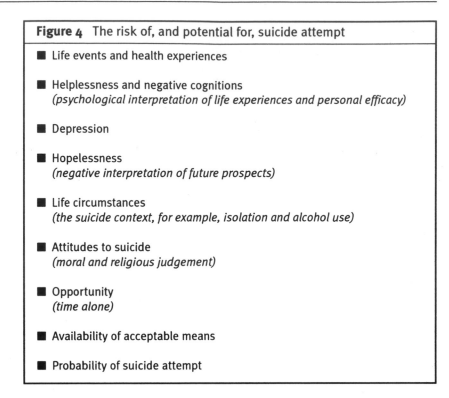

Figure 4 The risk of, and potential for, suicide attempt

■ Life events and health experiences

■ Helplessness and negative cognitions
(psychological interpretation of life experiences and personal efficacy)

■ Depression

■ Hopelessness
(negative interpretation of future prospects)

■ Life circumstances
(the suicide context, for example, isolation and alcohol use)

■ Attitudes to suicide
(moral and religious judgement)

■ Opportunity
(time alone)

■ Availability of acceptable means

■ Probability of suicide attempt

Depression or dementia – the diagnostic challenge of pseudo-dementia

Finally, there is the problem of differential diagnosis when a person presents with signs consistent with both dementia and depression. In this case, while it must always be borne in mind that people with dementia may also be depressed (Alexopoulos *et al*, 1988; Verhey *et al*, 1993), the two diagnoses are not mutually exclusive.

Some depressed people show impairments on cognitive testing – usually impaired concentration, attention and memory performance. McHugh and Folstein (1979) demonstrated the negative effect serious depression has on Mini-Mental State Examination scores in old age. Occasionally, a picture more like dementia is seen, and the condition is described as a reversible 'pseudo-dementia'. While the person may become disorientated, forgetful and unable to care for themselves, Woods (1996) believes the term is of little help as the impairments may not much resemble dementia (Poon, 1992) and the extent of their reversibility has been questioned (Abas *et al*, 1990).

Those with intellectual impairments also have more subjective memory complaints, particularly with regard to recent events and concentration (O'Boyle *et al*, 1990) although these concerns may have little relationship with performance on memory tests (Jorm, 1987). Furthermore, cognitive impairments may be more apparent than real ones; for example, answering 'don't know' may reflect a more conservative response bias, being less prepared to 'guess' the answer (Gainotti & Camillo, 1994).

While depression and dementia can be confused, Goudie (1990) outlines the key differences between the two conditions (**Figure 5** below).

Figure 5 The differences between depression and dementia	
The person with depression	**The person with dementia of the Alzheimer type**
● Often complains of a poor memory	● Is often unaware of memory problems
● Will say, 'I do not know' in answer to questions which require thought, concentration or effort	● Will 'confabulate' or make up answers to questions that require concentration or good memory and appear unaware that the answer is incorrect
● Shows fluctuating ability and uneven impairment on cognitive testing	● Tends to show consistent, global impairment on cognitive testing
● Gives up easily, is poorly motivated and uninterested	● Has a go
● May be slow but can complete complex tasks. Aware of errors	● Unsuccessful in carrying out tasks requiring skill and concentration
	● Appears unaware of errors

Summary

The most common mental health disorders in old age are dementia and depression, yet neither are the inevitable consequence of ageing. Neither are they to be viewed with therapeutic nihilism. Our contemporary understanding of the complex origins of both conditions enables us to pursue goals of rehabilitation and resolution, as distinct from policies of management and control. We are not presented with problems, but with people who have needs. Needs that may be difficult for us to interpret and for the older adult to articulate, but needs nevertheless.

References

Abas, M. A., Sahakian, B. J. & Levy, R. (1990) Neuropsychological deficits and CT scan changes in elderly depressives. *Psychological Medicine* **20** 507–520.

Addario, D. (1990) Treating Mental Health Conditions in the Rehabilitative Setting. In: B. Kemp, K. Brummel-Smith and J. W. Ramsdell (Eds) *Geriatric Rehabilitation.* Boston: College-Hill Press.

Alexopoulos G. S., Abrams, R. C., Young, R. C. & Shamoian, C. A. (1988) Cornell Scale for depression in dementia. *Biological Psychiatry* **23** 271–284.

Alzheimer's Disease Society (1995) *Services for Younger People with dementia. A report by the Alzheimer's Disease Society.* London: Alzheimer's Disease Society.

Ames, D., Ashby, D., Mann, A. & Graham, N. (1988) Psychiatric illness in elderly residents of Part III homes in one London borough: prognosis and review *Age and Ageing* **17** 249–256.

Baldwin, B. (1991) The outcome of depression in old age. *International Journal of Geriatric Psychiatry* **6** 395–400.

Barr, O. & Campbell, A. (1995) The link between Down's Syndrome and Alzheimer's disease. *Journal of Dementia Care* **3** 24–26.

Barraclough, B. M. (1971) Suicide in the Elderly. In: D. W. K. Kay and A. Walk (Eds) Recent Developments in Psychogeriatrics. *British Journal of Psychiatry*, Special Publication, No.6.

Beck, A. (1967) *Depression: Clinical, experimental and therapeutic Aspects.* London: Staple Press.

Berrios, G. E. (1987) The nosology of the dementias: an overview. In: B. Pitt (Ed) *Dementia* Edinburgh: Churchill Livingstone

Blazer, D. (1980) The diagnosis of depression in the elderly. *Journal of the American Geriatrics Society* **28** 52–58.

Blessed, G., Tomlinson, B. E. & Roth, M. (1968) The association between quantitative measures of dementia and of senile change in the cerebral grey matter of elderly subjects. *British Journal of Psychiatry* **114** 797–811.

Brown, G. W. & Harris, T. (1978) *Social Origins of Depression: A study of psychiatric disorders in women.* London: Tavistock.

Brun, A. (1987) Frontal lobe degeneration of non-Alzheimer type. I. Neuropathology. *Archives of Gerontological Geriatrics* **6** 192–208.

Bucks, R. (1990) *Depression: A new name for old.* Unpublished MSc Thesis, University of Birmingham.

Burns, A. & Hallewell, C. (1995) *Old age psychiatry.*Update, 15 March 341–346.

Burvill, P. W. (1993) Prognosis of depression in the elderly. *International Review of Psychiatry* **5** 437–443.

Busse, E. W. (1985) Normal Ageing: The Duke Longitudinal Studies. In: M. Bergener, M. Ermini and H. B. Strahelin (Eds) *Thresholds in Ageing.* New York: Academic Press.

Butler, R. N. (1963) *The life review: an interpretation of reminiscence in the aged. Psychiatry* **26** 65–76.

Byrne, E. J. (1987) Reversible dementia. *International Journal of Geriatric Psychiatry* **2** 73–81.

Byrne, E. J., Lennox, G., Lowe, J. & Godwin-Austen, R. B. (1989) Diffuse Lewy body disease: Clinical features in 15 cases. *Journal of Neurology, Neurosurgery & Psychiatry* **52** 709–717.

Cattell, H. R. (1988) Elderly suicide in London: an analysis of coroner's inquests. *International Journal of Geriatric Pyschiatry* **3** 251–261.

Cattell, H. R. (1990) Suicide in the elderly. *Psychiatry in Practice* **9** (2) 14–17.

Coleman, P. G. (1986) *Ageing and Reminiscence Processes.* Chichester: John Wiley.

Copeland, J. R. M., Gurland, B. J., Dewey, M. E., Kelleher, M. J., Smith, A. M. R. & Davidson, I. A. (1987) Is there more dementia, depression and neurosis in New York? *British Journal of Psychiatry* **151** 466–474.

Cummings, J. L. & Benson, D. F. (1983) *Dementia: A clinical approach.* Boston: Butterworths.

Folstein, M. F., Folstein, S. E. & McHugh, P. R. (1975) Mini-Mental State. A practical method for grading the cognitive state of patients for the clinician. *Journal of Psychiatric Research* **12** 189–198.

Friel McGowin, D. (1993) *Living in the Labyrinth: A personal account of dementia* Mainsail Press.

Gainotti, G. & Camillo, M. (1994) Some aspects of memory disorders clearly distinguish dementia of the Alzheimer's type from depressive pseudo-dementia. *Journal of Clinical and Experimental Neuropsychology* **16** 65–78.

Gallagher, D. & Thompson, L. W. (1983) Effectiveness of psychotherapy for both endogenous and non-endogenous depression in older adult outpatients. *Journal of Gerontology* **38** 707–712.

Goudie, F. (1990) Depression in Dementia. In: G. Stokes and F. Goudie (Eds) *Working with Dementia.* Bicester: Winslow Press.

Goudie, F. & Stokes, G. (1989) Dealing with confusion. *Nursing Times* **85** (39) 27th September, 35–37.

Hachinski, V. C., Lassen, N. A. & Marshall, J. (1974) Multi-infarct dementia: a cause of mental deterioration in the elderly. *Lancet* **2** 207–209.

Hebb, D. O. (1955) Drives and the CNS (conceptual nervous system). *Psychology Review* **62** 243–254.

Henderson, A. S. (1986) The epidemiology of Alzheimer's disease. *British Medical Bulletin* **42** 3–10.

Henderson, A. S. (1989) Psychiatric epidemiology and the elderly. *International Journal of Geriatric Psychiatry* **4** 249–253.

Henderson, A. S. (1990) The social psychiatry of late life. *British Journal of Psychiatry* **156** 645–653.

Henderson, A. S. (1994) Does ageing protect against depression? *Social Psychiatry and Psychiatric Epidemiology* **29** 107–109.

Heston, L. L. (1981) Genetic Studies of Dementia: with emphasis on Parkinson's Disease and Alzheimer's Neuropathology. In: J. A. Mortimer and L. M. Schuman (Eds) *The Epidemiology of Dementia.* New York: Oxford University Press.

Hodges, J. R. (1994) Pick's Disease. In: A. Burns and R. Levy (Eds) *Dementia.* London: Chapman and Hall.

Hofman, A., Rocca, W. A., Brayne, C. *et al* (1991) The prevalence of dementia in Europe: a collaborative study of 1980–1990 findings. *International Journal of Epidemiology* **20** (3) 736–748.

Holden, V. P. (1990) Dementia: some common misunderstandings. In: G. Stokes and F. Goudie (Eds) *Working with Dementia.* Bicester: Winslow Press.

Jagger, C. & Lindesay, J. (1993) The Epidemiology of Senile Dementia. In: A. Burns (Ed) *Ageing and Dementia: A methodological approach.* London: Edward Arnold.

Jolley, D. J. & Arie, T. (1978) Organisation of psychogeriatric services. *British Journal of Psychiatry* **32** 1–11.

Jorm, A. F. (1987) *Understanding Senile Dementia.* London: Croom Helm.

Jorm, A. F., Korten, A. E. & Henderson, A. S. (1987) The prevalence of dementia: a quantitative integration of the literature. *Acta Psychiatr Scand* **76** 465–479.

Kay, D. W. K. & Bergmann, K. (1980) Epidemiology of mental disorders among the aged in the community. In: J. E. Birren & R. B. Sloane (Eds) *Handbook of Mental Health and Ageing.* Englewood Cliffs: Prentice Hall.

Kay, D. W. K., Beamish, P. & Roth, M. (1964) Old age mental disorders in Newcastle-upon-Tyne, II. A study of possible social and medical causes. *British Journal of Psychiatry* **110** 668–682.

Kitwood, T. (1989) Brain, mind and dementia: with particular reference to Alzheimer's disease. *Ageing and Society* **9** 1–15.

Kitwood, T. (1990) The dialectics of dementia: with particular reference to Alzheimer's disease. *Ageing & Society* **10** 177–196.

Kitwood, T. (1993) Person and process in dementia. *International Journal of Geriatric Psychiatry* **8** 541–545.

Knight, B. G. (1996) *Psychotherapy with the Older Adult* (2nd edition). California: Sage.

Kral, V. A. (1962) Senescent forgetfulness: benign and malignant. *Canadian Medical Association Journal* **86** 257–260.

Kral, V. A. (1978) Benign senescent forgetfulness. *Ageing* **7** 47–51.

Kulawick, H. & Decke, D. (1973) Letze Aufzeichnungen – eine Analyse von 223 nach vollendeten Suiziden hinterlassenen Briefen und Mitteilungen, *Psychiat. Chin* **6** 193–210.

Ladurner, G., Iliff, L. D. & Lechner, H. (1982) Clinical factors associated with dementia in ischaemic stroke. *Journal of Neurology, Neurosurgery and Psychiatry* **45** 97–101.

Lewinsohn, P. M. (1974) A Behavioural Approach to Depression. In: R. Friedman and M. Katz (Eds) *The Psychology of Depression*. New York: John Wiley.

Lindesay, J. (1986) Suicide and Attempted Suicide in Old Age. In: E. Murphy (Ed) *Affective Disorders in the Elderly*. Edinburgh: Churchill Livingstone.

Lindesay, J. (1991) Suicide in the elderly. *International Journal of Geriatric Psychiatry* **6** 355–361.

Lindesay, J., Briggs, K. & Murphy, E. (1989) The Guy's/Age Concern survey. Prevalence rates of cognitive impairment, depression and anxiety in an urban elderly community. *British Journal of Psychiatry* **155** 317–329.

Livingston, G. & Hinchcliffe, A. C. (1993) The epidemiology of psychiatric disorders in the elderly. *International Review of Psychiatry* **5** 317–326.

Loebel, P. J., Loebel, J. S., Dager, S. R. & Centerwall, B. S. (1991) Anticipation of nursing home placement may be a precipitant of suicide among the elderly. *Journal of American Geriatrics Society* **39** 407–408.

MacDonald, A. J. D. (1985) Do general practitioners miss depression in elderly patients? *British Medical Journal* **292** 1365–1367.

Mann, D. M. A., South, P. W., Snowden, J. S. & Neary, D. (1993) Dementia of frontal lobe type: neuropathology and immunohistochemistry. *Journal of Neurology, Neurosurgery and Psychiatry* **56** 605–614.

Marsden, C. D. & Harrison, M. J. G. (1972) Outcome of investigation of patients with presenile dementia. *British Medical Journal* **2** 249–252.

Marshall, M. (1998) Therapeutic Buildings for People with Dementia. In: S. Judd, M. Marshall and P. Phippen (Eds) *Design for Dementia*. London: Hawker Publications.

McHugh, P. R. & Folstein, M. F. (1979) Psychopathology of Dementia: Implications for neuropathology. In: R. Katzman (Ed) *Congenital and Acquired Cognitive Disorders*. New York: Raven Press.

McKeith, I., Fairbairn, A., Perry, R., Thompson, P. & Perry, E. (1992) Neuroleptic sensitivity in patients with senile dementia of Lewy body type. *British Medical Journal* **305** 673–678.

McKeith, I., Galasko, D., Kosaka, K. *et al* (1996) Clinical and pathological diagnosis of dementia with Lewy bodies (DLB): Report of the CDLB International Workshop. *Neurology* **47** 1113–1125.

Miesen, B. M. L. (1993) Alzheimer's disease, the phenomenon of parent fixation and Bowlby's attachment theory. *International Journal of Geriatric Psychiatry* **8** 147–153.

Moniz-Cook, E. (1998) Psychosocial approaches to 'challenging behaviour' in care homes. *Journal of Dementia Care* **4** (3) 33–38.

Morris, E. (1995) This living hand. *The New Yorker* 16 January, 66–69.

Mortimer, J. A., French, L. R., Hutton, J. T. & Schuman, L. M. (1985) Head injury as a risk factor for Alzheimer's disease. *Neurology* **35** 264–267.

Murphy, E. (1982) Social origins of depression in old age. *British Journal of Psychiatry* **141** 135–142.

Murphy, E. (1983) The prognosis of depression in old age. *British Journal of Psychiatry* **142** 111–119.

Murphy, E. (1986) *Dementia and Mental Illness in Old.* London: Papermac.

Murphy, E. & MacDonald, A. J. D. (1993) *Mental Health Services for Elderly People.* London: Guy's and Lewisham NHS Trust.

Neary, D., Snowden, J. S. & Mann, D. M. A. (1994) Dementia of Frontal Lobe Type. In: A. Burns and R. Levy (Eds) *Dementia.* London: Chapman and Hall.

Nemiroff, R. A. & Colarusso, C. A. (1985) *The Race Against Time: Psychotherapy and psychoanalysis in the second half of life.* New York: Plenum Press.

Nussbaum, P. D. (1994) Pseudodementia: a slow death. *Neuropsychology Review* **4** 71–90.

O'Boyle, M., Amadeo, M. & Self, D. (1990) Cognitive complaints in elderly depressed and pseudodemented patients. *Psychology and Ageing* **5** 467–468.

O'Connor, D., Pollit, B., Hyde, J. *et al* (1988) Do GPs miss dementia in elderly patients? *British Medical Journal* **297** 1107–1110.

Oliver, C. & Holland, A. J. (1986) Down's syndrome and Alzheimer's disease: a review. *Psychological Medicine* **16** 307–322.

Pattie, A. (1988) Measuring Levels of Disability – the Clifton Assessment Procedures for the Elderly. In: J. P. Wattis and I. Hindmarch (Eds) *Psychological Assessment of the Elderly.* Edinburgh: Churchill Livingstone.

Pattie, A. & Gilleard, C. J. (1979) *Manual of the Clifton Assessment Procedures for the Elderly (CAPE).* Sevenoaks: Hodder and Stoughton.

Perry, E. K., McKeith, I. G., Thompson, P. *et al* (1991) Topography, extent and clinical relevance of neurochemical deficits in dementia of Lewy body,

Parkinson and Alzheimer type. *Annals of the New York Academy of Science* **640** 197–202.

Perry, R. H., Irving, D., Blessed, G., Fairbairn, A. F. & Perry, E .K. (1990) Senile dementia of the Lewy body type. A clinically and neuropathologically distinct form of Lewy body dementia in the elderly. *Journal of Neurological Science* **95** 119–139.

Pitt, B. (1982) *Psychogeriatrics: An introduction to the psychiatry of old age.* Edinburgh: Churchill Livingstone.

Pitt, B. (1987) Delirium and Dementia. In: B. Pitt (Ed) *Dementia.* Edinburgh: Churchill Livingstone.

Plopper, M. (1990) Evaluation and Treatment of Depression. In: B. Kemp, K. Brummel-Smith and J. W. Ramsdell (Eds) *Geriatric Rehabilitation.* Boston: College-Hill Press.

Poon, L. W. (1992) Towards an understanding of cognitive functioning in geriatric depression. *International Psychogeriatrics* **4** (2) 241–266.

Post, F. (1962) The significance of affective symptoms in old age. *Maudsley Monograph* **10**. London: Oxford University Press.
Reding, M., Haycox, J. & Blass, J. (1985) Depression in patients referred to a dementia clinic: A three-year prospective study. *Archives of Neurology* **42** 894–896.

Royal College of Nursing (1997) *Guidelines for Assessing Mental Health Needs in Old Age.* London: Royal College of Nursing.

Royal College of Physicians (1981) Organic mental impairment in the elderly. *Journal of the Royal College of Physicians* **15** 141–147.

Sacks, O. (1985) *The Man Who Mistook His Wife for a Hat.* London: Picador.

Seligman, M. (1975) *Helplessness: On depression, development and death.* San Francisco: W. H. Freeman.

Sixsmith, A., Stillwell, J. & Copeland, J. (1993) Dementia: challenging the limits of dementia care. *International Journal of Geriatric Psychiatry* **8** 993–1000.

Smith, J. S. & Kiloh, L. G. (1981) The investigation of dementia: results in 200 consecutive admissions. *Lancet* **1** 824–827.

Stenback, A. (1980) Depression and Suicidal Behaviour in Old Age. In: J. E. Birren and R. B. Sloane (Eds) *Handbook of Mental Health and Ageing.* New York: Prentice Hall.

Stokes, G. (1990) The Management of Aggression. In: G. Stokes and F. Goudie (Eds) *Working with Dementia.* Bicester: Winslow Press.

Stokes, G. (1992) *On Being Old.* London: Taylor and Francis.

Stokes, G. (1995) Incontinent or not? Person first, dementia second. *Journal of Dementia Care* Jan/Feb, 20–21.

Stokes, G. (1996) Challenging behaviour in dementia: A psychological approach. In: R.T. Woods (Ed) *Handbook of the Clinical Psychology of Ageing.* Chichester: John Wiley.

Stokes, G. (2000) *Challenging Behaviour in Dementia.* Bicester: Winslow Press.

Stokes, G. & Holden, U. (1990) Dementia: Causes and clinical syndromes. In: G. Stokes and F. Goudie (Eds) *Working with Dementia.* Bicester: Winslow Press.

Thase, M. E. (1982) Longevity and mortality in Down's Syndrome. *Journal of Mental Deficiency Research* **26** 177–192.

Tomlinson, B. E., Blessed, G. & Roth, M. (1970) Observations on the brains of demented old people. *Journal of Neurological Science* **11** 205–242.

Verhey, F. R. J., Rozendaal, N., Ponds, W. H. M. & Jolles, J. (1993) Dementia, awareness and depression. *International Journal of Geriatric Psychiatry* **8** 851–856.

Wade, J. P. H. & Hachinski, V. C. (1987) Multi-infarct Dementia. In: B. Pitt (Ed) *Dementia.* Edinburgh: Churchill Livingstone.

Woods, R. T. & Britton, P. G. (1985) *Clinical Psychology with the Elderly.* Beckenham: Croom Helm.

Woods, R. T. (1996) Mental Health Problems in Late Life. In: R. T. Woods (Ed) *Handbook of Clinical Psychology of Ageing.* Chichester: John Wiley.

Zemore, R. & Eames, N. (1979) Psychic and somatic symptoms of depression among young adults, institutionalised aged and non-institutionalised aged. *Journal of Gerontology* **34** (5) 716–722.

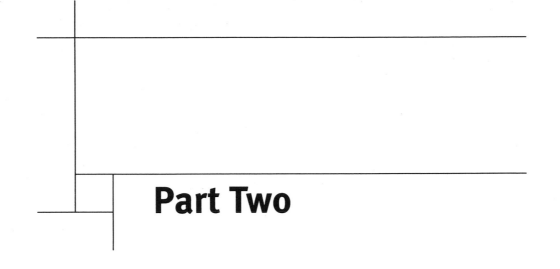

Part Two

Chapter 5

Mental Health Problems in Primary Care

Elizabeth Armstrong

Introduction

The majority of people with mental illness are cared for within the primary care system. This is nothing new – it was demonstrated more than 20 years ago by Goldberg and Huxley (1980) who described a series of levels and filters which influenced the ways in which people with mental illness obtained the care they required. Their model clearly showed that the vast majority of these people is treated by their general practitioner (GP) and are never referred to specialists.

The *National Service Framework for Mental Health*, published by the Department of Health in 1999, stated that in general, of every 100 people who consult their GP with a mental health problem, only 9 are referred on to specialist services. There is a strong primary care theme running through the whole document, though it is unfortunate that there was relatively little primary care input into its development. In particular there was no input at all from primary care nurses, which has meant that the contribution of practice nurses and district nurses – and even to some extent health visitors – continues to be under recognised and under valued.

The *Framework*, which focuses on adults of working age, sets out seven standards and defines service models for promoting mental health and treating mental illness. There are also milestones and performance indicators against which progress is to be measured.

The standards of particular relevance to primary care are:

- Standards 2 and 3 which are about assessment of need, effective treatment and access to care

- Standard 7 which is about the prevention of suicide.

Standard 1 – mental health promotion, contains important references to potential primary care roles, as does Standard 4 in relation to the Care Programme Approach (CPA), and Standard 6 in care for carers. For most primary care organisations, full implementation of Standard 2 would, in addition, mean that they had largely met their obligations under the other standards.

The key feature of primary care, and that which distinguishes primary care from the rest of the NHS, is that practitioners see the whole range of illness from mild to severe and both physical and psychological. Primary health care is a universally accessible service. The problem for primary care practitioners is how to provide a comprehensive service which meets the health care needs of all who consult: to treat those they can treat; to refer on those who need more specialist care, and to know the difference between them. There are also numbers of people consulting their GP with milder forms of distress and depression for whom medical interventions are inappropriate. Primary care staff need better strategies for signposting this group to other community-based helping agencies.

This chapter looks at the current state of primary health care and how it might begin to address these new standards. It will consider:

- the nature of primary health care

- mental health education and training for primary care professionals

- ways in which primary care groups (PCGs), trusts and individual practice interact with specialist and local authority services.

What is Primary Care?

There is a common belief that the role of the GP in the care of mentally ill people is new, and is mainly due to increasing numbers of mentally ill people being cared for in the community. The work of Goldberg and Huxley (*ibid*) clearly shows that this is not so. However, many GPs, especially in inner cities, complain of an increase in workload which they ascribe to increased care in the community, and some have been particularly concerned by an apparent increase in the numbers of homeless mentally ill people. It may not, in fact, be accurate to ascribe this latter increase to hospital closure. Craig and Timms (1992) reviewed a number of studies and concluded that the majority of homeless mentally ill people were not those who had been discharged as part of planned closure programmes. Most had never experienced long periods in hospital. These authors believed that what they called the *'crisis of visibility'* was more the result of long-term failures to provide adequate community services, and the closure of hostels which had previously acted as unofficial asylums for many mentally ill people.

Primary health care, as its name implies, is the first contact service. It is primary care professionals, most often the general practitioner (GP), to whom people go when they first consider themselves to be in need of help for their health. GPs are, in the main, accessible to members of the public without referral. Everyone is entitled to be registered with a GP, and any person on a GP's list may consult that doctor at any time. It is this accessibility and universality that distinguishes primary care from other parts of the National Health Service.

The average GP has about 1900 patients on his/her list. Only a relatively small proportion of these people will be requiring healthcare at any one time – but all are referred to by the GP as 'patients'. 'Service user' is not a term that is widely used in primary care. In the context of the *National Service Framework*, this is worth remembering. In Standard 2 the words 'service user' seem to mean 'user of primary care services', in other words 'patients' of the GP or 'clients' of the health visitor. Users of primary care services are the whole population.

Unlike secondary care professionals, GPs do not 'discharge' patients at the end of an episode of illness. Any patient may consult again at any time. This also applies to other primary care workers, such as practice nurses, whose potential clientele includes anyone on the practice list, and health visitors whose caseloads traditionally include all families with children under five, on the list of the practice to which they are attached. In inner city areas, where health visitors may work geographically, the caseload will be all families within the area, and anyone else requiring health-visiting help. District nurses usually take their referrals from the list of the GP practice to which they are attached, though in inner city areas they, like health-visiting colleagues, may work in geographical patches. Contact with a GP or practice nurse is generally initiated by the patient, though patients may attend special clinics (for example, Well Woman Clinics) by invitation from the practice. Health visitors usually work more pro-actively, frequently making the first contact with their clients.

General medical practice is a business, with GPs usually being independent contractors to the NHS. This has been the case ever since the beginning of the NHS and had nothing to do with fund-holding. Unlike other health service workers, most GPs are not salaried employees. Since April 1999, most practices have been organised into Primary Care Groups (PCGs) (Local Health Co-operatives in Scotland) with some now moving towards Primary Care Trust status. Trust status means that they will have full responsibility to commission local health services for their patient population, including those to meet mental health needs.

At present, practice nurses are usually employed directly by GPs although this will probably change as PCGs and PCTs (primary care teams) become established. Currently, however, these nurses are outside the normal NHS management structure and may have limited professional support, though arrangements do vary. The difference in employment conditions for practice nurses and other community nurses may cause tensions and mean that teamworking may suffer.

Not all primary care services are GP practice-based. Inner city geographically-based health visitors will see numbers of clients who do not have a GP, and occupational health services and the school health service might also be seen as part of primary care. It is important that other settings are not ignored. For example, school nurses may be well placed to identify and find help for children and young people experiencing mental health difficulties.

As well as providing the first contact service, primary care professionals, especially nurses, are also engaged in health surveillance (for example, cervical cytology), health protection (for example, immunisation) and health promotion (such as advising on smoking cessation and nutrition). In addition they also provide a large amount of ongoing care to people with existing illness and disability through chronic disease management clinics (especially for diabetes and asthma), in people's homes and in residential care of various types (Ross & MacKenzie, 1996). It is the last two of these activities that may be described as 'community care'.

Freeling and Kendrick (1996) have placed the tasks of primary care within a preventive framework, here applied to mental health but equally applicable to all aspects of health care:

- **Primary prevention** includes offering support to people at increased risk of mental illness, for example, the unemployed, the bereaved, new mothers, single parent families, isolated elderly and disabled people.

- **Secondary prevention** includes early identification and effective treatment for mental illness. The general practice setting offers a non-stigmatising environment in which this can happen, but it is also essential that there is rapid and easy access to specialist support when it is required.

■ **Tertiary prevention** is about the provision of ongoing care and support for those with chronic illness and persistent disability. In many cases this will necessitate effective joint working between specialist services, local authority services and the primary health care team (PHCT). There also needs to be rapid access to help for those whose conditions are likely to relapse or recur.

According to the 1989 White Paper *Caring for People*, community care means providing the right level of intervention and support to enable people to achieve maximum independence and control over their own lives. This White Paper envisaged a wide range of provision but also recognised that much 'community care' was, in effect, informal care by family members. The *National Health Service and Community Care Act 1990,* which followed the White Paper, sets out the responsibilities of health and social services to provide care appropriate to the client's needs. This seems to presuppose that clients in need of 'community care' will be those with existing illness and/or disability, whether physical, mental or both. Thus it is clear that community care is not the same thing as primary care, and that community care responsibilities form only part of the work of primary care teams.

The primary care of mental health

Most of the mental illness dealt with by GPs is non-psychotic illness such as depression and anxiety. It is inaccurate to characterise this population as the 'worried well'. People attending their GP surgery with depression have been shown to have as many symptoms as those attending psychiatrists, and depression is a serious illness from which people do die (Mann, 1992). It has been estimated that around 5% of GP attenders will have major depression with a further 5% having symptoms just a little below the threshold for major depression. Another 10% will have milder illnesses. This represents 300–400 patients per GP (Paykel & Priest, 1992).

Numbers of patients with psychotic illness on the average GP list are likely to be relatively small, varying from about 4 to 12 (Strathdee & Jenkins, 1996). The variability depends on a number of factors including the GP's interest in mental illness, but the most marked differences are between rural areas and the inner cities. In a survey conducted in the South West Thames region (Kendrick *et al*, 1991) those GPs with higher than average numbers tended to be working in inner London and near large psychiatric hospitals. They also tended to have worked in hospital psychiatry posts and had psychiatrists visiting their practices.

Recently there have been some research studies looking at the mental health-related roles of generalist community nurses, particularly practice nurses. A 1993 census of practice nurses (Atkin *et al*, 1993) estimated that about 40% were involved in the early detection of depression and anxiety. Significantly, this survey also showed that less than 2% of this group were qualified mental health nurses. Practice nurses are also quite heavily involved in giving depot neuroleptic medication to patients with schizophrenia. A South London study has suggested that about two thirds of all practice nurses in one district may be undertaking this task for at least one patient, on a regular basis (Burns *et al*, 1998). In an audit of patients receiving depot neuroleptic medication conducted in North Yorkshire (Hamilton, 1996), 59% of patients were receiving their injection from a practice nurse. The problem was therefore not confined to London.

Although many patients prefer to receive their medication in the relatively non-stigmatising setting of their GP surgery, Repper and Brooker (1993) have pointed out that many patients in this situation will have no contact with other health service professionals, and their carers may also be isolated. Kendrick (1996) confirms this, pointing to research which shows that up to a third of patients with psychosis lose contact with specialist services within a year of discharge from hospital, and rely totally on their GP for care. Many practice nurses may also be taking blood tests to monitor lithium levels in patients with bipolar disorder. Anecdotal evidence suggests that many nurses regard this as just another task, and again may be unaware of the needs of these patients.

One national survey of practice nurses (Gray *et al*, 1999) found that 61% of their respondents administered a depot neuroleptic injection at least once a month. More than half were also involved in screening for depression, monitoring anti-depressant medication and providing information on depression to patients and their families. Very few of these nurses had any involvement with arrangements under the Care Programme Approach and more than 70% had had no mental health training within the past five years. The authors concluded that side effects of anti-psychotic medication were rarely monitored and knowledge of treatment issues in depression was poor. Interestingly, they also found that the attachment of a community psychiatric nurse (CPN) to the practice made no significant difference to the numbers of patients with mental health problems seen by the practice nurse.

District nurse caseloads traditionally include large numbers of elderly people. Not only is depression more common in older than younger people and the suicide rate higher, but these nurses will also be caring for considerable numbers of patients with dementia. (See **Chapter 4**.) The district nurse may be the only professional with whom the carer has contact. Contacts between district nurses – who are usually general-trained nurses and may have little psychiatric experience or training – and their CPN colleagues may be limited. Co-ordination of care for people with dementia was a particular concern in the report of the Mental Health Nursing Review Team, *Working in Partnership* (Department of Health, 1994b), but the role of district nurses was not specifically acknowledged. An Audit Commission Review of District Nursing (1999) seems not to have acknowledged any mental health role for this group of nurses despite their high-risk caseload.

Health visitors have an important role in the recognition and care of mothers with postnatal depression, other mental illness in the postpartum period, and mental health problems in families in general. Although postnatal depression is, in the main, a primary care illness, in order for it to be adequately treated each district needs to have provision for those few mothers whose illness becomes more serious. There also needs to be an appropriate level of support and supervision for health visitors engaged in counselling for this condition (Cox & Holden, 1994).

Mental health training in primary care

Most primary care workers, including both doctors and nurses, are generalists who may have little or no formal training in psychiatry beyond that which they will have received in their basic professional education. Though many recognise the importance of mental health care for their patients, and may pay some lip service to concepts of the interdependence of physical and mental health, there may be little attempt in practice to bring them together. Many GPs and primary care nurses consider that they do practice in an holistic way but physical health care often takes precedence over mental health care. It is traditional to eliminate the physical before thinking about the psychological.

Jenkins (1992b) considers that it is the specialisation in medicine which occurred towards the end of the 19th century which led to the separation of mind and body in medical theory. This has encouraged the 'one patient, one diagnosis' model which may cause serious disadvantage for those with multiple problems. She points to research showing that people with emotional disorder are high consumers of general practice time, and that patients with identified psychiatric illness had illnesses in more categories per head than other patients consulting their doctors. She also believes that doctors miss disease because of a fixation with the 'one diagnosis' model. Psychiatrists miss physical illness and people with serious mental illness have higher death rates than the general population from the common killers such as heart disease and cancers (Department of Health, 1992).

Moreover, general physicians, including GPs, miss mental illness, especially emotional disorders.

Major concerns have been raised over many years about the ability of GPs to recognise depression. Research consistently shows that about 50% of those presenting to the GP with depression are not detected, though this is an average figure which varies widely and depends on many factors, including the interest of the GP (Tylee, 1996). Even people with recognised depression may receive sub-optimal treatment.

These concerns have led to the development of training programmes for GPs in the recognition and management of depression, but there have been some major difficulties with implementing such programmes and encouraging take-up. Turton and colleagues (1995) describe an assessment of the mental health training needs of general practitioners and point to a dichotomy between what they call *perceived competence* and *actual competence*. The GPs in their survey were confident of their ability to recognise depression, but felt least confidence in their skills of psycho-dynamic counselling and stress management. Unsurprisingly, they were most interested in further training in those areas in which they felt least confident. This survey also confirmed that most GPs had no formal experience or training in psychiatry beyond their basic education. There was also no apparent link between formal psychiatric experience (usually hospital-based) and the range of skills needed for mental health care in general practice. As these authors point out, there are challenges here to GP educators in motivating GPs to receive training in an area where research suggests there is a need, but where there is lack of awareness of that need. There is research demonstrating that appropriate training can lead to improvement in GP performance in both recognition and management of depression and also to better patient outcome (Gask, 1992).

In a more recent survey by Kerwick and colleagues (1997) of GPs' mental health training priorities in one inner London area, respondents again put psychological skills high on the list, but 'psychiatric emergencies' was the most frequently selected topic. This no doubt is a reflection of the geographical area in which the study was conducted.

Community nurse training needs in mental health have been less studied, but there are studies looking at practice nurse-assisted care of patients with depression (Mann *et al*, 1998). Health visitors, trained in fairly basic Rogerian person-centred counselling techniques, have been shown to improve the outcome for mothers with postnatal depression (Holden *et al*, 1989). Much of the research into improving the skills of general nurses in mental health care has been generated by psychiatrists and other non-nurses. It usually involves drafting new skills onto nursing practice, but the skills often derive from disciplines other than nursing and may therefore not fit easily into existing work patterns. There is a widespread perception amongst researchers that practice nurses have more time than GPs. This may not be borne out in practice and many practice nurses are restricted in the amount of time their employers will allow them to devote to individual patients.

Many nurses, especially practice nurses, complain that the attitude of GPs makes it hard for them to gain access to training. This is sometimes regarded by educators as a convenient excuse, but there is some support from at least two sources. Ross (1992) investigated the reason for poor take-up of a course in communication skills for practice nurses. Of the 18 nurses questioned, 10 said that their GP employers did not regard the course as a priority. Reported comments included *'You're paid to work, not go on courses'*. A survey of GP attitudes to practice nurses (Robinson *et al*, 1993) showed that less than half the respondents recognised the lack of training opportunities as a barrier to role development for practice nurses. These attitudes are by no means universal, and they may be slowly changing, but they are still sufficiently common to give primary care nurses considerable concern.

The Clinical Standards Advisory Group (CSAG) study into *Services for Patients with Depression* (2000) said that national and local training agendas should address the gaps in practitioners' knowledge, but there is little evidence of this happening in a planned way. Training for primary care nurses was particularly highlighted in the study and the need for identified budgets for training was clearly stated. The study also linked training issues to the clinical governance agenda in PCGs and suggested that the care of people with depression should be a priority for quality improvement.

Commissioning mental health services

One of the main priorities for the NHS in the '90s was the development of primary care-led commissioning, firstly under the GP fund-holding scheme and more recently through the newly established primary care groups (PGCs). The implementation of community care policies in mental health evolved alongside the development of fund-holding (Strathdee & Jenkins, 1996). Commissioning by PCGs is still in its early stages, and many PCGs still lack the necessary skills and knowledge. Planning by provider units remains a complex problem. Despite these issues, the White Paper, *Modernising Mental Health Services* (Department of Health, 1998) emphasised the integral role PCGs must play in the development of a safe, sound and supportive mental health service. The *National Service Framework for Mental Health* (1999) takes this further in looking at models for service delivery alongside the standards.

There is at least anecdotal evidence that many commissioning decisions are still based on inadequate assessment of need. Ford and Warner (1996) suggest that, with the then-state of development of mental health information systems, it was rarely possible to find out anything other than the number of inpatient episodes in a given district. Many GPs, even those actively involved in commissioning services, may still lack basic information such as the numbers of people with serious mental illness on their lists. The South West Thames survey by Kendrick and colleagues (1991) showed that although more than 40% of respondents indicated willingness to organise the care of these patients, with specialist back-up when necessary, almost none had specific practice policies by which this might be done. Most agreed that these patients usually only came to their attention when a crisis arose.

Problems are not all one-sided. GPs (and health authorities) may lack information on which to base rational purchasing decisions, but there is also evidence that some trusts have, in the past, adopted a 'take-it-or-leave-it' attitude to providing services, and expect to provide the same service to every practice in their district. This may be justified on grounds of equity but in reality it can be far from equitable. Not all practices are the same. Not only may different practices in the same locality have a completely different practice population in terms of factors such as deprivation and ethnic mix, but the levels of skill within the practice, and the interest of PHCT members in mental health, will also vary considerably. A practice where at least one partner has experience as a psychiatric registrar, where there are regular sessions from a clinical psychologist and perhaps a practice counsellor, will require a very different amount of input from the CMHT from the practice where no-one has ever done any psychiatric training and where the level of psychological awareness is low. Additionally, some services may still be provided 'because this is what we've always provided' rather than being based on good information about local need.

The Care Programme Approach in primary care

Secondary care services – including psychiatrists, community psychiatric nurses and social workers attached to community mental health teams – have been urged to prioritise the care of the most seriously ill. There is continuing debate about the definition of 'serious mental illness', but it is widely considered that diagnosis is only one of several criteria which should be taken into account. Others would include duration and level of disability and also safety and the need for formal or informal care (Department of Health, 1995).

The Care Programme Approach (CPA) was introduced in 1991 to provide a framework within which high quality care could be achieved. Though designed for people with severe mental illness, it was intended that its provisions should apply to:

■ all people accepted by specialist psychiatric services

■ all psychiatric patients being discharged from hospital.

This was to ensure that no vulnerable person was able to slip through *'the safety net of care'* (Department of Health, 1994a). It was never the intention that the CPA should apply only to people suffering from psychotic illness, though in some districts it has been interpreted in such a way that only those with a diagnosis of schizophrenia will qualify. Many psychiatrists and GPs are concerned that over concentration on diagnosis as the sole criterion for deciding eligibility for services means that many seriously disabled people with neurotic illness will not receive the care they need.

One of the responsibilities of the keyworker/care co-ordinator under the CPA is to ensure that the patient is registered with a GP, and to work closely with the primary care team. Where the patient was initially referred to the specialist services by their GP, this should not present too many difficulties, unless the patient is being discharged to a different area. It is undoubtedly working with GPs that causes the most difficulties to community mental health teams (CMHTs). There may be a number of reasons for this. Community psychiatric nurses may in fact have little community training and have moved into community work directly from hospital. It is therefore possible that many CMHT members give GPs little thought. One published description of the implementation of the Care Programme Approach in one district says only that care plan summaries and reviews were sent to GPs *'bearing in mind restrictions on the confidentiality of some information'* (Shepherd *et al*, 1995). There is no other mention that GPs were involved in any decision-making at all. Yet it is likely that, at least in some cases, GPs were expected to prescribe for these individuals, perhaps depot neuroleptics subsequently administered by practice nurses. There is no mention in this article of this aspect of care other than a very brief reference to treatment compliance.

In some geographical areas, primary care liaison teams have been established as a specialist variant of a community mental health team. Their brief has been to develop more effective liaisons with primary care partners. These developments, however, are patchy, and a lack of clarity about roles and responsibilities persists. There is also some degree of confusion as to how these teams link with the more generic community mental health teams. A lack of operational policies to support these developing services has added to this lack of clarity.

The interface between primary care and specialists

Strathdee and Jenkins (1996) contended that mental health research has consistently found that failure to communicate leads to poor patient care, and to misunderstandings about roles and responsibilities. They suggest a minimum amount of information required by primary care teams about their own area. This is summarised below, with some additional practical points:

- **How are local mental health services organised?** Sector names and boundaries are important, together with the names of key clinical and managerial staff.

- **A summary of the needs assessment for the area**, including number of patients on the CPA and supervision register, deprivation indices and any services which are planned.

- **Their own sector team names, roles and contact numbers,** including out-of-hours contact and crisis services. This is especially important in inner city areas where practices may often need to liaise with more than one provider. Such arrangements are cumbersome and may lead to 'inappropriate' referrals.

- **Directory of the services provided**, both at CMHT level, and by local hospital units.

- **Information booklets** about the various therapies available.

- **Named contacts** to advise on appropriate referrals. This function may be performed by a link worker, by regular meetings between PHCT members and the CMHT which serves their area, or by other means. Different models are evolving.

- **Process by which the PHCT will be updated when changes occur**; for example a regular trust newsletter, meetings or training events.

These authors also point to many studies showing that referral letters often do not contain information which is vital to decision-making, nor do replies from specialists necessarily contain information that the GP wants to know. They suggest the following is important to the CMHT in referrals:

- background information about family and social history

- presenting problem

- what has already been tried, and the outcome

- reason for referral – this may be for advice on management which the GP intends to continue, for the secondary care service to take over the care or even for the specialist to relieve the GP of care for a short time, for respite.

In a facilitation study in the early 90s (Armstrong, 1994), some GPs expressed dissatisfaction with letters they received from specialists in response to referrals. In particular, detailed assessments of family circumstances were said to be an unnecessary repetition of things that the GP, as the family doctor, already knew. What was actually required, it was suggested, was clear guidance on management. Strathdee and Jenkins (*ibid*) consider that some other pieces of information are essential:

- indication of suicide risk

- what the patient has been told about their condition

- prognosis and likely effect on lifestyle

- GP and PHCT role in management

- ■ what specialist team will do and when

- ■ who is responsible for prescribing and monitoring.

Models for change

A number of different models for improving communication between primary care teams and mental health specialists have emerged over recent years. Experiences in other fields of healthcare are also being used in mental health with some success.

Facilitation

A variety of primary care projects since the early 80s have demonstrated the value of facilitation methods in achieving change in primary care practice (Armstrong, 1992). Facilitators work by personal contact to help practices develop quality care. Important methods include building links between organisations and individuals and providing education and practical help to enable changes to happen as quickly and painlessly as possible. Practical help might include providing templates and support in designing practice-based clinical guidelines, and in audit of care (Wilson, 1994). Information about services can be disseminated via a facilitator and feedback can be encouraged. Increasingly, provider units and GP practices are seeing the facilitator role as a crucial element in helping to bring people together and improve the dialogue.

In the past, facilitators have been trust or health authority employees working on full-time projects. They usually have no clinical role, but most are experienced clinicians. Those currently working in primary care mental health come from a variety of professional backgrounds, with the majority being nurses, though not necessarily RMNs (Armstrong, unpublished). Others may combine a part-time facilitator role with clinical responsibilities. This can work very well provided there are clear barriers between the two roles, and protected time for facilitation activities. Facilitators are agents for change and it is vital, if change is to be accepted by all stakeholders and implemented, that the facilitator is able to maintain a neutral role, serving the interests of no single person or organisation. The purpose is to bring people together so that they can do things for themselves *'making it easier to understand others and effectively work with others'* (Thomas, 1994). If the facilitator is perceived as supporting the agenda of any single group, this purpose will not be achieved. They may again be found useful by PCGs and PCTs as these organisations struggle to bring disparate groups of GP practices up to the *National Service Framework Standards*.

Specialist attachments

Before the introduction of the Care Programme Approach, many CPNs were working with PHCTs on attachment, in much the same way as health visitors and district nurses do. One effect of these attachments was that many CPNs became drawn into providing care for people with less serious illness. This was often believed to be highly cost effective, but Gournay and Brooking (1995) contend that this belief was based on no good evidence. Their own study showed no difference in outcome for patients with depression cared for by a CPN or a GP. Further, there was no relationship between clinical improvement and the amount of contact the patient had with a CPN and patients seeing a CPN did not reduce their use of the GP. Though numbers in this study were very small, the authors state that there is very little other evidence that CPNs are cost-effective in generic rather that specialist roles.

Awareness that the CPN as a specialist is a scarce and valuable resource and may be best used in the care of the seriously mentally ill (Jenkins, 1992a), led to many CPNs being withdrawn from their general practice attachments, often to the dismay of GPs. Ironically, this withdrawal, whilst encouraging CPNs to prioritise people with serious illness, may also have adversely affected communication between specialists and PHCTs. It appears that some CPNs are now returning to GP practices, albeit with a much more clearly defined role, which may include acting as keyworker/care co-ordinator for patients of the practice who are subject to the CPA, and being a named link person with the rest of the CMHT. The link person does not have to be a CPN. Occupational therapists or social workers can also fulfil this role. Key features are:

- a named individual taking responsibility
- face-to-face meetings take place on a regular basis.

There are many more psychiatrists working at least part of the time with primary care teams than in the past, but nationally the situation is highly variable. Many GPs welcome input from a psychiatrist, particularly in assessment and perhaps short-term treatment (Strathdee & Kendrick 1996). However, it may be more important to most GPs that when they refer a patient to a specialist service, the patient is seen by an experienced practitioner, not a junior clinician who may have less experience than the referring GP (Strathdee & Jenkins, 1996).

A few GP practices are beginning to identify a need for a new kind of worker – a primary care mental health worker – whose role would be to support the GPs and other members of the primary care team in their mental health work. They would also do some clinical work, perhaps in assessment, patient education and follow-up of patients on medication. This role is developing in several different ways, sometimes as an extended practice nurse role, but in other instances as something between a CPN and a counsellor. It is not yet clear where this will lead.

Shared care

Diabetes and asthma specialists, and the maternity services, have long been involved in developing shared care systems with primary care teams. Shared care is said to be happening when *'the care of the patient is shared between individuals or teams which are part of separate organisations'* (Pritchard & Pritchard, 1994) Clearly this is the case for those with serious mental illness in the community. However, some of the reported attempts to introduce shared care systems for mentally ill people have been less than successful. Essex and colleagues (1990) considered that shared care records were acceptable to patients, improving autonomy and communication. Professional and managerial attitudes were the main barrier to further development, but these authors believed that the difficulties could be overcome.

Pritchard and Pritchard (1994) believe it to be fundamental that all teams involved should indeed be teams with common goals, not simply groups of people working from the same building. The need for teamworking in mental health care was also a fundamental conclusion of the facilitator in the Kensington & Chelsea and Westminster Family Health Services Authority (KCWFHSA) Mental Health Facilitator Project (Armstrong, 1994). My own, subsequent experience in leading practice-based courses in primary mental health care has tended to confirm the view that when teamwork is effective, patient care improves, but research is needed to properly evaluate such programmes.

Agreed guidelines, across all teams, also seem important, as is the evaluation of the systems set up. Clinical audit is an essential part of this process. Audit is not simply data collection, but should be seen as a cycle involving change and learning.

The comprehensive community-based approach to mental health care developed in Buckinghamshire and described by Falloon and Fadden (1993), involved working closely with primary care physicians, and seems to be the most highly developed form of shared care for mental health so far devised. The authors called their system 'integrated care'. They aimed to provide optimal clinical management for all the people who experienced mental disorders within a defined community. Key elements of the service were:

- early detection
- intensive interventions designed to:

- minimise impairment, disability and handicap

- minimise stress suffered by carers

- prevent future episodes as far as possible.

Their strategy involved a full range of community services including primary health care. The focus was on the provision of therapeutic interventions in a natural environment across biomedical, psychological and social management. They found that, with this intensive system they required minimal mental hospital provision and that specialist day hospitals and outpatient clinics were rarely needed.

However, for this approach to work, extensive, ongoing training of the specialist workforce in the latest, cost-effective clinical management was required, together with specific training for PHCT members, including GPs and community nurses.

Summary

The relationship between PHCTs and other services for mentally ill people, in both health and social services, may be an uneasy one, fraught with difficulty and misunderstandings. Cultural differences between different parts of the health service may lie at the root of at least some of the problems, but these are unlikely to change in the short term. They would matter less if they were openly discussed, accepted and understood. The most important elements of any strategy for change seem to be:

- **Communication** – which means not only improving the formal referral procedures between PHCTs and CMHTs, but also more face-to-face contact between members of both services. Better communication and real partnership between professionals and users/patients is also needed.

- **Teamworking** – this seems crucial. Modern healthcare is too complex for any one professional to think that they have all the answers, but the reality is that many teams are teams only in name, and do not work co-operatively.

■ **Education and training.** Deficiencies in the knowledge and skills of all professionals concerned in the care of mentally ill people are widely acknowledged.

■ **Information.** Lack of good information seriously hampers rational purchasing and meaningful planning. The means exist whereby information quality can be improved. Wider use of clinical audit could stimulate change relatively quickly.

The problems now being experienced in mental health care are the result of decades of neglect. This is not going to be turned round by one-off, short time-limited projects which can be terminated whenever health authorities or other bodies find themselves in financial difficulties. The *National Service Framework* provides a vision and a direction for change, and it is being introduced with a recognition on the Government's part that improvement is likely to take at least a decade. A similar view will need to be taken by health authorities, trusts, local authorities and PCGs if previous short term-ism is to be overcome. Moreover, primary health care needs to see more of the resources that are said to be attached to the *National Service Framework*, both for service improvements and for staff training.

References

Armstrong, E. (1992) Facilitators in primary care. *International Review of Psychiatry* **4** 339–342.

Armstrong, E. (1994) *The Kensington & Chelsea and Westminster Family Health Services Authority Mental Health Facilitator Project: Report of the project facilitator.* Unpublished.

Atkin, K., Lunt, N., Parker, G. & Hurst, M. (1993) *Nurses count: A national census of practice nurses.* York: Social Policy Research Unit, University of York.

Audit Commission (1999) *First Assessment: A review of district nursing services in England and Wales.* London: Audit Commission.

Burns, T., Millar, E., Garland, C., Kendrick, T., Chisholm, B. & Ross, F. (1998) Randomised controlled trial of teaching practice nurses to carry out structured assessments of patients receiving anti-psychotic injections. *British Journal of General Practice* **48** 1845–1848.

Clinical Standards Advisory Group (2000) *Services for Patients with Depression.* London: Department of Health.

Cox, J. & Holden, J. (1994) *Perinatal Psychiatry: Use and misuse of the Edinburgh Postnatal Depression Scale.* London: Gaskell.

Craig, T. & Timms, P. W. (1992) Out of the wards and onto the streets? Deinstitutionalisation and homelessness in Britain. *Journal of Mental Health* **1** 265–275.

Department of Health (1992) *The Health of the Nation: A strategy for health in England.* London: The Stationery Office.

Department of Health (1994a) *The Health of the Nation: Mental illness key area handbook.* Second edition. London: The Stationery Office.

Department of Health (1994b) *Working in Partnership: A collaborative approach to care. Report of the Mental Health Nursing Review Team.* London: The Stationery Office.

Department of Health (1995) *The Health of the Nation: Building Bridges.* London: DoH.

Department of Health (1998) *Modernising Mental Health Services: Safe, sound, supportive.* London: The Stationery Office.

Department of Health (1999) *National Service Framework for Mental Health: Modernising standards and service models.* London: DoH.

Essex, B., Doig, R. & Renshaw, J. (1990) Pilot study of records of shared care for people with mental illnesses. *British Medical Journal* **300** 1442–6.

Falloon, I. & Fadden, G. (1993) *Integrated Mental Health Care: A comprehensive community-based approach.* Cambridge: Cambridge University Press.

Ford, R. & Warner, L. (1996) Reasoning the needs. *Health Service Journal* **30** 24–25.

Freeling, P. & Kendrick, T. (1996) Introduction. In: T. Kendrick, A. Tylee and P. Freeling (Eds) T*he Prevention of Mental Illness in Primary Care.* Cambridge: Cambridge University Press.

Gask, L. (1992) Training general practitioners to detect and manage emotional disorders. *International Review of Psychiatry* **4** 293–300.

Goldberg, D. & Huxley, P. (1980) *Mental Illness in the Community: The pathway to psychiatric care.* London: Tavistock Publications.

Gournay, K. & Brooking, J. (1995) The Community Psychiatric Nurse in Primary Care: An Economic Analysis. In: C. Brooker and E. White (Eds) *Community Psychiatric Nursing: A Research Perspective* **3**.

Gray, R., Parr, A-M., Plummer, S., Sandford, T., Ritter, S., Mundt-Leach, R., Goldberg, D. & Gournay, K. (1999) A national survey of practice nurse involvement in mental health interventions. *Journal of Advanced Nursing* **30** (4) 901–906.

Hamilton, L. (1996) *Audit of Patients with Schizophrenia on Depot Neuroleptics.* York: North Yorkshire Medical Audit Advisory Group.

Holden, J. M., Sagovsky, R. & Cox, J. L. (1989) Counselling in a general practice setting: controlled study of health visitor intervention in treatment of postnatal depression. *British Medical Journal* **298** 223–226.

Jenkins, R. (1992a) Developments in the primary care of mental illness – a forward look. *International Review of Psychiatry* **4** 237–242.

Jenkins, R. (1992b) A Multi-axial Approach to the Primary Care of Schizophrenia. In: R. Jenkins, V. Field and R. Young (Eds) *The Primary Care of Schizophrenia.* London: HMSO.

Kendrick, T. (1996) Organising the Care of the Long-term Mentally Ill in General Practice. In: T. Kendrick, A. Tylee and P. Freeling (Eds) *The Prevention of Mental Illness in Primary Care.* Cambridge: Cambridge University Press.

Kendrick, T., Sibbald, B., Burns, T. & Freeling, P. (1991) Role of general practitioners in the care of long-term mentally ill patients. *British Medical Journal* **302** 508–10.

Kerwick, S., Jones, R., Mann, A. & Goldberg, D. (1997) Mental health care training priorities in general practice. *British Journal of General Practice* **47** 225–227.

Mann, A. (1992) Depression and Anxiety in Primary Care: The epidemiological evidence. In: R. Jenkins, J. Newton and R. Young (Eds) *The Prevention of Depression and Anxiety: The role of the primary care team.* London: HMSO.

Mann, A. H., Blizzard, R., Murray, J., Smith, J. A., Botega, N., MacDonald, E. & Wilkinson G. (1998) An evaluation of practice nurses working with general practitioners to treat people with depression. *British Journal of General Practice* **48** 875–879.

Paykel, E. S. & Priest, R. G. (1992) Recognition and management of depression in general practice: consensus statement. *British Medical Journal* **305** 1198–1202.

Pritchard, P. & Pritchard, J. (1994) *Teamwork for Primary and Shared care: A practical workbook.* Oxford: Oxford University Press.

At the Core of Mental Health © Pavilion 2000

Repper, J. & Brooker, C. (1993) Valuable insights. *Nursing Times* **89** (25) 28–31.

Robinson, G., Beaton, S. & White, P. (1993) Attitudes towards practice nurses – survey of a sample of general practitioners in England and Wales. *British Journal of General Practice* **43** 25–29.

Ross, F. (1992) Barriers to learning. *Nursing Times* **88** (38) 44–5.

Ross, F. & Mackenzie, A. (1996) *Nursing in Primary Health Care.* London: Routledge.

Shepherd, G., King, C., Tilbury, J. & Fowler, D. (1995) Implementing the Care Programme Approach. *Journal of Mental Health* **4** 261–274.

Strathdee, G. & Kendrick, T. (1996) The Regular Review of Patients with Schizophrenia in Primary Care. In: T. Kendrick, A. Tylee and P. Freeling (Eds) *The Prevention of Mental Illness in Primary Care.* Cambridge: Cambridge University Press.

Strathdee, G. & Jenkins, R. (1996) Purchasing Mental Health Care for Primary Care. In: G. Thornicroft & G. Strathdee (Eds) *Commissioning Mental Health Services.* London: The Stationery Office.

Thomas, P. (1994) *The Liverpool Primary Health Care Facilitation Project.* Liverpool: Liverpool Family Health Services Authority.

Turton, P., Tylee, A. & Kerry, S. (1995) Mental health training needs in general practice. *Primary Care Psychiatry* **1** 197–199.

Tylee, A. (1996) The Secondary Prevention of Depression. In: T. Kendrick, A. Tylee & P. Freeling (Eds) *The Prevention of Mental Illness in Primary Care.* Cambridge: Cambridge University Press.

Wilkinson, G. (1992) The role of the practice nurse in the management of depression. *International Review of Psychiatry* **4** 311–316.

Wilson, A. (1994) *Changing Practices in Primary Care: A facilitator's handbook.* London: Health Education Authority.

Chapter 6

Working with Offenders with Mental Health Problems

Aidan Houlders

Introduction

This chapter is a personal view and one which does not necessarily reflect the policies or practices of the author's place of work or his employing authority. The primary aim is to share an understanding of strategic, managerial and operational matters, and training issues as they specifically relate to mental health service users who come into contact with the criminal justice system. The author's references to the various publications are not meant to represent an exhaustive list of what is available in this growth area of care and public concern. They are included in the text for reference purposes and as an indication for further reading.

The chapter aims to provide a context for the current stage of developments in the services provided for mentally disordered offenders. The author draws upon his own experiences to help identify these developments and their application as they occur in his place of work as a social worker in a medium secure unit (MSU).

It is noted that there are a number of statutory and voluntary organisations that are directly involved in the care and management of mental health service users who come into contact with the criminal justice system. Each of these bodies will have workers who work directly with these people. They may not be called 'forensic social workers' but it is possible that they are practising this role under another job title. My references to 'forensic social workers' are meant to include all professional workers engaged directly in the delivery of a social work service to mentally disordered offenders.

It should also be noted that I am a White male who acknowledges the need for anti-discriminatory and anti-oppressive practices – especially in those services which provide secure accommodation for the treatment of men and women service users who are mentally disordered offenders or who require similar provision.

Overview

The following agencies may be involved in the management and care of mentally disordered offenders:

- Criminal Justice System including the Police, Home Office and Probation Service

- Department of Health including community mental health teams, general psychiatric hospitals, special hospitals and medium secure units

- local authority social services departments in concert with other appropriate departments eg housing and employment services

- voluntary organisations and the private sector have an important part to play in providing services in this specialised area of psychiatric care and management.

The role of the voluntary organisations are discussed in *Promoting Care and Justice* (Mental Health Foundation, 1994).

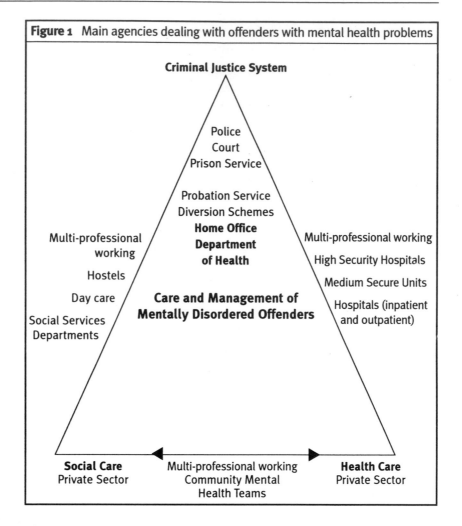

Figure 1 Main agencies dealing with offenders with mental health problems

Figure 1 illustrates the main agencies dealing with offenders with mental health problems. Ideally, the 'points' should be connected by multi-professional working based on joint service agreements and strategic planning.

The statutory organisations identified above all have partial responsibilties for the provision of services to deal with people who suffer from mental health problems and commit offences. The Criminal Justice System (CJS) plays a central role in the initial stages of a person's forensic psychiatric career. Gunn and Taylor, (1993) defined forensic psychiatry thus:

'.... At its simplest, forensic psychiatry can be defined as that part of psychiatry which deals with patients and problems at the interface of the legal and psychiatric systems. In many parts of the world it is a growth area of medicine. There are a number of factors which may have contributed to this growth. These include social pressures to reject chronically sick, the handicapped, the disruptive and aggressive, the development of new assessment and treatment skills for the behaviourally disordered, an increasing interest in institutions and what happens in them, and a rising concern with the problem of 'dangerousness...'

In *Offenders, Deviants or Patients?* (Prins, 1995) consideration is given to the issues relating to people with mental health problems and the responses of the CJS. Public concerns and attitudes towards the mentally disordered have played an important part in the management both of the CJS and the Mental Health System (MHS). Health and social care workers are affected by the public attitudes that are in turn reflected in Government policies and legislation. It is interesting to note that public concern about mentally disordered offenders living in the community and their treatment in institutions go back a long way, as the next section illustrates.

Background to significant legislation for the provision of services for offenders with Mental Health Problems

Legal system 15th century onwards

The following summary is based on *Secure Accommodation* (Gostin, 1985).

English law dealing with mentally disordered offenders can be traced back as far as the 15th century, when it was lawful to incarcerate a *'dangerous lunatic'* either at home or in a local Bridewell (the name given to any local prison). The *Vagrancy Act of 1714* dealt with *'furiously mad and dangerous... wandering lunatics...'* empowering two or more Justices of the Peace to direct that the 'lunatic' be kept safely locked up and (if the Justices found it necessary) chained.

One particular event appears to have had a very significant impact on the provision for the management and care of mentally disordered offenders...

On the 15th May 1880 James Hadfield fired a pistol at King George III as he was entering the Royal Box at Drury Lane theatre. Hadfield was found *'not guilty by reason of insanity'* but was considered dangerous and for his own sake and for that of the public, was returned to Newgate Prison. He was subsequently transferred to Bethlem Hospital.

The creation of Special Hospitals

The Hadfield case raised considerable public interest and concern about the safe management of people who were mentally disordered and deemed dangerous to self and others (It did not differentiate between the various mental states ie mental illness, impairment or personality disorders). The Lunacy Commission provided reports and recommendations that a separate asylum for *'criminal lunatics'* was needed. This led to the building of Broadmoor Hospital, which was opened in 1863 to accommodate 400 men and 100 women. This went some way to dealing with increasing concerns about the numbers of mentally disordered people who were in prison.

Legislation to enable transfer of prisoners to hospital

The *1808 Asylums Act* legislated for the transfer of prisoners to asylums. Subsequent legislation expanded provision for the transfer of prisoners who appeared to be mentally ill, and those with learning disabilities.

Further development of Special Hospital Provision

In 1912 Rampton Hospital was opened to meet the needs of mentally disordered people deemed to require 'high security' to manage their conditions and behaviours. A year later the *Mental Deficiency Act 1913* dealt with the needs of people with learning difficulties/disabilities. Moss Side Special Hospital and Park Lane, which have since merged to become Ashworth Hospital, were part of a Government programme to provide high security for the growing numbers of 'criminally insane' individuals – male and female.

Advances in psychiatry and its impact on legislation and healthcare policies

From the 1900s onwards, there have been significant developments in the understanding of mental disorder and its treatment. For example, the psycho-analytical schools had become well established. The inter-war period saw significant developments in psychiatry, brought about by the discovery of medication that could 'successfully' manage mental illness. These included various pharmaceutical discoveries and modes of administration, such as depots. These are injections of medication that have varying concentrations and chemical formulae which are fully absorbed into the blood stream over a given period of time. The rate of release is meant to ensure efficacy of the medication and obviates the need for oral medication. This has enabled psychiatrists to provide treatment and management of illness to patients who cannot be relied on to take their oral medication. Depots are a positive means of ensuring that patients are administered their prescribed medication and this, in theory, ensures some stability and control over the patient's mental state. These discoveries allowed for the opportunity for patients to be safely managed in the community for the first time.

The *Mental Health Act 1959*

These discoveries and advances in psychiatry led to a major change in Government policy reflected in the *Mental Health Act 1959*. This Act introduced the term 'mental disorder' covering the conditions of 'mental illness' (which was not defined), 'subnormality', 'severe subnormality' and 'psychopathy'.

The care and clinical management of psychiatric patients rested with responsible medical officers – consultant psychiatrists who employed the 'medical model' in the treatment of mental illness.

The same Act placed a greater emphasis on voluntary inpatient treatment, with an expectation that mentally disordered people should receive hospital services similar to those who suffered from physical disorders. Psychiatric patients could be admitted informally and were allowed to discharge themselves if they were receiving treatment on an informal basis. Emphasis was placed on the need to introduce community-based services to support people in the community and thus prevent or reduce the need for admissions into psychiatric hospitals. It was a revolutionary piece of social legislation.

This created the so-called 'open door' policy to the treatment of mental disorder. For the majority of people in need of psychiatric treatment this proved to be an appropriate arrangement.

Unfortunately the 'open door' policy became a revolving door for others and a closed door to some. Following the implementation of the *Mental Health Act 1959* it soon became apparent that there was a significant (but relatively small) number of people who could not be managed adequately in general psychiatric hospitals, either because they would not comply with treatment and follow-up and/or because they were a danger to themselves and/or others. For this smaller population of psychiatric patients there was the risk of either imprisonment or admission into one of the Special Hospitals (which are now referred to as High Security Hospitals) as a means of dealing with their mental disorder.

In 1961 a Government Working Party from the Ministry of Health reported on Special Hospitals, and the classes of people to be treated in them. Proposals were made for secure units for the diagnosis and treatment of psychiatric conditions in addition to existing hospital provision.

Regional (Medium) Secure Units

In 1974 the Glancy Report (DHSS, 1974) recommended that regional health authorities provide facilities for psychiatric patients who required conditions of security for their treatment.

In 1978, the Butler Report on Mentally Abnormal Offenders (DHSS) also reported on the urgent need to provide regional secure units to deal with the 'yawning gap' between NHS Hospitals with no secure provision and the overcrowded Special Hospitals. This was set against a background of increasing numbers of mentally disordered prisoners who were actively mentally ill. This committee recommended provision for 2,000 secure places. The then-Department of Health and Social Security accepted the need for 1,000 secure places, and made arrangements for regional health authorities to receive Government funds expressly for the provision of medium secure accommodation that would provide short-term care (less than 18 months) for people suffering from one or more of the classifications of mental disorder in the *Mental Health Act 1959*.

Since the 1960s there appears to have been a change in healthcare policies which has placed an increasing emphasis on treatment of the mentally disordered person in the community. There has been a nationwide closure of the Victorian psychiatric hospitals to redirect resources to support projects based in the community. The *National Health Service and Community Care Act 1990* reflects these changes in health and social care.

The Mental Health Act 1983

The *Mental Health Act 1983* (which replaced the 1959 Act) continued with psychiatric treatment based on the 'medical model'. However, it embodied the rights of individuals and the sanctity of human freedom. It revised the categories of mental disorder subject to compulsory treatment: 'mental disorder', 'severe mental impairment', 'mental impairment' and 'psychopathic disorder'. Part

III of the Act deals with people who are in prison, on remand or convicted, and in need of psychiatric inpatient treatment.

Diversion schemes

By the end of the 1980s it had become apparent that there was a need to deal with the growing numbers of people with mental health problems coming into contact with the Criminal Justice System. The 1990s began with Government recognition of the problem.

Central Government made the following responses.

The Home Office Circular No. 66/90 states:

'*...It is government policy that, wherever possible, mentally disordered persons should receive care and treatment from the health and social services... It is desirable that alternatives to prosecution, such as cautioning by the police, and/or admission to hospital, if the person's mental condition requires hospital treatment, or support in the community, should be considered first before deciding that prosecution is necessary...*'

The same circular provided a number of examples of diversion schemes. The following section considers suggested schemes of diversion.

Police powers

The police are very often the first statutory agency to be involved in dealing with the more acute or disturbed episodes in a person's mental condition. For example, Section 136 of the *Mental Health Act 1983* allows a police constable to take to a 'place of safety' a person who appears to be suffering from a mental disorder *and* is in a place to which the public have access. Removal is based on protecting the mentally disordered person and/or the public.

Diversion at the Point of Arrest (DAPA)

Ideally, the 'place of safety' should be a healthcare setting. In the author's experience, the place of safety has invariably been a police station where the person is detained in a police cell. To deal with this all-too-common practice, a scheme of Diversion at the Point of Arrest (DAPA) has been provided by community psychiatric nurses. The scheme aims to provide a service to people who appear to be suffering from mental disorder in police custody. Local services (where appropriate) assist in the provision of psychiatric assessment and further intervention, such as outpatient or inpatient treatment. If the local services are not appropriate, other assessments from the forensic services may take place for admission into secure accommodation.

Police and Criminal Evidence Act Code of Practice for mentally disordered people detained in police custody

It should be noted that police activity at the point of arrest and whilst in detention is dealt with in the Code of Practice, *Police and Criminal Evidence (PACE) Act*. The police are required to have an arrested person who appears to be suffering from a mental disorder medically examined and to have an 'appropriate adult' in attendance during a police interview. The 'appropriate adult' can be a relative, friend or suitably qualified person. The role of the appropriate adult is primarily to ensure that the person being interviewed by the police is in a fit state and is not answering questions under duress (Littlechild, 1995; Sheppard, 1996).

Magistrates Court Diversion

If a DAPA scheme is not available, another scheme, Court Diversion, may be employed. At this stage, the person will have been formally charged by the police and required to appear in court.

There are a number of Magistrates Court diversion schemes in operation around the country. These services are usually led by community psychiatric nurses who will have developed their own practice around agreed multi-agency procedures. One of the aims of these services is an initial screening of all people in custody. Priority is given to the examination of certain types of offending behaviours and those who have been identified by representatives of the CJS, including the Probation Service, which has a vital role in this stage of diversionary work.

In consultation with the Crown Prosecution Service, arrangements may be made by the CPN to arrange for admission into hospital under the provisions of the *Mental Health Act*. These arrangements may enable the magistrates to dispose of the case without recourse to custody or other punitive measures.

Bail hostels

The courts may make an order to allow a person bail providing he/she agrees to reside in a bail hostel. Elliot House Bail Hostel provides an exclusive service for mentally disordered offenders. The hostel, which is situated in Birmingham, is a national resource.

Application of the Mental Health Act (MHA) 1983 in the process of diversion

The *Mental Health Act* Parts II and III (patients concerned in criminal proceedings or under sentence) provides powers for people to be assessed and/or receive treatment (see below).

Diversion at the point of arrest and court diversion rely upon 'local health and social care' services to co-operate with the scheme and assist in the identified follow-up of a treatment, either in hospital (informally or compulsorily detained) or outpatient care.

Mentally disordered offenders may be directly admitted to a psychiatric hospital informally or under either Section 2 (Assessment) or Section 3

(Treatment). If the charges are of a serious nature, the defendant may be required to attend court again. Assessment and/or treatment may take place during the remand period either on bail or in custody. At the point of sentencing, magistrates courts may exercise a wide range of disposals. In addition to what might be used for a defendant who is not mentally ill, eg a fine, conditional discharge etc, the magistrates may make a Probation Order with or without conditions of medical treatment, or a Section 37 Hospital Order. This order can only be made for crimes that may be dealt with by way of a custodial sentence. It should be noted that probation orders and hospital orders are made on the basis of recommendations made by probation officers and medical practitioners respectively.

Mentally disordered offenders on remand

Prisoners on remand may be dealt with by the screening processes offered by some prisons. Community psychiatric nurses and prison doctors work with visiting psychiatrists to identify and refer prisoners who appear to be suffering from mental disorder. Depending upon the urgency, remanded prisoners may be transferred (under Sections 35, 36 or 48 of the *Mental Health Act 1983*) to a psychiatric hospital. Section 35 is for assessment and this may be ordered by either a Magistrates or Crown Court. Section 36 (for treatment) can only be made by a Crown Court. Section 48 is for urgent medical treatment. This is dealt with by the Home Office acting upon information from a doctor.

Typically, a person who requires treatment under Section 48 will also be subject to Section 49 which restricts the movement of patients who are not allowed to leave the hospital without Home Office permission. Dr Birmingham *et al* have reported on the problems of identifying prisoners with mental disorder (Birmingham *et al* 1996).

Crown Court and its management of mentally disordered offenders

Prisoners on remand who are due to appear in Crown Court may receive inpatient care to assess and/or treat their mental disorder. At their appearance in Crown Court they may be dealt with under various legislation including the *Mental Health Act* and the *Criminal Insanity and Unfitness to Plead Act.* If the patient is fit enough to stand trial and pleads guilty, or is found guilty, the court has to decide whether or not it is appropriate to impose a sentence or make an order that requires the patient to receive psychiatric treatment, either as an inpatient or outpatient. The Crown Court has a wide range of disposals, which are, as stated above, available to the Magistrates Courts. In addition, the Crown Court has the power to make a Hospital Order (Section 37) with restrictions (Section 41) (*Mental Health Act 1983*).

Hospital Orders with restrictions are made in cases when a serious crime has been committed and the courts are satisfied that at the time of the offence the convicted person was and remains mentally disordered and in need of treatment. At the time of making the Order, the Judge may indicate a time during which the restrictions should remain in force. Usually the Order is made without limit of time and may in theory last for the rest of the patient's life.

Criminal Procedure (Insanity and Unfitness to Plead) Act 1991 deals with those cases where a defendant is not fit to plead or stand trial. The Crown Court has the power to deal with a mentally disordered person in one of the following ways:

- an Order (an Admission Order)
- a Guardianship Order Section 37 (*MHA 1983*)
- a Supervision and Treatment Order requiring the accused to co-operate with supervision by a social worker or a probation officer for a period of not more than two years and with treatment from a medical practitioner
- an order for the absolute discharge of the accused.

Convicted prisoners

Within the provision of Part III (Patients Concerned in Criminal Proceedings or Under Sentence) *MHA 1983* the Home Office may authorise, under Section 47, transfer of convicted prisoners to psychiatric hospitals. Section 49 (Restrictions) are normally attached to ensure that the prisoner does not leave the hospital without the consent of the Home Secretary.

Assessment and support for sentenced prisoners

Sentenced or convicted prisoners who are mentally disordered, and remain in the penal system, present significant problems for the Prison Service. Direct work with sentenced prisoners may be seen in the Wessex Project *Crossing Boundaries* (Lart, 1997) which sets out an account of a project to provide multi-professional assessments and support for mentally disordered prisoners.

> *'The Project introduced the idea of planned discharge for the prison population with mental health needs, using the Care Programme Approach (1990) where appropriate...'*

The project identified prisoners who were actively mentally disordered.

It is interesting to note that Singleton reported on a survey of prisoners – remanded and convicted – who suffered from mental disorder. Singleton recorded an over-representation of black people and an under-representation of women in the survey, from a sample of the prison population. In July 1997 there were 61,994 prisoners in 131 penal establishments: 46,872 were male sentenced prisoners, 12,302 were male remands and 2,770 were women. Of the population surveyed the following incidence of psychosis was noted: 7% male sentenced, 10% male remanded and 14% for female prisoners (Singleton, 1998).

Victim support

Whilst the focus of this chapter is on the mentally disordered offender, it would be a serious omission not to consider the victim(s) of the crime(s) committed by the mentally disordered offender. The plight of the victim is officially recognised in Government policy eg *The Victim's Charter* and the Home Office Publication *Information for Families of Homicide Victims*. The Probation Service has been charged with the responsibility to interview victims and/or their families about plans to release the prisoner who perpetrated the crime. This activity is of special importance in the management and care of mentally disordered offenders. The Probation Service Circular 61/95 *Probation Service Contact with Victims* states its purpose as giving *'services...guidance about the arrangements of contact with victims of serious offences or their families...'*

The document concludes:

'Offenders subject to Hospital Orders 22, where probation officers are involved with the throughcare of offenders subject to hospital orders, whether or not with restrictions, no steps should be taken to contact the victims of offences except as directed by the responsible medical officer...'

Generally, victims are offered the services of the nationwide Victim Support Schemes, which are sponsored by the Government to provide support and care for victims of crimes and their families. The author takes the view that victims, who are not related to the perpetrator (mentally disordered offender), should be dealt with by a victim support scheme practitioner. The appropriateness of intervention or follow-up from a member of the clinical team looking after the patient to interview the victim, will be a matter of agreement between the victim and victim support worker.

Government responses to the impact of the psychiatric hospital closure programme

In addition to specific changes to the law, and to the collaborative schemes involving interagency working in the Criminal Justice to divert mentally disordered offenders away from the Criminal Justice System, there have been initiatives from the Department of Health and the Home Office to address the consequences of changes in hospital inpatient care. These previously dealt with the more seriously or severely mentally ill population, including mentally disordered offenders. These changes in Government policies were a reaction to public concerns about mentally disordered people living in the community who were committing serious crimes. These activities were taking place in the much publicised Government plan for Care in the Community, which appeared to be failing certain service users, in need of health and/or social care. People with mental health problems who have committed serious crimes or have demonstrated serious risk to themselves, have generated very specific pieces of Government guidance to health and social services to manage apparent deficiencies in the programme of Community Care.

Central Government policies and planning for mentally disordered people have changed significantly prior to and since the implementation of the *National Health Service and Community Care Act 1990* that came into force in 1993. There have been a number of circulars (see opposite) from both the Home Office and the Department of Health on the management of severely mentally ill people and mentally disordered offenders living in the community. There has also been an amendment to the *Mental Health Act 1983* which now has the power to make people subject to a Supervised Discharge Order (Section 25) referred to above (Jones, 1999).

As part of its raft of responses to deal with the issues raised by the management and care of mentally disordered offenders, the Government set up a committee under the Chairmanship of Dr John

Reed to undertake a 'review of health and social services for mentally disordered offenders and those who require similar provision' which has become known as the Reed Report. This report has been published and sets out a comprehensive framework to deal with mentally disordered people and others.

Other Government reports were published by the Department of Health: Mental Illness – *Key Area Handbook* (1994); *Building Bridges* (1993); and *Social Care Group Services for Mentally Disordered Offenders in the Community* (1997).

Care Programme Approach – Government Circular HC(90)23/LASSL(90)

In response to public concerns, the Government produced a number of circulars on the management of severely mentally ill people living in the community or those ready for discharge from inpatient treatment to return to the community. For example, in 1991 the Care Programme Approach (CPA) was introduced to provide a systematised and co-ordinated programme of care for severely mentally ill people. The CPA also applies to mentally disordered offenders in the high security hospitals and those serving prison sentences. It is a health service-led arrangement that should directly link into social care provision. CPA is available to all patients who are deemed to be at serious risk of harm to self or others (or of neglect).

In 1999 the Department of Health revised the Care Programme Approach. This document does not exclusively deal with mentally disordered offenders but makes the point that patients in high security hospitals and prisoners with diagnosed mental disorders should be managed within an integrated health and social care service. This has implications for health and social care workers to develop systems of collaboration to monitor, review and assess a segment of the psychiatric population that has hitherto been overlooked.

Section 117 aftercare

It is the duty of local health and social services, in co-operation with relevant voluntary agencies, to provide aftercare services for discharged mental health service users who have received treatment under Sections 3, 37, 47 and 48 of the *Mental Health Act 1983* (Jones, 1999 *ibid*) Sheppard (1996). Note that Section 37 is a Hospital Order made by the courts. Sections 47 and 48 deal with the treatment of prisoners, who have respectively been convicted or are on remand in custody. It follows that aftercare should be available to prisoners upon their release from prison.

The next section considers matters which local authority social services departments need to address in providing services for mentally disordered offenders and those who require similar provision.

Interagency collaboration

Government publications such as the *Health of the Nation* series, including *Building Bridges* (Department of Health, 1995) emphasise the need for interagency schemes to manage the complex area of human suffering experienced by mentally disordered offenders and their victims. There are examples of good practice around the country which demonstrate what can be achieved when statutory and voluntary organisations and the private sector come together to provide a co-ordinated programme of care and support (Department of Health, 1999).

Despite changes in the law and guidance from both the Home Office and the Department of Health, tragedies in the care and management of mentally disordered people still occur. The Zito Trust's publication *Learning the Lessons* (Sheppard, 1996) details the numerous mental health inquiries into the tragic deaths of innocent victims and patients because of failures in the mental health system to provide proper psychiatric care and supervision in the community. The question of lessons learned is to be regarded with some caution because the same mistakes appear to recur with alarming frequency. Interagency working and the multi-professional approach to the assessment, treatment and rehabilitation of mentally disordered offenders appear as regular recommendations from these various inquiries.

Social work with the mentally disordered offender and those who require similar provision

Social work with mental health service users who come into contact with the Criminal Justice System has formed a significant part of the workload for probation officers and approved social workers (mental health specialist social workers). This is well documented in the Central Council for Education and Training in Social Work document *Training for Work with Mentally Disordered Offenders* (1993).

In the wake of the Butler Report (1978) and the creation of interim and regional secure units (RSUs), a distinct body of professional workers has developed who practise alongside health service workers in the specialism of forensic services. These services reflect the specialist nature of working with mentally disordered people who commit crime as a consequence of their disorder. Such criminal activities can and do cover the spectrum of all types of crime. Inevitably, to ration the service and direct it effectively, forensic services have concentrated on the more serious offending behaviour that threatens the safety of the public and which results in serious damage to property. It is interesting to note that the Department of Health reported that people with mental health problems are more likely to harm themselves than others (Department of Health, 1999).

Since 1990 there have been numerous mental health inquiries that have raised awareness of the needs of mental health service users who commit serious criminal offences as a consequence of their disorder, and the effects that the offending behaviours have had upon the victim, family, carers and the public.

Over this period various attempts have been made by professional workers in 'social work' to come together to provide support and act as a reference group for individual practitioners who may be working in professional isolation. The British Association of Social Workers (BASW) established a Special Interest Group to deal with this situation.

As previously mentioned, in 1993 the Central Council for Education and Training in Social Work published *Training for Work With Mentally Disordered Offenders* (Hudson *et al*, 1993). This publication addressed training needs and availability of training for probation officers and social workers. This document was followed by the National Association for the Care and Rehabilitation of Offenders (NACRO) publication, *Working with Mentally Disordered Offenders* which is a training pack designed to assist workers in a variety of settings which deal with mentally disordered offenders. It should be noted that it has long been recognised that there are workers (who are neither probation officers nor social workers) in the statutory, voluntary and private sectors who deal directly with mental health service users who are currently being, or have in the past been, dealt with by the criminal justice system. These staff also require training and guidance. This should be dealt with in any training programme that attempts to reach all those who are involved in the social care of mentally disordered offenders.

In 1994 the Department of Health commissioned the Central Council for Education and Training to:

'*...undertake a project to produce a package of guidance material to enhance post qualification training in forensic social work...in light of the findings from the Department of Health/Home Office Review of Health and Social Services for Mentally Disordered Offenders and others with similar needs*'. (The Reed Review, 1991)

In 1995 CCETSW published *Forensic Social Work Competence and Workforce Data* which '*... describes the competencies required for best practice* *in the range of settings where social work with mentally disordered offenders is undertaken...'* (CCETSW, 1995) and provided the following definition:

'Forensic Social Work is social work with mentally disordered people who present, or are subject to, significant risk and, as a consequence, are, or could be, in contact with the criminal justice system.'

The following key purpose was established:

'The key purpose of forensic social work is to hold in balance the protection of the public and the promotion of the quality of life of individuals and by working in partnership with relevant others to:

- *identify, assess and manage risk*
- *identify and challenge discriminatory structures and practices*
- *engage effectively with mentally disordered offenders and other people with similar needs*
- *identify, develop and implement strategies.'*

The same document refers to **key tasks**, which are:

1 assessment

2 care planning and management

3 report writing

4 working with individuals and families

5 managing crisis and trauma

6 maintaining effective social supervision

7 managing external systems

8 complementary professional activity.

CCETSW has published a companion booklet to *Forensic Social Work: Achieving competence in forensic social work* (CCETSW, 1995). This document sets out guidance on how social work practitioners may qualify for the Advanced Award in (Forensic) Social Work.

Forensic social work: implications for service delivery

Forensic social work interventions should be part of an integrated service provided within a framework of agreements between the NHS mental health services, social services departments and the probation service, in collaboration with and supported by the voluntary and private sectors. The delivery of these services should be set against regional or national 'standards' for research and monitoring purposes.

Risk assessment and its management is not an essential element of forensic services. Social workers have their part to play in the process of risk assessment but this must not be an exclusive role. On the contrary, this activity should be part of an agreed integrated strategy determined within multi-professional teams; working in co-ordination with other related services providing care for the same service user. Joint planning – for example, between social services departments, the Probation Service and victim support schemes – is required to assess the needs of service users' families and his or her victim(s). Family support and victim support should be seen in terms of helping people to come to terms with what has happened and also provides valuable information for risk assessment purposes.

Service users who need 'secure provision' either in the criminal justice system or mental health systems become a part of a population which over or under represents the general population in terms of gender, race, culture or ethnicity. There are significant issues for anti-discrimination and anti-oppressive practices in these institutional secure settings. The Social Services Inspectorate Report (Reaside, 1994) refers to the over representation of Black male service users and the under representation of women in psychiatric secure units. Also there is a need to take into account the provision for mental health service users who also suffer from sensory impairments and/or physical disabilities.

Service users in the forensic services typically have been part of other mental health systems or probation services. This has implications for planning and purchasing of locally based forensic services. This would certainly appear to be the case in managing anticipated movement of patients from special hospitals to less secure settings and in diverting mental health service users from the criminal justice system. (The Prison Service has a long history of managing prisoners with mental health problems. Fluctuations in the prison population could be examined in the context of changes in local and national policy regarding caring for mental health service users.)

In the more extreme cases it is inevitable that service users and others will receive media attention which has to be managed by the health authorities and social services departments. The impact of media reporting and ongoing interest should never be underestimated. Adverse publicity or sensationalised reporting of events may leave deep and lasting impressions on the public, who will understandably be alarmed about the prospect of the mentally disordered offender being returned to the community and possibly, living in their neighbourhood.

Following the Fallon Report (*ibid*) there is a further dimension to the role of the forensic social worker. This role relates to the contact between patients and children. Access between patients and children now requires careful scrutiny and approval. Local authority social services departments are required to investigate a patient's request to have access to a named child irrespective of the relationship. This is another example of the need to have arrangements in place between social care staff based in the community and their social work colleagues in psychiatric settings.

This serves to underline the importance of developing a multi-agency co-ordinated strategy to respond to the needs of mentally disordered offenders, and of those who have been affected by the crimes committed.

With these themes and considerations in mind, the remainder of this chapter will outline social work activities with services users at various stages of the forensic psychiatric career from pre-admission, admission and pre-discharge, discharge and aftercare.

Criminal Justice System

Forensic Social workers may also undertake the roles of ASW and Appropriate Adult to deal directly with mentally disordered offenders in the initial stages of contact with the criminal justice system, ie police arrest and appearance in court.

Social workers and probation officers should not lose sight of the importance of their role in working with mentally disordered offenders in the Criminal Justice System which can use Part II of the *Mental Health Act* and other legislation (see previous pages) without recourse to the forensic services.

Mental health specialist social workers occupy a very important position in the process of diversion not only from the Criminal Justice System but also from forensic services.

Interagency working and multi-professional health, social care and probation service strategies are vital at these initial stages of contact and should of course be available throughout a person's psychiatric career if this is required.

Social work with families, who are so often the victims of the crimes committed by mentally disordered offenders, should also take place in this initial stage. Agreements between the Probation Service and Victim Support appear to be of vital importance to ensure that victims receive their own support and therapeutic management. In the more extreme cases of offending behaviour, such as homicide, special provision and arrangements should be available to immediately deal with bereaved relatives, carers and significant others. Social workers should be part of a network of support to assist victims and/or their families.

Risk assessment and risk management: the role of a forensic social worker

In my view, social work risk assessment and its management should be based on a thorough and comprehensive understanding of a service user's offending or challenging behaviours viewed from, and openly discussed within, an agreed multi-professional approach to the assessment, treatment and rehabilitation of mental health service users. Social work assessment should not be a professionally isolated activity. Clinical and community-based multi-professional teams should work together to accept collective responsibility for the formulation of risk assessment and its management – an *ongoing* process. This responsibility implies the need for teamworking and for developing standards of assessment and management, which are appropriate and responsive to the local conditions.

It is therefore the responsibility of each individual practitioner to ensure that risk assessment is carried out according to an agreed approach, based on multi-professional working. It is the responsibility of health and social services managers to ensure that practitioners have proper support to conduct their work in a structured way, one which is set within a framework of agreed standards, and which is complementary to the approach adopted by fellow professional workers engaged in the same activity. Risk assessment matters should be recorded, stating the practitioners' opinions about risk and its management. In addition, a written account of proposed action and anticipated outcomes is necessary to justify the action which is subsequently taken, or not as the case may be. This aspect deals with some of the issues raised by Kemshall and Pritchard (1996) on the matter of litigation in cases where professional workers are accused of neglect of duty to care.

Risk assessment should also be seen as a positive process calculated to improve the quality of life for the service user (Davis, 1996). Risk-taking should be seen as a positive action, which should be aimed at enhancing a person's quality of life.

Essential information to base a risk assessment upon

R isk assessment is a process which requires thorough examination of all aspects of a service user's mental state, familial and social relationships, employment activities and the evidence produced in criminal proceedings. Detailed examination appears to be an obvious prerequisite to such activity, but systems, particularly those which uphold the fundamental right of confidentiality, can seriously jeopardise the full and complete understanding of a person's 'riskiness' and the management of the risks he or she poses.

Pre-admission

Initial contact with mentally disordered offenders who are living in the community usually takes place either in police custody or before a court appearance. Social work activity is confined to the urgent matters of Mental Health Act assessments and organising hospital inpatient treatment. This activity should not be isolated but part of an agreed multi-professional response to appropriately managing a situation and offering realistic, sustainable alternatives to further detention and diversion from court. These situations obviously relate to minor offending behaviour where the service user is not deemed a risk to self and/or others. As already indicated above, Diversion at the Point of Arrest and Court Diversion schemes have developed across the country to provide this service.

Health authorities and social services departments, in partnership with probation services, should continue to work together and further develop schemes of partnership to address the needs of mental health services, to ensure that they do not find themselves in another form of revolving door – in and out of the criminal justice system.

Admission

Social work activity during this period is an opportunity to further assess the service user's personal circumstances, in terms of researching his or her personal development, viewed from the perspectives of the service user, family carers and significant others, including other agencies which have, or have had, contact. This process provides an opportunity to put in a social context the process and effects of the mental disorder on the service user and his or her 'social situation'. Within this context, issues which relate to a person's culture, belief systems, religion, language, dietary needs and customs should be observed in the framework of anti-discriminatory and anti-oppressive practices.

Family work and support for victims or others forms another important part of social work activity. As already indicated, these processes aim to provide support for others and assist in the risk assessment formulation. Family attitudes, injury and the suffering of the victim or damage to property need to be properly understood if the formulation has any real or meaningful basis. Time should be set aside to read the legal documents produced for court hearings which dealt with the offending behaviour.

This period also includes the operation of any **protocols** which exist between the Medium Secure Unit (MSU) and appropriate local authority. There should be an agreement between MSU-based staff and the purchasers/providers in social services departments and district health authorities to prepare for the service user's eventual discharge. This planning takes place within the context of 'care management' which is now incorporated in the revised Care Programme Approach (DOH, *ibid*).

Pre-discharge/aftercare and follow-up

It would be unwise to differentiate the requirements for follow-up arrangements based on a person's legal status. All patients will require their own particular packages of care and agreed levels of supervision and support. For restricted patients (Sections 37/41), Mental Health Review Tribunals (MHRTs) or the Home Office will need to be satisfied that the proposed arrangements are satisfactory and afford protection for the public. These arrangements, if accepted, become part of the conditions laid down by the tribunal and, if broken, may result in a person's recall to hospital.

A person's dangerousness is seldom tested out in the psychiatric secure setting. The real test is when the person is returned to live in the community or a less secure/structured environment (Prins, 1995). Social workers (SWs) and community (forensic) psychiatric nurses (CPNs) will be the main contact between the service user and the clinic. Effective follow-up in the community will be based on the working relationship developed between SW/CPN and the service user and his/her family. Supervising social workers will need to have developed that relationship during the admission period.

Monitoring of community-based activity should be rigorously applied through direct one-to-one supervision and team supervision (Outpatient Reviews in Clinical Team Meetings), with impartial observers in attendance to note, in a detached way, significant shifts in clinical management, and to enquire, and be satisfied that, these changes are appropriate and represent safe practice.

Supervision and support of patients living in the community is a labour intensive activity which requires supervising health and social care staff to have limited and protected caseloads.

Supervision of mentally disordered offenders who have been conditionally discharged to live in the community

Social workers and probation officers may take on the role of 'social supervisors' to those patients who are subject to Section 37/41 (see above), when they have been conditionally discharged either by a Mental Health Review Tribunal or the Home Office.

Social supervisors are required to liaise with the responsible medical officer (RMO) and provide the Home Office with reports on the patient's progress whilst living in the community. The Home Office has a checklist to examine the reports submitted by the psychiatric and social supervisors. If the patient's mental state deteriorates s/he may be re-admitted informally, compulsorily (sections 2, 3 or 4) or recalled by the Home Office, which issues a warrant of arrest to be executed by the police.

Before a social worker or probation officer accepts the responsibility of being a social supervisor s/he should have information about:

- the circumstances and consequences of the index offence taken from official records: court depositions and press/media coverage

- the patient's pre-morbid personality and personal history, including education, employment, hobbies and interests

- the patient's willingness to discuss, and attitudes shown towards, the index offence

- the patient's acceptance that the index offence was committed by him/her

- the patient's participation in, and responses to, therapeutic interventions which should be clearly stated in their clinical file

■ reports from hospital-based staff about the patient's progress and his/her management

■ previous presentations of mental illness (to assist in the assessment of early warning signs)

■ whether the patient has insight into his/her mental condition

■ the family and social networks' attitudes – negative and positive; assessment of the part they might play in the management of risk

■ victim(s) perspective(s)

■ community support and likely responses from the public to the patient.

Summary

'It is government policy that mentally disordered offenders, wherever possible, should receive care and treatment from the health and social services.'
(Rees, 1991)

Since the implementation of the *Mental Health Act 1959* there has been an emphasis on caring for psychiatric patients in the community. This has remained central to government policies and planning strategies. Mentally disordered offenders who commit serious crimes have exposed some of the inadequacies of service provision. The programme of hospital closures has seriously affected the availability of effective care and support. Secure psychiatric accommodation has been provided to manage mentally disordered offenders who could not be adequately supported by local services. The prison service, however, continues to receive and imprison people with active mental illness.

Government policies have focused on the need for rigorous arrangements to ensure proper follow-up and care of seriously mentally ill people living in the community. Legislation has strengthened the

Mental Health Act 1983 to place stricter controls on patients who do not comply with treatment whilst living in the community.

Working with offenders with mental health problems requires a co-ordinated, multi-professional, interagency partnership approach. Mental health service users who commit crimes face a variety of statutory agencies whose job it is to assess and appropriately manage their situation. Where the statutory departments fail to meet the needs of mental health service users, tragedies have frequently followed.

Underpinning the work with offenders who have mental health problems is the requirement to have an effective means of risk assessment, risk formulation and risk management. Practitioners involved in this work require peer support and agency commitment to provide training and ongoing supervision to deal with typically complicated and stressful situations.

Offenders who have mental health problems do not automatically require the services of a regional forensic psychiatric service. Commonly, mental health service users who commit crimes can be managed by local provision. Their criminal behaviour might be a symptom of an external failure within the systems of community care rather than a profound failure in their own mental state.

References

Alberg, C., Hatfield, B. Huxley, P., Bowers, L., Bingley, W., Ferguson, G., Oban, A. & Maden, A. (1960) *Learning Materials on Mental Health Risk Assessment.* DOH: University of Manchester.

Birmingham, L., Mason, D. & Grubin, D. (1996) Prevalence of mental disorder in remand prison: consecutive Study. *British Medical Journal* **313** 1521–1524.

Brown, L., Christie, R. & Morris, D.(1990) *Victim Support Families of Murder Victims Project Final Report.* Liverpool: University of Liverpool, Social Studies Department.

Brown, V. A. (1995) *Psychiatric Assessment Pre and Post Admission Assessment: Forensic Focus* **8.** London: Jessica Kingsley.

CCETSW (1995) *Forensic Social Work Competence and Workforce Data* London: CCETSW.

Coid, J. (1996) Dangerous patients with mental illness: increase risk warrant new policies, adequate resources, and appropriate legislation. *British Medical Journal* **312** 965–966.

Davis, A. (1996) Risk Work and Mental Health. In: H. Kemshall and J. Pritchard (Eds) *Good Practice in Risk Assessment and Risk Management*. London: Jessica Kingsley.

Department of Health and Social Services (1978) *The Butler Report*. London: DHSS.

Social Services Inspectorate (1994) *Report of an inspection of management and provision of social work in the three special hospitals*. London: DoH.

Department of Health (1999) *Effective Care Co-ordination in Mental Health Services: Modernising the Care Programme Approach*. London: DoH.

Department of Health and Social Services (1974) Revised report of the working party in security in NHS hospitals: unpublished report.

Department of Health/Home Office (1991) The Reed Report. Review of Health and Social Services for Mentally Disordered Offenders and Others Requiring Similar Services. London: DoH.

Department of Health (1995) *Building Bridges: A guide to arrangements for interagency working for the care and protection of severely mentally ill people*. London: The Stationery Office.

Department of Health (1994) *Mental Illness – Key area handbook*. Second edition. London: The Stationery Office.

Department of Health (1994) *Guidance on the Discharge of Mentally Disordered People and their Continuing Care in the Community*. London: DoH.

Department of Health (1994) *Mental Illness – Key area handbook*. London: The Stationery Office.

Department of Health (1999) *Safer Services: National Confidential Inquiry into Suicide by People with Mental Illness*. Summary Report. London: The Stationery Office.

Department of Health (1997) Social Care Group Services for Mentally Disordered Offenders in the Community – an Inspection Report. London: DoH.

Health Service Guidelines (HSG(94)27).

Gostin, L. (Ed) (1985) *Secure Provision: A review of special services for mentally ill and mentally handicapped in England and Wales*. London: Tavistock.

Greek, J. (1997) *Occupational Therapy and Mental Health* (Second Edition). London: Churchill.

Gunn, J. & Taylor, P. (1993) *Forensic Psychiatry: Clinical, legal and ethical issues*. Oxford: Butterworth-Heinemann.

HC(90)23/LASSL(90)11 (The Care Programme Approach)

Home Office (1995) *Information for Families of Homicide Victims.* London: The Stationery Office.

Home Office (1990) *Victim's Charter: A statement of the rights of victims of crime.* Available from the Home Office.

Home Office (1990) *Provision for Mentally Disordered Offenders. Circular 66/90.* London: The Home Office.

Hudson et al (1993) *Training for Work with Mentally Disordered Offenders.* London: CCETSW.

Jones, R. (1999) *Mental Health Act Manual: 6th Edition.* London: Sweet and Maxwell.

Kemshall, H. & Pritchard, J. (1996) *Good Practice in Risk Assessment and Risk Management.* London: Jessica Kingsley.

Lart, R. (1997) *Crossing Boundaries: Accessing community mental health services for prisoners on release.* Bristol: Policy Press.

Littlechild, B. (1995) The social worker as appropriate adult. *British Journal of Social Work* **7** (2).

Mental Health Foundation (1994) *Promoting Care and Justice: Report of the Mental Health Foundation's regional conferences on improving services for mentally disordered offenders.* London: MHF.

Moore, B. (1996) *Risk Assessment: A practitioner's guide to predicting harmful behaviour.* London: Whiting and Birch.

Prins, H. (1995) *Offenders: Deviants or Patients?* Second Edition. London: Routledge.

Prins, H. (1996) Risk assessment and management in criminal justice and psychiatry. *Journal of Forensic Psychiatry.* **1** (7).

Reaside (1994) DoH/SSI Report of an Inspection of Social Work in Medium Secure Units: The Reaside Clinic. London: DoH.

Ritchie, J., Dick, D. & Lingham, R. (1994) *The Report of the Inquiry into the Care and Treatment of Christopher Clunis.* London: The Stationery Office.

Sheppard, D. (1995) *The Appropriate Adult: A review of the case law 1988.* Norfolk: The Institute of Mental Health Law 1995.

Sheppard, D. (1996) *Learning the Lessons.* Second Edition. London: Zito Trust.

Sheppard, M. (1990) *Mental health: the role of the Approved Social Worker. Social Services Monographs: Research in Practice.* University of Sheffield/Community Care.

Singleton, N. (1998) *Psychiatric Morbidity among Prisoners: Summary Report.* London: The Stationary Office.

Snowden, P. (1997) Practical aspects of clinical assessment and management. *British Journal of Psychiatry* **170** (l.32) 32–34.

Chapter 7

Mental Health Issues for People who Use Substances

Di Bailey

The dilemmas and challenges facing practitioners working with people with both mental health and substance needs are illustrated by the two cases outlined below. (The names of these individuals have been changed in order to ensure their anonymity.)

Joint assessments under the *Mental Health Act 1983* involving a GP, approved social worker (ASW) and psychiatrist were undertaken (Jones, 1996) with:

1. **Ranjit**, a 22-year-old Asian man who was taken to the Accident and Emergency department of the local hospital by his mother and father because of increasing concerns about his behaviour

and

2. **Phil**, a 17-year-old White male, adopted at the age of six months who was referred to the community mental health team because of frequent mood swings, accompanied by repeated absences from home when he would live rough on the streets of Oxford.

The assessments revealed that both of these young men presented similar difficulties, including:

- paranoid thoughts that they were being constantly watched and their behaviour reported upon

- disorientation to the extent that they were confused about days, times, where they were and events that had taken place over the past 48 hours

- reports of hearing voices commenting upon their behaviour

- expressions of agitation, anxiety and mood swings

- inappropriate laughing and sniggering to themselves as though they were engaged in some private exchange

- problems in employment due to stealing or rude behaviour, and the use of offensive language with customers with the resulting loss of jobs

- fragmenting social and familial relationships due to a combination of the above.

In an attempt to try and preserve relationships within the family, Ranjit had been sent to stay with relatives in Canada 'for a break'. On return his parents reported he was *'in a worse state than when he left'*.

Phil's parents were farm owners and had recently moved into a purpose-built barn conversion which they had financed on the farm's site. This development included a self-contained flat for Phil. Despite this arrangement Phil continued to reject his parents' attempts to help. He trashed the flat and refused to stay there, preferring to live with his 'mates' on the street.

There was evidence that both young men were abusing substances. Phil's mother had found empty syringes in the flat and Phil had admitted to recreational use of cannabis and ecstasy whilst living on the streets.

Ranjit's parents were aware that their nephew in Canada used cannabis and were concerned that their son had been smoking marijuana whilst on holiday with his cousin. Ranjit however denied that he had taken any illicit substances.

Both young men reported smoking heavily and drinking alcohol to excess on a regular basis.

The initial mental health assessments in both these cases were inconclusive. Whilst it was apparent that symptoms of mental ill health were evident, self-reports from both men were vague regarding the extent to which they were using illicit substances. This made it difficult to discern whether interventions should be targeted at the presenting psychiatric symptoms or alleged substance abuse. In both cases the psychiatrist was not convinced of an underlying mental disorder and compulsory treatment in hospital was felt to be an inappropriate option at such an early stage in the assessment process. Ranjit did however agree to stay in hospital voluntarily. It was acknowledged that this would give the professionals a chance to observe any behavioural changes in the absence of substance abuse. In contrast, Phil ended up on remand due to repeated offending. This raised some concern as to whether his mental state and possible abuse of substances would merit any further indepth investigation within the criminal justice system.

The difficulties involved in establishing a way forward with these two individuals and others like them is due to a complex interrelationship between mental health problems and substance abuse. Decisions about how to intervene are also compounded by:

- a lack of clarity in Government policy about how people with dual mental health and substance misuse needs should be treated

- issues around definitions and diagnosis

- the increased concerns around risky behaviours and their management

- lack of agreement and research about assessment and treatment methods.

This chapter explores these issues before attempting to suggest how a more comprehensive assessment may be undertaken in respect of both Ranjit and Phil and before arriving at an intervention strategy. It also looks at the ways in which staff training and integrated services may provide some opportunities for a more co-ordinated approach in the future.

Policy implications for people with mental health and substance misuse needs

To date there has been no specific Government guidance or legislation outlining how people who have both mental health and substance misuse problems should receive care and treatment. Instead, key messages must be teased out through an appraisal of existing Government policy in the domains of mental health, drug misuse and community care.

Specialist services for people misusing substances have striven to remain separate from the psychiatric services in order to avoid the labelling of their clients as mentally ill. The *Mental Health Act 1983* Section 1 (3) provides the ultimate authority for the separation of these two issues (Jones, 1996). However, according to Rorstad and Checinski (1996), these efforts have disadvantaged a group of people who have combined needs in relation to their mental health and substance misuse problems.

Rorstad and Checinski (*ibid*) argue that the introduction of the *NHS and Community Care Act 1990* and the accompanying contract culture have highlighted the gap in services for this client group for two reasons:

- Firstly, the failure of services to cope with people with a dual diagnosis is more open to scrutiny. Thus, care managers – by having to follow up the substance misuse client who has been asked to leave the residential facility for inappropriate behaviour – could discover that the client has a mental health problem. The health authority extra-contractual referral panel will then have to consider the whole range of needs presented by the client when deciding whether to fund a treatment package.

■ Secondly, the growing emphasis on the need to provide adequate care for mentally disordered offenders (MDOs) has indirectly raised the profile of people with mental health difficulties and substance misuse needs in the criminal justice system. The Reed Report (1992) calls for 'active links' to be made between services for MDOs and those for substance misusers. The SSI report (1995) also recognises the link between chronic mental ill health and alcohol and/or substance misuse in defining the mentally disordered population. Unfortunately, the report has nothing to say about joint working across the ASW/drugs work interface for this group of people, even though joint working is advocated as a way of improving services for MDOs throughout.

Recent developments in mental health policy and Government strategies to tackle drugs misuse reveal two areas where some recognition is given to people with dual needs. Firstly, through policies aimed at risk minimisation:

The *Progress Report of the National Confidential Inquiry into Suicide and Homicide by People with a Mental Illness* (1997) found that 45% of the sample were reported to have a history of mental disorder including alcohol or drug dependence and personality disorders.

HSG (94) 27: 9 contends that it is likely that an individual will present with an increased risk *'when a person who has previously offended under the influence of alcohol or drugs starts drinking again or enters and environment where drugs are commonly available'.*

The circular also highlights that *'serious mental disorder and alcohol misuse greatly increase lifetime suicide rates'.*

The *Guidance on Supervision Registers* (HSG (94) 5) allows for people to be registered if they are suffering from a severe mental illness and likely to be at significant risk. Misusing drugs or alcohol are factors seen to contribute to such risk (Department of Health, 1995).

Tackling Drugs to Build a Better Britain (Department of Health, 1998c) acknowledges that for drug misusers significant health risks *'include a wide range of psychiatric and psychological problems'*.

A number of mental health inquiry reports have also emphasised the increased risk posed to members of the public from people with combined mental health and substance misuse needs (Ward & Applin, 1998). Given the current Government emphasis on public protection (Department of Health, 1998a) it is perhaps surprising that policies have not been more prescriptive in respect of working on a day-to-day basis with this client group.

The second theme continues to make the link in respect of aftercare provision.

The *Mental Health (Patients in the Community) Act 1995* (Jones, 1996) outlines the procedures for providing Aftercare under Supervision to ensure people who are most at risk receive the aftercare package of which they are deemed in need. Whilst people have to be suffering from one of the four forms of mental disorder (mental illness, mental impairment, severe mental impairment and psychopathic disorders) (MHA, 1983), exposure to the risks of drug misuse is identified by Jones (1996) as one of the factors which would render a person at risk of being seriously exploited, and therefore eligible to be subject to the legislation.

Government guidance on the Care Programme Approach (Department of Health, 1995) – the recognised framework for providing care planning on discharge – claims that wider networks should be established between mental health and specialist drug and alcohol misuse services. The *Effectiveness Review* published in May 1995

(Stimpson *et al*) as part of the Government's Drugs Strategy
recommended that:

*'purchasers and providers should ensure that people working in both drugs and
mental illness services are aware of the need to identify and respond to problems
of combined psychiatric illness and drug misuse'.*
(paragraph 8.72)

The Department of Health (1998a) reiterates the need for integration
of health and social services as part of the modernisation framework.
This theme is echoed in respect of people with drugs and mental
health problems in *Tackling Drugs to Build a Better Britain* (*ibid*).

The call for an integrated response in terms of service delivery to
people with dual needs is a relatively recent phenomenon. Johnson
(1997) points out that traditionally there has been a preoccupation
with trying to identify the primary disorder in people presenting
symptoms of both. Such confusion seems to add to the risk that
people with combined mental health and substance misuse difficulties
will slip through the net of health and social care provision.

Goldberg *et al* (1997) point out that many people with mental health
problems experience social pressures and disadvantage and may turn
to illicit substances in an attempt to find release or to cope with such
difficulties, with addiction as the outcome of such attempts.
Alternatively, they claim it is well documented that people who use
substances such as cannabis, hallucinogenic or amphetamine type
drugs have a greater chance of developing a psychotic illness.

Dilemmas in diagnosis and definitions

Government policy is also unhelpful in clarifying which people
should be grouped together under the **'dual diagnosis'** label –
an issue which mirrors some of the policy dilemmas outlined above
and in many respects contributes to them. This lack of clarity presents

practitioners and service providers with uncertainties about which individuals are eligible for their services.

Practitioners liberally refer to people with both mental health and substance misuse needs as people with a 'dual diagnosis' which may mask some of the underlying difficulties. Evans and Sullivan (1990) define a 'dual diagnosis person' as *'an individual with both a substance abuse or dependency problem and a co-existing psychiatric disorder'*. Yet as Schmidt (1991) points out, *'dual diagnosis also refers to the fact that the problems crosscut two distinct and specialised treatment systems'*.

Indeed, Rorstad and Checinski (*ibid*) debate the accuracy of the term 'dual diagnosis' although concede that *'at the moment the "label" is a useful marker to draw attention to a real problem which is not being addressed'*. They are of the view that whilst the term is likely to be misunderstood it does *'crystallise ideas about the combination of substance misuse and severe mental illness'*.

Watkins (1997) provides a useful review of the different terminologies used to define people with dual needs such as **'multiple diagnosis'** (Read, Penick & Nickel, 1993), **'mental disorders with chemical dependency'**, (Alterman, 1985) and **'mentally ill chemical abuser'** (Cohen & Levy, 1992). However he settles for the terminology used by Ryglewicz and Pepper (1992) who use the term **'dual disorder'** and **'substance use or use/abuse'** in order to provide a broad conception of the population being referred to. Indeed, Watkins (*ibid*) points out that *'both mental illness and substance abuse disorders vary over a spectrum from mild to severe and overlap with normal behaviour'*.

In an attempt to deal with the issue of diagnostic heterogeneity, some writers have delineated different groupings of individuals under the umbrella category of the 'dually diagnosed'.

El-Guebaly (1990) outlines the four main groups of people that they agree the term alludes to:

1. people who have a primary mental illness with subsequent (including consequent) substance use (eg depressive disorder, self-treating with alcohol)

2. a primary substance misuse with psychiatric consequences (eg amphetamine-induced psychosis)

3. a dual primary diagnosis (eg LSD misuse and manic depressive illness)

4. a common aetiological factor causing mental illness and substance misuse (eg post traumatic stress disorder (PTSD) leading to both alcohol misuse and depressive disorder).

A similar breakdown is provided by Ryglewicz and Pepper (*ibid*) who identify four sub-groups within the population of people with a dual diagnosis. Their classification is much more an attempt to describe the contributory effects of each problem and to utilise the American Diagnostic Statistical Manual (DSM) classification system in an attempt to be more specific about the presenting issues for each sub-group. For example, their first sub-type includes people with a major mental illness who have intermittent psychotic episodes even without the use of drugs but more frequent and severe episodes when substances are used. The second sub-type includes people with severe personality disorders who experience psychotic episodes only under the influence of alcohol or drugs. Their third sub-type includes people whose addiction and dependency on drugs and/or alcohol may lead to *'persistent personality immaturity and dysfunction'* compared to the fourth group whose most apparent problem is drug use but who may experience problematic symptoms and behaviours during the withdrawal phase.

It is apparent that whilst all groups are in need of interventions, each would be accorded different priorities and require an approach with a slightly different focus, depending upon whether access to services was via the mental health or substance misuse route.

The issue of diagnosis is further complicated by the availability of evidence which indicates that people with severe mental health problems may be especially vulnerable to only small amounts of substances (Drake *et al*, 1998), which jeopardise their mental and emotional stability (Watkins *ibid*). Possible motivations for substance misuse also differ in people with mental health problems as would be expected within the general substance misusing population. Some people with mental health problems use substances to self-medicate against positive or negative symptoms of the disorder. Others use substances as a relief from boredom and to provide access to social groups or as a coping strategy in stressful situations, relationships and lifestyles (Johnson, 1997).

In order to begin to address some of the difficulties associated with diagnosis, it is therefore important that practitioners explore the underlying motivational factors affecting the individual as part of the initial stages in building a therapeutic relationship.

Problems related to concurrent misuse and psychosis

Why is diagnosis so difficult?

In an attempt to gain a more complex understanding of mental ill health and distress, there has been a shift away from the traditional medical model concepts of disease and illness towards an appreciation of mental disorder as a biopsychosocial condition. According to Watkins (*ibid*), chemical dependency can be understood in a similar way.

By using this conceptualisation, mental health and substance misuse workers may be in a better position to understand why people with dual diagnosis experience the problems they do, and this may be the first step towards providing an appropriate response.

For example, one explanation for the susceptibility to illicit substances mentioned above is that people with mental health problems experience biochemical changes within their brain chemistry. This can mean that even social use of drugs or alcohol can upset the biochemical imbalance even further, thereby destabilising their mental health and causing psychotic episodes. Similarly, drug users, by using alcohol and/or street drugs, risk interfering with biochemical processes and may render themselves vulnerable to more transient psychiatric problems.

People with mental health and emotional problems are also likely to experience difficulties in perception, making judgements and controlling their behaviour. They are also likely to experience social problems as a result of society's response to their mental disorder or through other forms of oppression and discrimination, such as racism and homophobia. As a consequence of these pressures, in addition to their mental distress, they are increasingly likely to be vulnerable in relationships and a range of life situations, which in turn may compound difficulties in decision-making and other psychological processes.

Because of this complex interrelationship between substance use, mental distress and behaviour, it is necessary for practitioners to be able to take account of such multi-faceted phenomena in their approach to assessment. They may also be able to offer a combination of approaches and interventions geared at tackling the problem from any number of different starting points, depending upon the concerns of the individual with whom they are working.

Practitioners need to acknowledge that people's understanding and concerns about mental illness and substance misuse will differ in the degree of stigma and fear they associate with the disorder. This will also influence the discussion between worker and service user about diagnosis and the route through which an individual is encouraged to access services.

The quest for a conclusive diagnosis is therefore hindered by factors which arise in the diagnostic process, the individual themselves and the level of understanding and expertise of the worker. There is thus a need for practitioners to consider carefully how the issue of diagnosis should be dealt with. For example, if this is merely a labelling process in order to gain access to services, are other longer term difficulties being created for the individual in terms of self-esteem and stigma by having to regard oneself as having a mental illness or as being a substance abuser? Alternatively, if the individual and their family are in need of a diagnosis in order to begin to make sense of the difficulties they are experiencing, and move forward to accept assistance from the services available, what issues might be raised if the diagnosis changes over a period of time?

Despite the difficulties in diagnosis there is a growing body of evidence that the population of people with dual needs is increasing and posing a new set of challenges for the delivery of services.

The scope of the problem

Although the estimates of the scope of the problem vary across studies due to methodological differences, Graham (1998) reviews the literature and suggests that somewhere between 10 and 65% of people in the USA with psychiatric problems, especially schizophrenia, have concurrent problems with substance abuse during their lifetime. Johnson (1997) cites similar prevalence rates of between 20 and 65%, with most recent estimates for people living in the community or attending outpatients departments standing at between 30 and 50%. (Mueser *et al*, 1990). Hein *et al* (1997), who studied a group of outpatients with either mental health or substance misuse issues, found that nearly two-thirds in each setting had a dual diagnosis.

Rates of active substance use disorder are also higher amongst certain sub-groups of the mentally disordered population. Not surprisingly, Galanter *et al* (1988) report higher rates among people with mental health problems in crisis settings such as hospitals, gaols, emergency rooms and homeless shelters.

Blowers (1998) reports that in a two-day survey of 31 inpatients, 29 had a history of drugs misuse; also that 60% of people detained under the *1983 Mental Health Act* had a similar history. Menezes *et al* (1996) found that 40% of people with alcohol abuse problems also had some form of mental illness. Similar studies show that the prevalence of substance misuse among mentally disordered offenders is also high (Barker, 1998).

This analysis accords with Minkoff and Drake (1991) who argue that *'substance use disorder is the most common comorbid complication among severely mentally ill persons'* (cited in Drake *et al*, 1998). According to Regier *et al* (1990), people with psychiatric disorders were more prone to substance use disorder than the general population. However, those with severe mental illness were especially vulnerable with lifetime prevalence rates of approximately 50%. To illustrate this point, people with schizophrenia are more than four times more likely to have a substance use disorder than a member of the general population.

Surprisingly, despite the empirical evidence to support the increase in people with a dual disorder, and the anecdotal evidence that practitioners are being increasingly exposed to people with dual diagnosis who present a particular challenge to the service (Barker, 1998), there remain significant problems of non-detection for this group.

Non-detection exists for a number of reasons and therefore needs to be tackled at different levels. Ryglewicz and Pepper (1992) emphasise that *'we are trying to address ourselves to a mixed population with various symptom profiles and with multiple causative factors'*. It is often difficult – as illustrated by the presentation of Ranjit and Phil at the start of this chapter – to determine whether the symptoms are due to substance abuse, or to an underlying mental health problem. Symptoms of depression may present like symptoms that are the secondary effects of long-term substance abuse. Alternatively, if an individual claims to be hearing voices but also admits to being intoxicated, the assumed treatment strategy may be detoxification. However, if the voice-hearing continues following detox this is an indication that the problem is perhaps more complex than initially presumed.

According to Ananth *et al* (1989), rates of undetected and under-diagnosed substance use disorders in acute psychiatric settings are as high as 98%.

In their review, Drake *et al* (*ibid*) cite factors which contribute to non-detection as:

- clinicians' lack of awareness of the high rates of substance disorders in psychiatric problems

- inattention to substance abuse as a problem

- the inadequacy of standardised assessment tools

- individuals' denial or minimisation of the problem and failure to see the relationship between their substance use and problems of adjustment and psychological impairment.

Problems with detection are also compounded by separate services for people who use substances and those who have mental health problems. For example, mental health workers often do not subscribe to the goal of abstinence that may be needed by people whose illness is exacerbated by even minor amounts of substance (Watkins, *ibid*). Conversely, staff working with drug users may be unfamiliar with contemporary approaches in mental health aimed at recovery and relapse prevention. This may lead them to the fear that people with mental health problems are always dangerous and difficult, with intractable mental disorders.

Johnson (1998) argues that workers in CMHTs may lack the training, experience and confidence to help people with addictions whilst staff in addiction services may lack confidence in working with people with a psychotic illness, particularly when active symptoms are present. As a way forward, Johnson calls for closer links between generic mental health and addiction services by facilitating cross referrals and joint discussions. She cites training in addiction interventions for all community mental health staff as one of a number of strategies to bridge the gap.

Thorley (1997) identifies co-morbidity of mental illness and substance misuse as a constant predictor of poor prognosis, often associated with poor compliance with medication, higher rates of violence, homelessness and suicidal behaviour. There is an increasing body of evidence that inadequate assessment and unco-ordinated, inappropriate treatment leads to these repeatedly poor outcomes, which absorb disproportionate resources. Other negative outcomes include increasing relapse and readmission rates (Carey & Correia, 1998), increasing use of services under emergency conditions, and increasing problems with acting-out behaviour (Watkins, *ibid*).

To begin to address some of these difficulties, the assessment undertaken by either mental health or substance misuse workers needs to be robust enough to include information relevant to both agencies and about both types of difficulties. It is to the process of assessment and intervention that this chapter now turns its attention.

Assessment and interventions

Increasingly, reference is being made in the literature to a useful distinction between the different functions of assessment (Drake *et al*, 1998; Carey & Correia, *ibid*). They argue that assessment is undertaken in order to:

- detect the existence of a problem

- provide a diagnosis

- indicate the need for a more specialised assessment to aid treatment planning.

Practitioners, managers and indeed those responsible for the training of staff would be advised to pay heed to this distinction as it can assist in reaching agreement about what level of assessment can realistically be achieved at the point of referral. It can also help to show that the process of assessment needs to be adapted when mental health and substance misuse services are operating separately, compared to where integrated services are in place with a particular focus on working with the dually diagnosed.

There have been some recent suggestions within the literature about how practitioners might set about an assessment particularly geared towards establishing the existence and extent of the problem. According to Carey and Teitelbaum (1996), assessment methods for this 'screening stage' should include a combination of:

- observation

- obtaining collateral information from friends, family members, other treatment providers and any record or reports

- biochemical tests

- self-report methods.

Used in combination, this approach increases the likelihood of a realistic assessment, which can assist in determining the next steps with regard to diagnosis, further specialist assessment and intervention.

However, in using these methods there are certain findings to bear in mind.

The value of collateral information varies depending upon the degree of contact with the client and the confidence in the accuracy of the information being provided. Some people with severe mental health difficulties may not have reliable collateral informants due to the fragmentation of their social networks and relationships.

Self-report methods tend to provide an under-representation of substance use, especially in the acute crisis phase or in psychiatric hospitals. Yet stable outpatients can provide quite reliable and valid reports of their drinking behaviour.

Whilst biological tests, such as urine screening for drugs, may increase the accuracy of individuals' self-reports of drug use, they only provide a limited indication of the amount and frequency of drug use (Drake *et al*, 1998). Tests for alcohol consumption, such as analyses of blood chemistry and breathalysers, are less satisfactory than urine analyses for substances, again due to the short time-intervals during which detection can occur and only moderate sensitivity. Cox and Crifasi (1990) advocate using a simple, inexpensive saliva test to detect the presence of alcohol. Any biological test should also be consolidated by a full medical history and examination.

In terms of a more specialised assessment which attempts to explore the interrelatedness of mental health problems and substance abuse disorder, there are now an increasing number of assessment tools available to practitioners which utilise the different sources of information outlined above. These include the Alcohol Use Scale (AUS) and the Drug Use Scale (DUS), both of which are 5 point scales which incorporate ratings by clinicians (Drake, Meuser & McHugo, 1996).

Self-report methods include the CAGE (Teitelbaum, 1998) which, according to Carey and Correia (1998), has shown adequate criterion validity in predicting relevant substance use disorders. Recently, a new screening tool – the only one specifically designed to identify substance use disorder in people hospitalised for mental health problems – has been designed by Rosenberg *et al* (1998). This is called the Dartmouth Assessment of Life Instrument or DALI, and although it relies on self-reporting, it is administered by an interviewer. Early reports indicate it is more reliable over time and across interviewers than other tools such as the CAGE.

Once the assessment is underway, the issue of how to intervene becomes increasingly important. The innovative services developed for people with dual disorders in the USA revolve around philosophies and approaches that regard the maintenance and continuity of care as pivotal to the intervention process. Treatment approaches are integrated for people with severe mental health problems and addictions and are delivered by the same team (Drake *et al*, 1993).

It is well accepted that there are stages within the intervention process which really begin with the engagement stage where the objective is to establish a *'helping relationship'* or *'treatment alliance'*. This is often referred to as the **persuasion phase** where individuals are encouraged to begin to understand the relationship between substance use and problems in daily living, including mental distress.

Intensive case management promotes the continuity of care and often combines techniques for dealing with addiction and the management of the symptoms of mental distress. This approach also includes relapse prevention, psycho-education (individual or group) and motivational interviewing. The philosophy of intervention revolves around 'gentle confrontation' and frequent relapses do not result in rejection from the service. In addition, as part of the case management role, attention is paid to basic needs such as housing and finances, and to developing activities and networks which involve community-based services rather than specialist substance abuse or mental health services (Johnson, 1997). A model of integrated treatment is provided by Drake *et al* (1998), accompanied by a more in-depth review of the research into the effectiveness of such approaches.

Implications for training and service development

One of the difficulties in achieving an integrated response to intervention that has already been referred to is the lack of interprofessional training for mental health and drugs workers, where a shared understanding and approach to people with dual disorders can be consolidated. In the UK, integrated services are still the exception rather than the rule, which makes a co-ordinated approach to assessment and intervention difficult to achieve, especially in the absence of joint training initiatives.

According to Lucas (1996):

'In localities where there is good communication and information exchange between workers and agencies users always get a better service...' as *'...resources are not wasted on duplication...'* and *'...skills and resources are harnessed to the same, or at least similar outcomes'.*

An opportunity to promote joint training is suggested by current Government policy that locates the training and development of staff as a key building block in the modernisation agenda.

Significant financial resources are earmarked for investment in the training of psychiatrists, mental health nurses and other clinical and care staff (para 5.5:5). The focus of this investment is specifically to support service developments such as Assertive Outreach and 24-hour crisis support. Indeed, the Health Service *Guidance on the Modernisation Fund and Mental Health Grant* (MHG) (1999) calls for health authorities to focus on the skills necessary to deliver *'Assertive Outreach and engage with patients and service users, particularly those with a dual diagnosis'* (para 14 (ii):6).

A similar theme of improving the extent of training in the drugs field is found in *Tackling Drugs Together* (1995) although the specific need for mental health training for drugs workers remains unmentioned. Nevertheless, the recognition of training and staff development as a way forward is echoed by the professional context with priority given to staff development (Department of Health, 1998b) linked to improved performance and quality standards. This will be achieved through the setting up of the General Social Care Council (GSCC) (Department of Health, 1998b: para 5.6) with the National Training Organisation (*ibid*: para 5.34) responsible for the development and promotion of training at all levels linked to occupational standards.

To support these developments an extra £19.7 million is to be allocated through the Training Support Programme (TSP) 1999/2000 (LAC (99) 10) which continues to accord ASW training a priority for TSP spend. Training in relation to drug and alcohol misuse is also mentioned (*ibid*: para 20:15).

Increasingly, post-registration training is having to shape up to the needs of employers who require workers to be *'fit to undertake the duties for which they are being trained'* (Borland & James, 1999).

Unfortunately, the lack of explicit direction regarding dual diagnosis, in both the political and professional contexts, is paralleled by the lack of a competence framework for staff practising in this area. However, several frameworks do exist in relation to mental health practice; these include:

- ASW competencies and performance criteria (CCETSW paper 19.19, revised 1993)

- *Forensic Social Work Competencies* (CCETSW, 1995)

- core competencies for specialist staff working with adults with severe mental illness (Sainsbury Centre for Mental Health, 1997).

All of these frameworks embrace the skills, knowledge and attitudes relevant to working with people with dual diagnosis needs, such as the ability to collect and interpret information from a variety of sources at the point of assessment, and to be able to intervene in situations where risk is a feature.

The current developments in respect of education and training thereby pose a challenge to both employers and training providers to look creatively at the opportunities for developing an integrated training response for both mental health and drugs workers. In the interim phase, before such training programmes are developed, the implications for practice are that it will largely depend upon the efforts of individual practitioners involved as to the degree to which co-ordinated response is adopted with people like Ranjit and Phil who have dual needs, as outlined at the start of this chapter.

Implications for practice

Given the dilemmas and difficulties highlighted above, it is not surprising that the initial assessments with Ranjit and Phil provided only a limited understanding of their difficulties. In accordance with the functions of assessment outlined earlier, the professionals involved were able to detect the existence of a problem but were unable to move towards agreeing a diagnosis. Indeed, a much longer period of ongoing specialised assessment is necessary before any decisions can be made about intervention. Drawing upon the literature reviewed during this chapter and a model for integrating a cognitive behavioural approach with this client group (Graham, 1998), the chapter now concludes by making some suggestions as to how an integrated approach with both Phil and Ranjit could be pursued in an endeavour to maximise the chances of a positive outcome in each of their situations.

Assessment

Any worker–client relationship which commences with a formalised assessment under the mental health legislation runs the risk of hindering the engagement process because of the power dimension associated with statutory involvement. Whilst the initial assessment conducted under the *Act* would serve the purpose of gathering together relevant information from the two men themselves, their families and other professionals, it could do little to promote engagement and harness motivation for change, mainly because of the legal constraints which come into play. On a positive note, neither Phil nor Ranjit were subject to a compulsory admission which increases the likelihood of their co-operation in a longer ongoing period of assessment which should be tailored to relationship-building and encouraging them to think about changing their behaviour.

In addition to this, whilst the initial assessment conducted was a joint assessment as defined by the *MHA Code of Practice 1983* (Jones, 1996), a crucial perspective from a specialist drugs worker was missing. This then raises the issue of how the ongoing assessment should be conducted and who should be involved. In the absence of an integrated service with workers trained in both mental health and substance abuse, the continuing assessment is likely to require joint involvement from both the ASW and a worker from the substance misuse field.

Further information is required, which may not be forthcoming until the engagement process is underway, in terms of more detail about the substance use behaviours of both men including:

- the types of substance used

- their reasoning behind their use

- any problems resulting from it.

More needs to be known about the mental disorder component, particularly the signs and symptoms they experience and their own understanding of any links between the two areas of difficulty. Of particular significance with Ranjit is the role that cultural factors will play in his acceptance and understanding of mental disorder and substance abuse. Only when information is available relating to both aspects of the disorder can an assessment of risk be undertaken, both in terms of the risky behaviours and their consequences for both men and also in terms of the coping or safety strategies which Ranjit and Paul are able to implement to lessen the chances of these risky behaviours occurring (see **Chapter 9**).

Continued information-gathering will rely heavily on Ranjit and Phil's self-reports of their thought processes, behaviour and experiences. It will need to be consolidated with collateral information from other sources wherever possible – in Ranjit's case, from staff at the hospital where he was a voluntary patient; for Phil, workers in the criminal justice system may be able to offer useful insights into his presenting difficulties.

Assessment tools such as the CAGE should be used to supplement any information obtained, and the use of the DALI should be considered for Ranjit if his stay in hospital confirms the presence of mental health problems. Consideration must also be given to the use of biological tests mentioned earlier in this chapter, if the information obtained about substance misuse conflicts and requires further validation.

Care planning

Once the assessment process has achieved the initial objectives of engagement and information-collection, a decision needs to be taken in respect of continued care planning. Whilst the Care Programme Approach (CPA) (see **Chapter 8**) is not a recognised vehicle for care planning in the drugs field, consideration should be given to its implementation in these two cases, especially if it is apparent that both mental health and substance misuse difficulties are evident.

By adopting the CPA with both Phil and Ranjit, the chances of a co-ordinated approach to care planning across the mental health–drugs interface are increased. Discussions will need to take place involving the service providers, and indeed Ranjit and Phil as receivers of the service, as to who is the most appropriate person to undertake the role of keyworker, and co-ordinate the delivery of care.

Intervention

As part of the care planning process, whether formalised under the CPA or not, a decision will need to be reached as to the intervention strategy to be adopted with both Phil and Ranjit, and will depend to some extent on whether they are institutionalised or living in the community at the time the intervention strategy is implemented.

The model outlined earlier in this chapter is routed in an integrated intensive case-management service designed specifically for people with dual disorders. In the absence of such a service an intervention which draws upon cognitive behavioural techniques in addition to the use of medication is likely to be the preferred option. If this is to be provided as part of each individual's care plan, it is important that the role of the care co-ordinator providing practical support and advice – in relation to finance, housing and day time activities – is kept distinct from the role of the worker, and focuses specifically upon the cognitive behavioural intervention. The skills of the workers involved will depend upon whether one worker undertakes both tasks, or whether these are shared between the mental health and drugs workers. This choice may also hinge upon whether the focus of the intervention is targeted primarily at the management of signs and symptoms of mental distress or the substance abuse.

Irrespective of the primary focus, the ultimate objectives of the Cognitive Behavioural Approach will be to:

- enable Phil and Ranjit to understand the mediating role of dysfunctional beliefs about their substance abuse and psychotic symptoms

- identify alternative beliefs and coping strategies.

In order to meet these objectives the following areas will form the focus of the interventions (adapted from Graham's model, 1998).

(a) identifying beliefs surrounding substance abuse and mental distress, testing these beliefs and identifying alternatives

(b) exploring and developing strategies for the prevention and management of relapse including issues of compliance with any prescribed neuroleptic medication

(c) monitoring symptoms and substance use particularly in relation to the early signs of mental disorder and the links with substances used

(d) giving psycho-educational information, either individually or in the context of family work, covering both areas of mental disorder and substance abuse

(e) developing strategies to improve self-esteem and non drug-related activities

Delivering this programme of intervention is likely to occur at a slow pace, taking a long-term perspective. In the case of both Ranjit and Phil it is unlikely that there will be a 'quick fix' to their difficulties; rather they will require a response from both mental health and substance abuse services over a prolonged period of time.

Conclusion

Given the separateness of services for people with mental health needs and those for people with drugs and alcohol problems, there is a danger that services will compound the problems for people like Ranjit and Phil, exacerbating their mental distress and increasing the likelihood that their dependence on substances will remain an integral coping strategy.

Attempts are needed to develop an integrated response from services that build upon a common biopsychosocial model of understanding both mental distress and substance misuse; one that also capitalises on systems already in existence for improved communication, assessment and care planning.

Such an approach will optimise the chance of services dealing with interrelatedness of needs for people with both mental health and substance misuse issues and only then will outcomes begin to improve for people like Ranjit and Phil.

References

Ananth, J., Vanderwater, S., Kamal, M., Broksky, A., Gamal, R. & Miller, M. (1989) Missed diagnosis of substance abuse in psychiatric patients. *Hospital and Community Psychiatry* 4 297–299.

Alterman, A. I. (Ed) (1985) *Substance Abuse and Psychopharmacology.* New York: Plenum Press. Cited in: T. R. Watkins (1997) Mental Health Services to

Substance Abusers. In: T. R. Watkins and J. W. Callicutt (Eds) (1997) *Mental Health Policy and Practice Today*. California: Sage.

Barker, I. (1998) Mental illness and substance misuse. *Mental Health Review* **3** (4).

Bartholomew, A., Davis, J. & Weinstein, J. (1996) *Interprofessional Education and Training: Developing new models*. London: CCETSW.

Blowers, A. J. (1998) Drugs and mental health. *Mental Health Review* **3** (4).

Borland, J. & James, S. (1999) The learning experience of students with disabilities in higher education: a case study of a UK university. *Disability & Society* **14** (1) 85–101.

Carey, K. B. & Correia, C. J. (1998) Severe mental illness and addictions assessment considerations. *Addictive Behaviours* **23** (6) 735–748.

Carey, K. B. & Teitelbaum, L. M. (1996) Goals and methods of alcohol assessment. *Professional Psychology: Research and practice* **27** 460–466.

CCETSW (1993) Requirements and Guidance for the Training of Social Workers to be considered for approval in England and Wales under the *Mental Health Act 1983* (Paper 19:19 revised). London: CCETSW

CCETSW (1997) *Assuring Quality for Post Qualifying Education and Training-1. Requirements for the post qualifying and advanced awards in Social Work*. London: CCETSW.

Cohen, J. & Levy, S. J. (1992) *The Mentally Ill Chemical Abuser: Whose client?* Lexington: Lexington Books.

Cox, R. A. & Crifasi, J. A. (1990) A comparison of a commercial micro-diffusion method and gas chromatography of ethanol analysis. *Journal of Analytic Toxicology* **14** 211–212. Cited in: R. E. Drake, S. D. Rosenberg and K. T. Mueser (1998) Assessing Substance Use Disorder in Persons with Severe Mental Illness. In: R. E. Drake, C. Mercer-McFadden, G. McHugo, K. Mueser, S. Rosenberg, R. Clark and M. Brunette (Eds) (1998) *Readings in Dual Diagnosis*. Columbia.

Department of Health (1994) *Introduction of Supervision Registers for Mentally Ill People from 1 April 1994 HSG (94)5*. London: Department of Health.

Department of Health (1994) *Guidance on the Discharge of Mentally Disordered People and their Continuing Care in the Community*. London: DoH.

Department of Health (1995) *Health of the Nation: Building Bridges: A guide to the arrangements for interagency working for the care and protection of severely mentally ill people*. London: DoH.

Department of Health (1997) The Progress Report of the National Confidential Inquiry into Suicide and Homicide by People with Mental Illness. In: NACRO (1998) *Risks and Rights: Mentally disturbed offenders and public protection.* London: NACRO.
Department of Health (1998a) *Modernising Mental Health Services: Safe, sound, supportive.* London: The Stationery Office.

Department of Health (1998b) *Modernising Social Services: Promoting independence, improving protection, raising standards.* Cm 4169. London: DoH.

Department of Health (1995) *Tackling Drugs Together: A strategy for England 1995–1998.* London: HMSO

Department of Health (1998c) *Tackling Drugs to Build a Better Britain: The Government's 10-Year strategy for tackling drug misuse. Cm 3945.* London: The Stationery Office.

Department of Health (1999) *Modernising Mental Health Services: NHS Modernisation fund for mental health services & Mental Health Grant 1999/2002 HSC 1999/038: LAC (99)8.* London: DoH.

Department of Health (1999) *Social Services Training Support Programme. LAC (99)10* London: DoH.

Drake, R. E., Mueser, K. T. & McHugo, G, J. (1996) *Using Clinician Rating Scales to Assess Substance Abuse Among Persons with Severe Mental Disorders.* Cited in: R. E. Drake, S. D. Rosenberg and K. T. Mueser (1998a) Assessing Substance Use Disorder in Persons with Severe Mental Illness. In: Drake *et al,* 1998. Columbia MD International Association of Psychosocial Rehabilitation Services.

Drake, R. E. Rosenberg, S. D & Mueser, K. T. (1998) Assessing Substance Use Disorder in Persons with Severe Mental Illness. In: R. E. Drake, C. Mercer-McFadden, G. McHugo, K. Meuser, S. Rosenberg, R. Clark and M. Brunette (Eds) (1998) *Readings in Dual Diagnosis.* Columbia.

Drake, R. E., Mercer-McFadden, C. Mueser, K.T., McHugo, G. J. & Bond, G. R. (1998b) Review of integrated mental health and substance abuse treatment for patients with dual disorders. *Schizophrenia Bulletin* **24** (4) 589–608.

El-Guebaly, N. (1990) Substance abuse and mental disorders: the dual diagnosis concept. *Canadian Journal of Psychiatry* **35** 261–267. Cited in: P. Rorstad & K. Checinski (1996) *Dual Diagnosis: Facing the Challenge The Care of People with a Dual Diagnosis of Mental Illness and Substance Misuse.* Guildford: Wynne Howard Publishing.

Evans, K. & Sullivan, J. M. (1990) *Dual Diagnosis: Counselling the mentally ill substance abuser.* New York: Guilford Press.

Galanter, M. Casteneda, R. & Ferman, J. (1988) Substance abuse among general psychiatric patients. *American Journal of Drugs and Alcohol Abuse* **14** 211–235.

Goldberg, D., Benjamin, S. & Creed, F. (1995) *Psychiatry in Medical Practice.* London: Routledge.

Graham, H. L. (1998) The role of dysfunctional beliefs in individuals who experience psychosis and use substances: implications for cognitive therapy and medication compliance. *Behavioural and Cognitive Psychotherapy* **26** 193–208.

Hein, D., Zimberg, S., Weisman, S., First, M., Ackerman, S. (1997) Dual diagnosis sub types in urban substance abuse and mental health clinics. *Psychiatric Services* **48** (8) 1058–1063.

Johnson, S. (1998) The implications of dual diagnosis for service provision. *Mental Health Review* **3** (4).

Johnson, S. (1997) Dual diagnosis of severe mental illness and substance misuse: a case for specialist services? *British Journal of Psychiatry* **171** 205–208.

Jones, R. (1996) *The Mental Health Act Manual.* (Fifth Edition.) London: Sweet and Maxwell.

Lucas, J. (1996) Multidisciplinary Care in the Community for Clients with Mental Health Problems: Guidelines for the Future. In: M. Watkins, N. Hervey, J. Carson and S. Ritter (Eds) *Collaborative Community Mental Health Care.* London: Arnold.

Mental Health (Patients in the Community) Act 1995.

Mercer, C. C. Mueser, K. T. & Drake, R. E. (1998) Organisational guidelines for dual disorders programmes. *Psychiatric Quarterly* **69** (3) 145–168.

Menezes, P. R., Johnson, S., Thornicroft, G., Marshall, J., Prosser, D., Bebbington, P. & Kuipers, E. (1996) Drug and alcohol problems among individuals with severe mental illness in South London. *British Journal of Psychiatry* **168** 612–619.

Minkoff, K. & Drake, R. E. (Eds) (1991) Dual Diagnosis of Major Mental Illness and Substance Disorder. Cited in: Drake *et al* (1998) *op cit.*

Mueser, K. T., Yarnold, P. R. & Levinson, D. F. (1990) Prevalence of substance abuse in schizophrenia. demographic and clinical correlates. *Schizophrenia Bulletin* **16** 31–56.

NHS and Community Care Act (1990)

Read, M. R., Penick, E. C. & Nickel, E. J. (1993) *Treatment for Dually Diagnosed Clients*. Cited in: T. R. Watkins (1997) *op cit.*

Reed, J. (1992) *A Review of Health and Social Services for Mentally Disordered Offenders and Others Requiring Similar Services*. London: HMSO.
Regier, D. A. Farmer, M. E. Rae, D. S. Locke, B. Z. Keith, S. J., Judd, L. L. & Goodwin, F. K. (1990) Co-morbidity of mental disorders with alcohol and other drug abuse. *Journal of the American Medical Association* **264** 2511–2518.

Rosenberg, S. D., Drake R. E., Wolford, G. L., Mueser, K. T., Oxman, T. E., Vidaver, R.,M., Carrieri, K. L. & Luckoor, R. (1998) Dartmouth assessment of lifestyle instrument DALI: a substance use disorder screen for people with severe mental illness. *American Journal of Psychiatry* **155** 232–238.

Rorstad, P. & Checinski, K. (1996) *Dual Diagnosis: Facing the Challenge: The care of people with a dual diagnosis of mental illness and substance misuse*. Guildford: Wynne Howard.

Ryglewicz, H. & Pepper, B. (1992) The Dual-disorder Client: Mental Disorder and Substance Use. In: S. Cooper & T. H. Lentner (Eds) *Innovations in Community Mental Health*. Sarasota: Professional Resource Press.

Sainsbury Centre for Mental Health (1997) *Pulling Together: The future roles and training of mental health staff*. London: Sainsbury Centre for Mental Health.

Schmidt, L. (1991) Specialisation in alcoholism and mental health residential treatment: the dual diagnosis problem. *Journal of Drug Issues* **21** 859–874.

Social Services Inspectorate (1995) *Mentally Disordered Offenders: Improving Services*. London: Department of Health.

Stake, R. E. (1995) *The Art of Case Study Research*. London: Sage.

Stimpson, G., Hayden, D., Hunter, G., Metrebian, N., Rhodes, T., Turnbull, P. & Ward, J. (1995) *Drug Users Help Seeking and Views of Services*. Centre for Research on Drugs and Health Behaviour.

Teitelbaum, L. M. (1998) *Reliability of Self-Reported Alcohol Use in Psychotic Settings*. Syracuse University, Unpublished Doctoral Thesis.

Thorley, A. (1997) Dual Diagnosis: The Challenge of Comorbid Psychiatric Disorder and Substance Misuse. Cited in: I. Barker (1998) *op cit.*

Ward, M. & Applin, C. (1998) *The Unlearned Lesson: The role of alcohol and drug use perpetrated by people with mental health problems*. London: Wynne Howard.

Watkins, T. R. (1997) Mental Health Services to Substance Abusers. In: T. R. Watkins and J. W. Callicutt (Eds) (1997) *Mental Health Policy and Practice Today*. California: Sage.

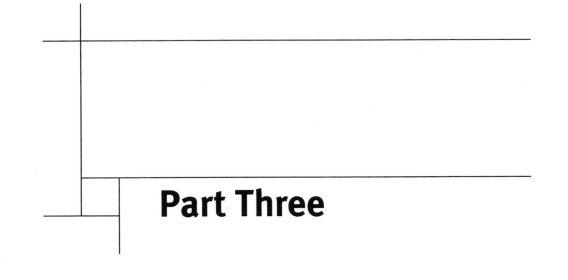

Part Three

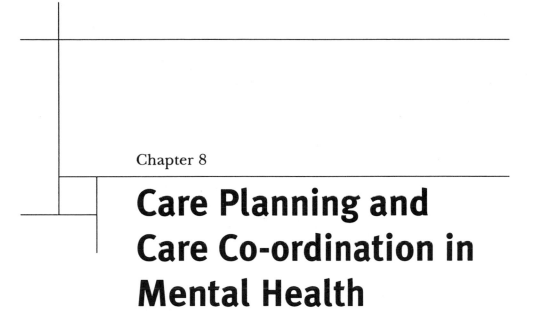

Chapter 8

Care Planning and Care Co-ordination in Mental Health

Di Bailey

Introduction

The concept of care planning in the field of mental health continues to present a range of difficulties to practitioners for whom this should be the 'bread and butter' of everyday practice. The same old questions keep being asked over and over again as practitioners strive to make sense of a framework for care delivery that in principle they support but in practice struggle to implement. Such questions include:

- How does the Care Programme Approach fit with care management?

- How does my role as a care co-ordinator link to the role of the care manager?

- Am I individually accountable if the care plan goes wrong?

- How does the Care Programme Approach fit with mental health legislation in respect of aftercare?

...and the list goes on.

The recent launch of the *National Service Framework* (Department of Health, 1999) re-emphasises that despite these difficulties, the Care Programme Approach (CPA) will remain the vehicle for ensuring that people with severe mental health problems receive the care they need in a co-ordinated and planned way.

In an attempt to help service providers and practitioners to continue to implement the Framework, standards are at last set for providing written care plans alongside a requirement that specific arrangements be put in place to integrate care management and the CPA (*ibid*). For people on a CPA there is now also a formal recommendation that individuals who provide care for these people should have an assessment and written care plan to reflect their own needs as a care giver (*ibid*).

This chapter will attempt to provide some practical suggestions as to how practitioners can rise to the challenges of implementing the CPA effectively. It will describe the framework for the CPA – what it is and also, importantly, what it is not. Discussion will follow about how it can be linked with care management and the role of the care 'co-ordinator' – a term which has replaced that of keyworker in the *National Service Framework*. A flow chart will be introduced, which has been tried and tested by the author on a number of mental health training programmes; this chart depicts diagrammatically the integration of the care planning process and the mental health legislative framework. Feedback from recipients indicates that the flow chart has been helpful in clarifying the interconnections. Finally, the process of formulating a care plan will be described, outlining what might be covered as part of the assessment, and the design of the plan itself, including how to write objectives and to measure outcomes.

I make no apology for having several key messages to communicate when it comes to care planning. These will become apparent from the text and are intended to reflect best practice. They stem from my own experience in receiving numerous incomplete care plans and my attempts to redress the balance by basing my own practice around a set of guiding principles.

The historical development of care planning

Community care for people with mental health problems is not a new concept. Originally introduced by the *Mental Treatment Act 1930* (Rogers & Pilgrim, 1996) it was supported by the developments in neuroleptic medication in the 1950s which meant that people did not need to be in hospital to receive care and treatment for mental disorder. As a consequence, the old institutions built of bricks and mortar have been gradually replaced by the institution of care planning which is constructed using documentation, processes and systems.

One of the difficulties in making sense of the care planning framework is that two developments which emerged from this new paperwork and systems 'institution', occurred relatively close together. This left those key agencies involved in the purchasing and commissioning of mental health services somewhat bemused about which system they should implement and how to do it most effectively.

In 1988 the *Griffith Report's* Community Care Agenda for action expounded the principle that *'community care should be directed towards obtaining the best quality of life possible for people leaving hospital'* (Rogers & Pilgrim, *ibid*). The notion that people who use services should have a choice in the type, range and level of services they use was placed firmly on the agenda. The ideas of users as consumers and a market place of services were born (Social Services Inspectorate, 1991).

In 1990 the *NHS and Community Care Act* was introduced in an attempt to translate the principles of the Griffith's Report into statutory care planning for all potential users of services.

The key effects of this piece of legislation were:

■ the separating of the commissioning function (in some authorities referred to as the purchasing, contracting or assessing function) and the providing function in service delivery

■ the demise of generic social work which was replaced by specialisation within social work departments where social workers were divided into adult teams to deal specifically with the implications of the Act. Children's teams were set up specifically to deal with the *Children Act 1989*. This occurred in response to the local authority becoming the lead agency implementing changes in respect of the community care legislation

■ the focus on 'needs led' as opposed to 'service led' assessments with subsequent care plans being drawn up in full consultation with service users and their family

■ the setting up of independent inspection units and complaints procedures.

The general thrust of the legislation was to make providers of services more accountable for delivering better quality care. This was based upon the premise that the market place of community care would provide a wide range of services which could be selected in order to match identified needs more appropriately. Underpinning service delivery was a value base that emphasised the rights of citizenship, independence, privacy, dignity and choice for service users in pursuing the realisation of their aspirations and abilities (Social Services Inspectorate, *ibid*).

Local authorities were required to publish information on services available, and the eligibility criteria were used to target services at those most in need.

Translated into practice, the legislation gave rise to the role of **care manager** with responsibility for assessing individuals' care needs and drawing up a care plan to meet those needs **in consultation with the service users and their family/carers.**

The care manager would then commission the services to meet the needs and, in some authorities, hold the budget to pay for these services.

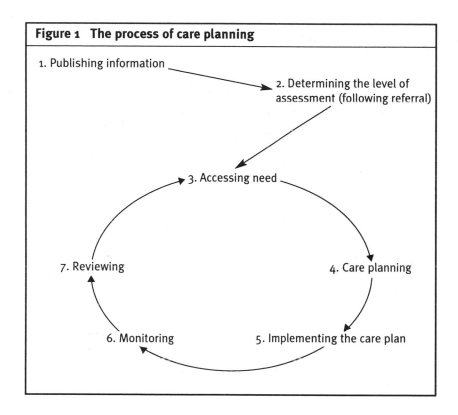

Figure 1   The process of care planning

1. Publishing information

2. Determining the level of assessment (following referral)

3. Accessing need

4. Care planning

5. Implementing the care plan

6. Monitoring

7. Reviewing

The final stages in the process would be to review and monitor the care plan – including service input – on a regular basis to ascertain whether the needs remained the same and whether the services provided were still in a position to meet them (Social Services Inspectorate, *ibid*).

At the time of its inception it was suggested that this process constituted a major shift in ways of thinking and working with people in the community. However, for those of us who had been involved with hospital social work and discharge planning since the early 80s, this framework did little more than formalise what was already being promoted as best practice.

The legislation did not specifically relate to people with mental health problems and the NHS retained the responsibility for community mental health services.

Shortly after this major piece of legislation, in 1991, the Department of Health introduced the Care Programme Approach in the form of circular HC 90(23)/LASSL (90) 11. An American import, it was originally intended as a screening system to prevent people with severe mental health problems falling through the net of psychiatric care. In the early days of its inception the consultant psychiatrist decided which individuals were 'suitable' for the CPA, usually at the point of discharge planning.

According to Shepperd *et al* (1995) both the CPA and care management were variants of the *'case management interventions which appeared in the United States some 15–20 years earlier'*. In the UK, the introduction of Government guidance in relation to CPA was patchy (Audit Commission, 1994) especially in the wake of a care management process couched in legislation as opposed to guidance. The fact that these two policy imperatives came close together raised dilemmas between health and social services staff as to how they were working jointly with people with mental health problems, as the two approaches reflected the different responsibilities being placed on the host agencies (Shepperd *et al, ibid*).

In the early days of the CPA, most people with mental health disabilities who moved from hospital to residential or nursing home care probably did so through the care management framework. Whilst this was perhaps a more structured approach to acquiring the services of which they were deemed in need (and the financial support to pay for them) it is probably one of the factors that has contributed to the lack of integration of the two approaches.

Because the original response to the CPA was so patchy (Social Services Inspectorate, 1995; Audit Commission, 1994) the Government of the 1990s introduced a number of initiatives to encourage mental health providers and practitioners to apply the CPA framework to any individual in contact with the psychiatric services at *any* stage, not purely on the point of discharge (Department of Health, 1995b).

These persuasive approaches came in the form of the *Health of the Nation Mental Illness – Key area handbook* (1994) and *Building Bridges* (1995). The message was that the CPA was an approach, a process. Whilst the Government was willing to leave the details of its implementation locally to mental health purchasers and local authorities, the essence of the process was as follows:

- Everyone in contact with the specialist psychiatric services should have a systematic assessment of their health and social care needs.

- A care plan should be drawn up in consultation with the individual and their family/carers and also with members of the multidisciplinary team, including care managers and GPs.

- A keyworker should be nominated who would keep in close contact with the service user and their family and co-ordinate the contributions to the care plan.

- There would be a regular review and monitoring of the care plan to assess and respond in an ongoing way to any changes in need or circumstances.

The subsequent Government circular focusing on discharge (HSG [94] 27) required that, prior to discharge, each individual must have a thorough multidisciplinary assessment put together by those responsible for their care in hospital and those taking on the responsibility in the community. It also introduced the notion that some individuals would need a more complex care plan than others, and terms like 'simple' and 'complex' or 'full' and 'minimal' CPA began to be bandied about. The desirable outcomes from a CPA were identified by the CPA Training Pack produced jointly by the Open University and the Department of Health (1996). They were detailed as follows:

- All needs for health and social care will be identified by competent assessors.

- Needs will be addressed through a well designed care plan agreeable to clients and carers which co-ordinates the service involves.

- Someone will take responsibility for co-ordinating care planning and care delivery.

- The client and carer will know who to contact as their keyworker.

- Someone will be responsible for convening reviews.

The success of the care plan and the changing needs of the client will be reviewed, and plans amended as necessary.

If the Care Planning process was effectively implemented, all of these elements should be in place, clearly documented and communicated to all parties involved.

These repeated attempts to provide guidance and clarity on the CPA as a recognised framework for care planning have recently been consolidated through the *National Service Framework*.

The two levels of CPA are now clearly delineated (*ibid*, 53) in addition to the areas of care that should be covered by the care plan. Whilst it is unfortunate that it has taken eight years for the Government to be more prescriptive about the approach, this level of detail can only be helpful to practitioners and must surely maximise the chances of the CPA being implemented in a more systematic way, nationally, in the future.

One of the common misconceptions about the CPA that has unfortunately been translated into practice is the misinformed belief that it only applies to people at the point of discharge. Over the years the guidance has attempted to make it clear that the CPA is the care planning framework for anyone in contact with the specialist psychiatric services at any stage.

Unfortunately, the *National Service Framework* does not help in clearing up this ambiguity as whilst it states that *'all mental health service users on CPA should .... have a written care plan'* it does not reiterate that access to the CPA is synonymous with access to specialist mental health services. It also states that those users *'who are assessed as requiring a period of care away from their home should have a copy of a written aftercare plan agreed on discharge'*. So what of the person whose contact is made at the point of admission – is the CPA ruled out? The answer should obviously be 'of course not'. The author would argue that the assessment at the point of admission should be delivered as part of the CPA framework focusing upon the health and social care needs of the individual alongside an assessment of risk and safety behaviours.

Following on from the assessment it may be decided that the needs identified can only be met in a hospital setting, either as an informal patient whereby the individual accepts the need to receive their care and treatment in this way, or on a formal basis where a Compulsory Order is used. Irrespective of the legal status of the individual, part of the care planning process is to identify the best place to provide the care. At this juncture, what nursing and hospital staff require from the assessment is information about the individual's needs so that they can begin to meet them. These can then be met on an inpatient basis. This is a specific example of the CPA where the subsequent care plan is delivered within the hospital setting.

For the duration of the process there should be someone specifically allocated to co-ordinate the care. In this instance it is likely to be either the named nurse on the ward who will be responsible for co-ordinating the hospital input, or the responsible medical officer (RMO).

A review should be held in readiness for discharge to reassess the needs, which, by this time, should be met in the community or through a combination of community/hospital-based care. The role of care co-ordinator will now sit more easily with a member of staff from the community team and can be transferred as a result of the review meeting. Effectively, the elements of the CPA remain the same – it is just the location of the care plan delivery that is different.

Thinking about the CPA in this way seems logical, given that in recent times with the emergence of home treatment and Assertive Outreach teams, care and treatment for people with severe and enduring mental health problems is more likely to take place in the community. These developments will increasingly render 'artificial' the separation of hospital and community services, and for this reason the operation of the CPA must be sufficiently portable to deliver a care plan which embraces a range of settings, workers and services.

Links with care management

Thus far the links between care management and the CPA have been identified in terms of the evolution of the *NHS and Community Care Act* and Government guidance on CPA in the form of HC (90) 23/LASSL (90) 11.

Since the introduction of the two approaches, parallels have become evident in terms of the level of care planning people were deemed to need. Hence there has been a large degree of overlap between 'simple' assessments for care management and 'simple' or 'minimal' CPA. Likewise, at the other end of the spectrum, those receiving 'complex' or 'full' CPA were also likely to be considered 'complex' care management cases by the local authority (Newton, *et al* 1996).

Table 1 (above) depicts the differences and similarities between the CPA and care management.

Table 1 A comparison of the CPA and Care Management Frameworks for Care Planning

CPA	Care management
■ Department of Health Guidance HC(90)23 plus *Building Bridges*	■ Legislation NHS plus CCA 1990
■ Patient-centered	■ User-centered
■ Needs-led assessment for people being discharged/in contact with psychiatric services. (Contact with services)	■ Needs-led assessment and care planning for people who qualify for the level of support offered (eligibility)
■ Keyworkers have a role in:	■ Care manager has a role in:
– making assessments	– assessment
– making care plans in consultation with others	– care plan in consultation
– co-ordinating/monitoring/renewing implementation	– seeking out outside resources
– Keyworker may also provide therapeutic support	– may provide support
	– allocation of finance for residential care, day care, domicillary care and so on
Adapted from Bleach & Ryan (1995)	

Thus in 1995 the Social Services Inspectorate (SSI) reported that there was still much work needed on procedures to integrate the CPA and care management. In the same year, the Department of Health emphasised that *'it is essential that health and social services departments co-ordinate the implementation of the two processes to avoid duplication and the waste of precious resources'* (*Building Bridges* para 1.3.8 page 15). This message has now been very clearly reiterated and to some extent demystified by the *National Service Framework for Mental Health*.

At this point it is worthwhile reflecting on ways of managing the different agendas with regards to the integration of CPA Care Management and asking the key question, *'Which stakeholders have a vested interest?'*. Very often, service users tend to be more concerned about the quality and relevance of the care plan they receive than in whether their care plan is couched in the terms of care management or CPA. Alternatively, practitioners may require integration of the systems for bureaucratic reasons, usually because of the documentation they are attempting to complete. If organisations are endeavouring to respond to Government guidance and dovetail the two systems in respect of people with mental health problems, this needs to have some beneficial effect for the users of the service and should not be primarily about managing budgets and bureaucratic procedures.

During the process of integrating the two systems it is therefore important that any debates and potential disagreements between health and social services should take place behind the scenes of the care plan meeting. My experience is that if such a debate is part of an open dialogue during the care plan meeting, during which a user is attempting to contribute to the discussion about their care, this only serves to undermine and devalue the care planning process, particularly for themselves and their families.

It is also worth acknowledging that, in general, we, as practitioners, do at times find this whole approach confusing. Therefore we need to reflect upon what it must be like for people who (a) don't use the language of care planning in common parlance, and (b) may find it difficult to grasp why meeting basic human needs has to be described in terms of a complex process. The symptoms of mental health problems are often compounded, or in many cases accounted for, by significant social disadvantage. For those people struggling with these problems, debates about bureaucratic procedures, responsibility and accountability may only exacerbate their frustration by detracting from the issues that they consider important. Care must be taken not to confuse the organisation's agenda with that of the service user's. According to Carpenter and Sbaraini (1996), *'whilst staff appeared sympathetic to the idea of involving users and carers in planning the users' own care and empowering them to take greater control over their own lives, they lacked the knowledge and sometimes skills to make this a reality'.*

From research, we know that users are more concerned about having an appropriate place to live, adequate income, employment, something meaningful to do during the day/social activities, and help and support, including medical assistance when needed, rather than a care plan which satisfies organisational standards but does little to promote the realisation of their individual goals and aspirations (Mental Health Foundation, 1994).

In attempts to address these and other issues, different authorities have implemented the two systems in different ways (SSI, 1995). Newton *et al* (1996) found that a joint services approach, where CPNs as well as social workers acted in the capacity of care manager, greatly increased the numbers of care managers, enabled health workers to gain access to community support for their clients and resulted in the caseloads of both social workers and CPNs being equally focused upon people with severe and enduring mental health problems.

In some geographical areas, these links may be supported by inter-organisational procedures which have been jointly agreed by health and social services, whilst in others, practice may still be in a vacuum of organisational policy, whilst agencies are in the process of modernising their mental health services.

The *National Service Framework* makes reference to innovative services in different parts of the United Kingdom where the two systems have been integrated effectively.

Obviously, such integration will have implications for the care co-ordinator role, and it is to this topic that the discussion will now turn.

The care co-ordinator role

Although it is perhaps obvious, it is worth stating at the outset that the care co-ordinator role will only be effective where the person responsible agrees that they have the skills and capacity to do so. Co-ordinating care by coercion is not the best way to implement the CPA, yet time and again practitioners complain they have been nominated as the care co-ordinator at a meeting at which they weren't present, or because theirs was the only caseload with space – even though they may have little legitimate input to the care plan.

The decision about who should be the care co-ordinator was initially discussed in para. 3.1.18, page 50 of *Building Bridges* and a number of factors are outlined that should be taken into account, including:

- users' needs and wishes

- workloads

- authority to undertake the role

- adequate training.

Despite the recent changes in terminology, there is no indication from the *National Service Framework* that the role will change significantly.

When the person has been admitted to hospital, Ryan *et al* (1991) claim that *'it is not clear whether the hospital based multidisciplinary team will supply the keyworker or whether they will more frequently be drawn from CPNs or CMHTs'*. With the increasing integration of hospital and community-based services it is likely that all workers will be able to develop the skills, knowledge and attitudes to undertake the role. Thus the location of the worker will progressively become less significant.

The core function of the keyworker is spelt out quite clearly in *Developing the Care Programme Approach* (NHS Training Division, 1995). It is:

- *'to monitor and review the package of care agreed in the care plan*

- *to liaise, co-ordinate and keep in regular contact with the service user and so be able to respond effectively and quickly to changing circumstances and needs*

- *to be the focal point of contact for the other professionals involved with the GP and with any carers who may also be involved*

- *to identify unmet need and communicate unresolved issues to appropriate managers.'*

Despite the recent changes in terminology, there is no evidence within the *National Service Framework* that redesignating the keyworker as a care co-ordinator will effect any change in these core functions.

Essentially there are two inter-related but specific parts to this role that require a slightly different mix of skills and knowledge:

- In order to co-ordinate the care plan, the care co-ordinator needs to be able to have a wide span of responsibility and networks with other professionals and services. They need to be a key point of information about services and how to access them, and about the user, such that information flows in a two-way process.

- They also need a basic knowledge of the legal framework in which they are operating together with the skills and authority to be able to negotiate with other professionals and agencies (Gupta, 1995).

To be an effective care co-ordinator, as far as the service user is concerned, workers must be able to engage with them and obtain their trust and have frequent and meaningful contact, as well as some freedom to act as an advocate on their behalf at CPA meetings, and in negotiating about how their needs will be met (Gupta, *ibid*).

The *National Service Framework* has also stated explicitly how carers should be involved in the CPA (*ibid*, 69). Thus care co-ordinators need to ensure that carers' needs are also taken into account as part of the care planning process.

Given the potential involvement of so many stakeholders, practitioners need to think carefully about who they are undertaking the role of care co-ordinator for? In the past there has been a tendency for care co-ordination to take place to satisfy the CMHT, rather than to improve the delivery of care to the service user. However, the *National Service Framework*, despite its lack of emphasis on user involvement generally, does make explicit the standards of care that users can expect to receive in relation to care planning. This provides an impetus for care co-ordinators to fulfill their role in a creative way with improving service delivery as an agreed priority. Nevertheless, it becomes apparent, as identified by the Open University (1996), that keyworking and care plan co-ordination are not necessarily the same thing, and the recent introduction of the term 'care co-ordinator' should not be used to confuse the roles and responsibilities.

Links with legislation

As stated previously, the CPA is Government guidance as opposed to legislation. However, when it becomes the framework for the planning of hospital discharge it does become linked with the *Mental Health Act 1983* (Wilkinson & Richards, 1995). If a person with a mental health problem has been admitted to hospital either informally or under a Section 2 – Admission for assessment – a care plan should be drawn up prior to discharge that will assist the individual to transfer successfully back into the community. There are certain decisions that must be made as part of this discharge planning process. These include decisions about which members of the community mental health and primary care teams need to be involved in the care plan.

The *National Service Framework* now states quite clearly that people with multiple needs who are in contact with more than one professional or agency require an 'enhanced CPA' (*ibid*, 53) compared to the standard CPA for people who *'require the support or intervention of one agency or discipline, who pose no danger to themselves or to others, and who will not be at high risk if they lose contact with services'.*

In relation to an assessment of risk, another question must be considered – is the individual at risk of mistreatment or exploitation from others? If it is felt to be a risk issue then a decision can still be taken to place the individual's details on a Supervision Register administered by the mental health trusts. Supervision registers were introduced by the Department of Health on the 1st of April 1994 through HSG (94) 5. Criteria for inclusion comprise whether the person is suffering from severe mental illness and at significant risk of suicide or serious self-harm, serious violence towards others or severe self-neglect.

According to *Building Bridges* (1995), supervision registers are a *'sub-section of the CPA'*. Registration does not ensure that people whose details are included will receive a difference in service but it *'may mean greater prioritisation'* of their needs. Registration *does* mean that information can be shared between those who 'need to know' and the contents of the individual's care plan and can be transferred between mental health trusts if the individual moves area.

To date there have been very few instances of registration nationally, although the people who are most likely to be subject to registration are those who have complex needs, such as a need for a risk management plan to address the areas of risk identified (see **Chapter 9**). These people are also likely to be subject to statutory aftercare as a consequence of their complex needs.

The status of the Register *vis à vis* the *Mental Health Act 1983* and the Code of Practice was debated by Spolander (1996). He queried whether its inception would promote the management of risk and protection of individual rights or whether the Register is a potential instrument of oppression. Given these dilemmas it is not surprising that the Government will allow trusts to phase out the Register over the next two years provided that they are able to demonstrate that procedures are in place for the appropriate assessment and management of risk as part of the CPA and discharge planning process.

When people are admitted under the longer term sections of the *Mental Health Act* (Sections 3, 37,47 and 48), they are entitled to statutory aftercare under Section 117 at the point of discharge. This Section places a statutory duty on both health and social services to provide a package of aftercare which cannot be removed or revised unless both agencies are in agreement and sign documentation to authorise any change. For some people, even though they may be entitled to an aftercare package under Section 117, there is a need to strengthen this entitlement, as they may be reluctant to accept services once they are discharged into the community.

The *Mental Health (Patients in the Community) Act 1995* was designed to do this in addition to changing arrangements for leave from hospital. Supervised Discharge or Aftercare Under Supervision provides professionals with powers to gain access to the service user, and to require them to reside at a particular place and attend for treatment. Finally, it sets out the power to convey the person to a place for receiving such treatment using reasonable force if they are reluctant to go. Those practitioners who are familiar with the *Mental Health Act 1983* in some detail will recognise that these powers are very similar to those of guardianship with the added power of conveyance.

The decision to place someone on Aftercare Under Supervision rests with the RMO with recommendations from an approved social worker and a second doctor (not the same as the RMO). A supervisor will be appointed (not to be confused with a social supervisor for people on Section 37/41 of the *Mental Health Act*) who will have regular contact with the person, and who can authorise their return to hospital if the aftercare plan is not working.

The flow chart shown in **Figure 2** opposite demonstrates these links and hopefully clarifies the interconnections described above. It can be seen that the CPA framework provides the mechanism for the decision-making process including whether the professionals are considering statutory aftercare. The key difference is that if Section 117 and or Supervised Discharge are invoked, the case should automatically require an enhanced CPA, and the *Mental Health Act Code of Practice* (paragraph 27.8) states explicitly that these decisions must be made by a multidisciplinary team of professionals – and even goes so far as to list who should be included.

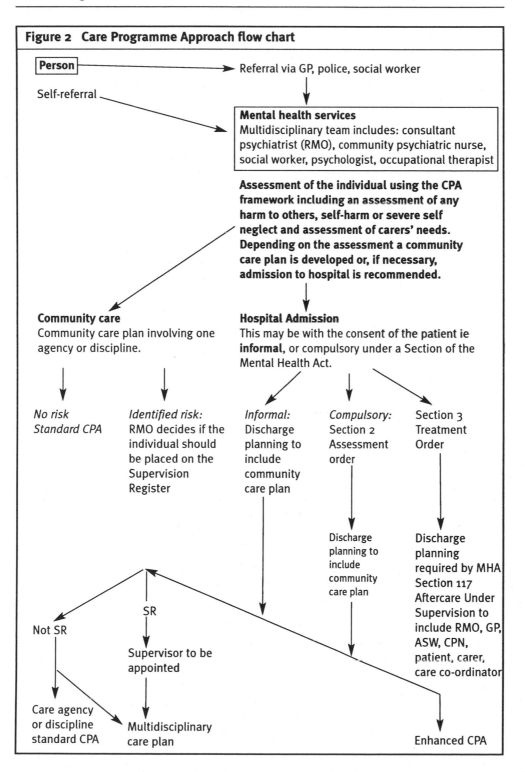

Figure 2 Care Programme Approach flow chart

Person → Referral via GP, police, social worker

Self-referral

Mental health services
Multidisciplinary team includes: consultant psychiatrist (RMO), community psychiatric nurse, social worker, psychologist, occupational therapist

Assessment of the individual using the CPA framework including an assessment of any harm to others, self-harm or severe self neglect and assessment of carers' needs. Depending on the assessment a community care plan is developed or, if necessary, admission to hospital is recommended.

Community care
Community care plan involving one agency or discipline.

Hospital Admission
This may be with the consent of the patient ie **informal,** or compulsory under a Section of the Mental Health Act.

No risk Standard CPA

Identified risk: RMO decides if the individual should be placed on the Supervision Register

Informal: Discharge planning to include community care plan

Compulsory: Section 2 Assessment order

Section 3 Treatment Order

Discharge planning to include community care plan

Discharge planning required by MHA Section 117 Aftercare Under Supervision to include RMO, GP, ASW, CPN, patient, carer, care co-ordinator

Not SR

SR

Supervisor to be appointed

Care agency or discipline standard CPA

Multidisciplinary care plan

Enhanced CPA

Care planning: how to do it

The discussion above has outlined the links between the CPA and care management. The role of the care co-ordinator has been established and the interconnections with the mental health legislation outlined. How then are practitioners to demonstrate best practice in respect of the CPA? A key message here is any CPA documentation practitioners must complete should not be allowed to constrain best practice. As stated in *Building Bridges* (para 3.0.2, page 45) the *'CPA should not be a form-filling bureaucratic exercise'*. If practitioners only record what the documentation allows for, then crucial information will very often be missed. This is borne out by my own experience in scrutinising documentation from a number of mental health trusts and local authorities. It seems most organisations have opted for the minimalist approach and have ended up with documentation which is a recording device rather than a tool to aid the assessment and care planning process.

The first stage is assessment spanning health and social care needs, and risk (Department of Health, 1999). To aid this part of the process there are some extensive checklists available and the practitioner's attention is drawn to Bleach and Ryan (1995). The crux of the matter is this – how do practitioners document the assessment if there is insufficient space on the form? This is where some practitioners might be tempted to turn to their care management documentation (which may provide a much better model) whilst other workers devise their own. It is worth spending some planning time with colleagues in the CMHT and in the trust and local authority to decide what information should be collected as *part* of the initial assessment, as one cannot assume that all practitioners' information needs will be the same irrespective of discipline. It is also important to agree as a team with support (maybe in the form of guidelines and procedures from the trust and local authority) at what stage a more specialist assessment is needed. It is my view that specialist assessment means involving more than one worker from the mental health team depending upon where the key concerns lie (Bleach & Ryan, *ibid*).

Having completed the assessment, the next stage is to write the aim of the care plan and the means by which this will be achieved.

The aim is to make an overarching statement about what the care plan endeavours to do. For example:

> *'To prevent further hospital admissions and promote an increase in the individual's quality of life.'*

Or, being more specific and measurable:

> *'To promote continued independent living in the community and increase the social networks of the individual using generic community-based resources rather than specialist mental health services.'*

Table 2 Care plan: specific and vague objectives	
Ambiguous/vague objectives	**SMART objectives**
Henry will be provided with support to get out more.	By the next review in 6 weeks' time Henry will have attended the drop-in centre at least twice. Once supported by his care co-ordinator, and once by himself, to establish whether the centre can offer a social outlet.
Henry will be encouraged to attend the local day centre and take his medication.	Henry will receive two hourly sessions over the next two weeks with the community psychiatric nurse to specifically discuss his concerns and questions about his medication. By the end of the two sessions Henry will be able to describe the side-effects of his medication and will know how to contact his GP and RMO if he is concerned.
By the next review Henry's housing problems will have been sorted out.	Within the next week Henry will visit his local housing department accompanied by his care co-ordinator and will complete an application to be placed on the housing association's waiting list.

The objectives are the means by which the aims will be achieved. Objectives should focus on what the person will be able to do as a result of the care plan, under which conditions of support and guidance and to which standards. For someone who has never engaged with specialist services, it is likely that, realistically, the maximum attendance at consultant appointments will be 70%. Striving for 100% attendance is unrealistic.

Objectives should follow the SMART rule in that they should be: Specific, Measurable, Achievable, Relevant and Time-limited. They will need to be amended as the individual's needs change. When writing objectives as part of a care plan it is worth reflecting whether they fit with these guiding principles. The table below shows examples of specific and vague objectives for a fictional service user, Henry Hooper.

On reflection, it can be seen from the above objectives that the more specific they are the more chance practitioners and users have of seeing, at the point of review, whether they have been successful in their efforts and whether the outcomes for the plan have been achieved. In terms of best practice, and now in accordance with the *National Service Framework*, it is important for the service user to have their own individual copy of the objectives and to be asked to comment either verbally or in written form what has helped or hindered their realisation. This information is of paramount importance at the review stage in deciding how objectives might be amended to become more achievable and realistic.

Summary

The CPA is a framework for care planning which is similar to that for care management except it is specific to people with mental health problems and is invoked because of Government guidance rather than as a consequence of legislation. One way of looking at the CPA is as a specialist variant of care management for a specific client group – thus integrating both systems in accordance with recent government guidance should in no way detract from the key elements of the care planing process being in place, namely assessment, care planning, care co-ordinator allocation and review. The CPA should be used as the framework for care planning for all people in contact with specialist mental health services. Hospital admission can be part of the CPA; it is merely a change in location of the provision of care and the care plan will need to reflect this.

The care co-ordinator role should be allocated in full agreement with the person concerned and the service user. Keyworking and care co-ordination are not necessarily the same thing, as different skills are required and thought should be given as to the emphasis on the different parts of the role in terms of whose needs are being met.

The CPA provides a framework for discharge planning which currently links with statutory aftercare, supervision registers and supervised discharge. It should provide the mechanism for making all decisions connected with discharge for anyone who has been in hospital. Depending on the complexity of the individual's needs, the level of CPA will differ.

A care plan should be needs-led and have a clear aim and a set of objectives that are measurable such that at the point of review it can be seen whether the outcomes of the care plan have been met and if not, then why not. Documenting the assessment and care plan should not be constrained by minimalist paperwork, but must reflect the information needs of the multidisciplinary team involved with care provision for the individual.

References

Audit Commission (1994) *Finding a Place: A review of mental health services for adults.* London: HMSO.

Bleach, A. & Ryan, P. (1995) *Community Support for Mental Health: A training resource pack for the care programme approach and care management: trainers' notes.* Brighton: Pavilion Publishing in association with The Sainsbury Centre for Mental Health.

Bleach, A. & Ryan, P. (1995) *Community Support for Mental Health: A training resource pack for the Care Programme Approach and Care Management* (Handbook). Pavilion Publishing in association with The Sainsbury Centre for Mental Health.

Carpenter, J. & Sbaraini, S. (1996) Involving service users and carers. *CPA Journal of Mental Health* **5** (5) 483–488.

Department of Health (1994) *Introduction of Supervision registers for mentally ill people from 1 April 1994. HSG (94) 5 D.H.*

Department of Health & The Welsh Office (1999) *Code of Practice Mental Health Act 1983.* London: HMSO.

Department of Health HC 90(23)/LASSL (90) II *The Care Programme Approach For People with a Mental Illness referred to the Specialist Psychiatric Services.*

Davis, A. (1996) Risk Work and Mental Health. In: H. Kemshall and J. Pritchard (Eds) *Good Practice in Risk Assessment and Risk Management.* London: Jessica Kingsley.

Department of Health Social Services Inspectorate (1994) *Report of an inspection of management and provision of social work in the three special hospitals.* London: DoH.

Department of Health (1994) *Health of the Nation: Mental illness – key area handbook.* Second edition. London. HMSO.

Department of Health (1994) *Guidance on the Discharge of Mentally Disordered People and their Continuing Care in the Community.* London: DoH.

Department of Health/SSI (1995a) *Social Services Departments and the CPA – an Inspection.* DoH London.

Department of Health (1995b) *Health of the Nation: Building Bridges.* London: HMSO.

Department of Health (1999) *National Service Framework for Mental Health: Modernising Standards and Service Models.* London: DoH.

Griffiths, R., (1998) *Community Care Agenda for Action.* London: HMSO.

Gupta, N. (1995) Keyworkers and the care programme approach the role and responsibilities of community worker. *Psychiatric Care* **1** (6).

Mental Health (Patients in the Community) Act 1995

Mental Health Act 1983

Mental Health Foundation (1994) *Creating Community Care.* London: Mental Health Foundation.

Newton, J., Carmen, A., Clarke, K., Coombs, M., Walsh, K. & Muijen, M. (1996) *Care Management: Is it working?* London: The Sainsbury Centre for Mental Health.

NHS & Community Care Act 1990.

NHS Executive (1994) HSG (94) 27 *Guidance on the Discharge of Mentally Disordered People and the Continuing Care in the Community.* London: NHS Executive.

NHS Training Division (1995) *Developing the Care Programme Approach: Building on Strengths.* Bristol.

Open University (1996) *Co-ordinating Community Mental Health Care – The Care Programme Approach: A training pack for social services staff and others caring for mentally ill people.* Milton Keynes: Open University, DoH. & SSI OU.

Rogers, A. & Pilgrim, D. (1996) *Mental Health Policy in Britain: A Critical Introduction.* Basingstoke: Macmillan Press.

Ryan, P., Ford, R. & Clifford, P. (1991) *Case Management and Community Care.* London: Research and Development for Psychiatry.

Shepperd, G., King, C., Tilbury, J. & Fowler, D. (1995) Implementing the Care Programme Approach. *Journal of Mental Health* **4** 261–274.

Social Services Inspectorate (1995) *Social Services Departments and the Care Programme Approach*: an Inspection. London: DoH.

Spolander, G. (1996) The Supervision Register: its use in care management. *Practice* **9** (1) 59–63.

Wilkinson, E. & Richards, H. (1995) Aftercare under the *1983 Mental Health Act. Psychiatric Bulletin* **19** 150–160.

Wilson, J. (1996) Power games. *Community Care* **9** May, 22–23.

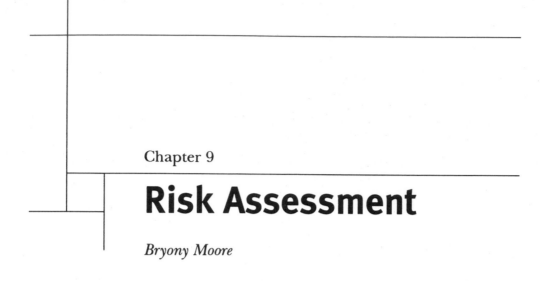

Chapter 9

Risk Assessment

Bryony Moore

'Risk assessment' must be one of the most overworked terms of the decade, and is justifiably viewed with deep suspicion. Most mental health professionals, first encountering it as a new heading in their paperwork, have wondered, *'Does this refer to what I have been doing all along, or perhaps* (plunge into self-doubt) *some new skill of which I am negligently ignorant? And if the latter, why haven't I been offered the relevant training by those who are asking me to do it?'*

Firstly, be reassured; it's almost certainly what you have been doing since you qualified. On the other hand, there have been some important recent advances in the prediction of harmful behaviour, as well as in the decision-making process itself. Secondly, those who are asking you to provide 'risk assessments' almost certainly know as little as you do about the actual process involved. Finally, you are undoubtedly correct in your morbid imaginings that you could in future be held more directly responsible for your clients' misdemeanours than previously. The Care Programme Approach (CPA) (1990) particularly, in identifying a named keyworker, signals the dawn of an era when individual professional answerability is becoming a central feature of psychiatric case management.

At the Core of Mental Health © Pavilion 2000

The assumption underlying current public thinking on mental health and offending appears to be that the absence of harmful acts is the natural status quo, and that any deviation from this norm is somehow the fault of individual professionals or systems. Until fashions in policy-making swing back towards a more realistic position, it falls to those in the frontline of mental health work to protect themselves and their agencies, while at the same time ensuring that their practice continues to be informed by the soundest principles, strongest theory and most rigorous research.

Key principles of decision-making about risk

1 Always remember the fundamental ethical dilemma inherent in prediction

Whenever we attempt to predict harmful behaviour, we are potentially in the position of punishing someone for acts which they have not yet committed, and indeed may never go on to commit. Given the limited accuracy of our predictions, and the huge cost to those falsely identified as dangerous, we should never forget that we are ourselves at high risk of preventing possible harm by inflicting certain harm.

2 Be aware of the most likely sources of error

The accuracy of prediction is largely the result of the information available (its type, amount and quality), and of the distortions arising from the decision-making process. This is considered in more detail later.

3 Define the behaviour to be predicted, not the person

It is essential to focus assessment on the potentially harmful behaviour rather than the 'dangerous' individual.

It is also crucial that each target behaviour is assessed individually, as each is likely to involve different risk factors. It is unsafe to assume, for instance, in the case of a person having committed both sexual and violent offences, that both types of behaviour are the result of identical drives and influences; each requires separate assessment. Even if a series of similar actions (eg violence) is involved, where they occur in more than one setting and against very different victims, grouping them together inevitably reduces predictive accuracy.

4 Distinguish between the probability and cost of the behaviour recurring

When an event is said to be 'low-risk', do you mean that it's unlikely to happen, that it wouldn't matter much if it did happen, or that there's not enough information to conclude much either way? There is a huge difference between a low-cost, high-probability act (eg indecent exposure to a resilient subject) and one which is of low probability but high cost (eg the accidental killing of a child). Unless the assessor distinguishes between the seriousness of the anticipated conduct and the likelihood of its happening, they are unlikely to be able to weigh the facts appropriately or provide any reliable basis for decision-making.

5 Take into account both internal and external factors

Almost all behaviour is the result of interaction between characteristics of the individual (eg attitudes, needs, skills, controls) and those of the environment (eg demands, constraints, stressors etc). An understanding of these two sources of influence on the target behaviour, as well as the balance between them, is crucial to any prediction.

Error is likely to arise in the assessor's assumption:

- that individuals who are very different from her/himself are largely driven by internal factors (eg illness, personality)

■ that those with whom they identify are primarily motivated by external influences (eg deviant sub-culture, marital stress etc).

In offences which arouse especial revulsion, the active deviance of the perpetrator is likely to be over-rated, and any influence of the victim tends to be underrated. By contrast, those individuals already perceived as disadvantaged (eg women who have previously been the subjects of abuse) are likely to be attributed with least deviant internal drive, regardless of clear evidence to the contrary. In other words, professionals' viewpoints significantly affect the quality of their judgements about risk, a very human failing but one which needs to be suspended in the interests of accuracy.

6 Check whether all necessary historical information has been gathered

Most professionals would accept that *'the best predictor of future behaviour is past behaviour'*, yet many risk assessments are carried out using only a fraction of the historical data potentially available. A sound framework for the assessment will identify the types of information necessary for a confident prediction: this not only serves to prompt a systematic search for the material, but helps to explain the limitations of an assessment which has necessarily been based on inadequate or patchy facts.

The lamentable practice, often statutorily imposed on institutions and agencies, of destroying professional records after a few years has made the task of informed risk assessment unnecessarily difficult. Special schools and child guidance teams, whose accumulated observations, assessments and opinions regarding the early life of a troubled and troublesome child would provide vital insights into later deviancy, are required to shred their files after a minimal period, disregarding the evidence that some offending behaviours tend to re-emerge cyclically throughout the life cycle. Probation departments have to dispose of all but a skeleton of their old notes and reports. Frequently, crucial facts are gained only by virtue of the inefficiency of individual teams in adhering to the shredding policy or of the capacity of their storage shelves.

It should go without saying that restrictions on the access to such material has to be established and applied rigorously if civil rights are to be protected. However, there is an equally powerful argument in favour of ensuring the protection of the information, if later developments in the individual's life are to be understood fully and informed decisions made.

7 Avoid interpreting information from other professions

Past reports from other disciplines may not be limited to clear-cut facts whose meaning is evident. In cases where summaries, inferences and interpretations must be made about others' work, it is rarely appropriate for this to be done by anyone except the original author. If the person in question is not accessible, someone from their profession should be consulted, in order to ensure that the intended meaning is retained. The author (or their colleague) will also be able to advise on the validity of applying their old conclusions to the current situation. (Check too that the confidentiality constraints applying to this new information are not violated by its inclusion in your report. Anyone who has suffered the experience of having their views distorted into an unrecognisable 'summary' by someone else, whose assessment is misapplied to a quite different situation, or who has been quoted in a report which is then circulated to people who were never intended to be privy to the original, will appreciate the importance of these professional courtesies.)

Accounts gathered from individuals who have known the client and/or victim for some time are often invaluable in corroborating or contradicting their views of events. Some agencies such as social services, probation and the police tend to collect such accounts as a matter of course; mental health workers, including psychologists, seem to be among the worst culprits in ignoring these invaluable, independent sources of information. As well as providing a crucial insight into the historical context of the behaviour, these significant others can also act as monitors of change once intervention has begun.

The assessed individual should also be encouraged to provide as much information as possible about their target behaviour. This may seem too obvious to need mentioning, but in reality it is too often assumed that the client will be so motivated to appear acceptable that their accounts will be useless in prediction. A number of studies have shown that self-report, for example, of violent assaults, significantly improves predictive accuracy. This is likely to be the case, particularly in a continuing, rather than snapshot, assessment.

8   Be theory-driven

The collection and analysis of past and present information about a behaviour and its context only becomes fully meaningful when placed within its theoretical framework.

A conscientious worker will often amass huge quantities of information about an assessed individual, much of which may seem highly unusual, worrying and obviously significant. Without background knowledge against which to measure the new information, however, its true predictive value remains unclear.

Relevant theory may have identified, for example, the various motivational drives for the behaviour, how common it is among those who do not go on to offend, its functions, the types of individual most likely to act in this way, what distinguishes them and the range of indicators for successful clinical intervention. Without well-supported theory, any attempt at assessment can only be a collection of descriptions, impressions and hunches.

9   Be aware of the actuarial (statistical) basis for the behaviour in question

In assessing the probability of a given individual acting in a certain way, it is important to have an accurate idea of the likelihood of the behaviour occurring in the group to whom that individual belongs.

Imagine that you were asked to make a prediction about a psychiatric inpatient who has committed several acts of arson, and who is soon to be discharged from hospital. Imagine too that, in all previous cases of people with this diagnosis and offence history, 80% have been recorded as setting a fire within a week of discharge. Your assessment would then start from the assumption of high probability, and would go on to establish the extent to which this individual resembles the majority who set fires or the minority who do not. On the other hand, research may show that only 1% of such patients go on to set a fire after discharge: you would then start from an assumption of low probability, and consider whether there is any evidence that this individual represents a higher risk than that of the majority.

Clearly, where the true base-rate for the behaviour is not known, or has only been established in relation to groups very different from the target individual, predictive accuracy will be greatly weakened.

10 Identify those factors likely to increase/decrease the risk in the future

It is inevitable that any assessment of the risk represented by an individual will in some sense be a snapshot picture, describing the situation at a specific moment in time. If the basic drive and significant influences behind the behaviour have been identified, however, it should be possible to offer a prediction of how the risk could change over time.

Where the key factor in a series of angry assaults has clearly been the time elapsed since the last anti-psychotic depot injection, for example, any prediction would need to take this into account. If on the other hand the necessary and sufficient trigger was the behaviour of the victim, it would be important to identify the likelihood of this behaviour being encountered (or provoked) again in the future.

Where a certain combination of events has led to the assault on this occasion but not in the past, and no additional factors can be

At the Core of Mental Health © Pavilion 2000

identified to explain the different reaction, this should be stated. It is tempting to imply a greater degree of confidence in one's assessment than is actually the case, but this is unwise. Quite apart from the ethical implications of over-prediction, when new information subsequently comes to light, as it invariably does, the lack of substance for the original view becomes embarrassingly transparent.

11 Identify key interventions

Where a sound assessment of risk will be based on the formulation of the mechanisms underlying the behaviour, it will automatically identify those processes which appear to be key elements in increasing or reducing such risk.

In cases where the resources needed to address the identified issue are not available, the professional should nevertheless state the requirement in their recommendations, so that a realistic picture of clients' needs continues to be generated.

12 Recognise your own limitations in carrying out the assessment

One of the most common weaknesses identified in risk assessment is the tendency for it to be carried out by single disciplines, or even individuals. The range of information necessary is rarely to be found within the training and expertise of one profession, and predictive accuracy is likely to be compromised as a result.

If, having worked through the above principles, it becomes clear that the key issues underpinning the target behaviour are not the province of your profession, say so. If a risk assessment is required of you notwithstanding, make it plain where contributions from another discipline are essential or desirable. State clearly the limitations of your own report, precisely what else is needed, and what such a contribution would add to the overall predictive accuracy.

It may be that yours is the appropriate profession to complete the full assessment, but that your own existing role in the case restricts your ability to carry out the wider task. Often a supervising social worker's policing responsibilities create a tension between them and the assessed individual/s which understandably compromises full objectivity and trust on both sides. When it becomes clear that the same worker will be required to complete (rather than contribute to) the overall risk assessment, it is important that they acknowledge the degree to which close involvement is likely to have distorted their capacity for detached analysis of the issues. As professionals, it is easy for us to be persuaded that we should be able to remain objective, but we accept this fantasy at our own peril.

The Risk Assessment Framework

Possible sources of error

No assessment can ever be error-free. Maximum accuracy can be achieved, however, by:

- being aware of the ways in which your prediction could be weakened

- controlling or adjusting for probable error where you can

- identifying where the other limitations lie

- stating which measures could improve confidence in your prediction.

Error related to the information available

Do you actually know which facts would indicate greater risk? (For example, in the case of a convicted rapist, would the number of previous offences, the degree of violence used, or the relationships to previous victims be most significant? Are you qualified to judge whether past episodes of violence are consistent with epilepsy rather than anger? Would denial of responsibility signify a greater future risk than seriousness of past acts?)

In other words, are you familiar with the relevant theory and research, and qualified to interpret the evidence, or are you responding to your own 'gut feelings' about the information available?

Error related to the client/patient

- Which sources of bias are most likely to apply to the individual being assessed?

- Do they appear particularly likeable/unlikeable, hostile/compliant, defensive/open, powerful/powerless, damaged/sadistic, like you/unlike you?

- Would they tend to evoke strong positive or negative reactions in the minds of the general public and other professionals?

- What emotions have they aroused in you, which could influence the starting point of your attitudes and judgement in the case?

Error related to the assessor

- Are there any external or internal constraints on you to reach a particular conclusion?

- Have you had previous experience of this sort of behaviour, either personally or professionally?

- Would it be particularly inconvenient/expensive/painful/ unwelcome to decide one way or another?

- Do you know in general about the sorts of error which tend to apply in this kind of decision-making? Can you afford to be wrong (ie to over or under-predict)?

Error related to the agency/climate

- Are you aware of any biases in your organisation/team predisposing it towards or against certain decisions (eg a highly critical view of suspected 'collusion' with alleged perpetrators, or a resistance to perceiving risk from members of disadvantaged racial groups)?

- Have recent events (locally or nationally) made some reasonable courses of action more difficult to justify?

- Does the lack of genuine multi-professional teamworking mean that you are regularly asked to make decisions without the necessary information or skills?

- Do other deficits in resources (eg scope for full case discussion, inadequate time allowed for assessments) compromise your accuracy in predicting risk?

Assessment of individual risk

Definition of the target behaviour

Where more than one harmful behaviour requires assessment (eg physical abuse and neglect), each must be considered separately. It may transpire that all are the result of the same factors, and are equally likely to occur in risky situations, but this is actually rarely the case, and should never be assumed.

Probability of recurrence

Past behaviour

- **Type & frequency.** Precisely what has occurred in the past, when and how seriously?

- **Actuarial prediction.** In the research on this type of behaviour, what are the identified predictors of high risk in the future?

Motivational drive (theory-based formulation)

- Why is this behaviour happening, and why now?

- What are the underlying drives leading to this type of behaviour, as identified by research and theory?

- Which best seem to fit the evidence in this particular case? In other words, which factors are necessary and/or sufficient to explain the behaviour, and which factors appear to be merely influential, somehow related or even coincidental?

Mental illness

Has it been reliably established that the individual does or does not suffer from mental illness? Is the illness connected to the behaviour in the form of

(a) the sole, direct and necessary cause (eg through delusional drive)

(b) a necessary but not sufficient cause (ie other factors must also be present)

(c) an exacerbating influence (eg through disinhibition), or is it entirely irrelevant?

Deviant v normal drive

While the behaviour is clearly deviant (unusually and knowingly harmful) in its effect, is the same necessarily true of the drive behind it? (For example, someone who commits rape because they cannot achieve intimate relationships any other way presents a very different risk from someone who is highly aroused by the victim's suffering.) Is there clear evidence of a need to cause harm, or does it appear to be incidental to the main purpose? What are the individual's realistic alternatives for achieving the same end in a non-harmful way?

Influence of previous learning

- Has the individual been exposed to unusual learning experiences in the more impressionable stages of developing this behaviour (eg parental modelling, childhood abuse)?

- To what extent have appropriate influences also been available?

Necessary triggers/conditions

- Does the behaviour invariably occur at every opportunity?

- If not, what combination of conditions seems necessary to bring it about?

- Are there identifiable high-risk situations?

Sources of reinforcement

- What function does the behaviour play?

- What are the necessary/intended consequences, as opposed to the coincidental (even regretted) ones?

- Does the behaviour bring about desirable additions to the situation or merely relief from an intolerable state (often the most powerful drive)?

Controls & disinhibitors

The motivational drive to commit an act is not in itself sufficient to explain why it occurs. Every person's daily life contains thousands of opportunities for action, some highly appealing, which they fail to carry out. (Our outrage at harmful acts committed by others is often flavoured with resentment that we managed to resist a similar temptation while they clearly did not.) It is necessary to explain behaviour not only by its attraction and function, but also by the failure of the controls which normally prevent it.

Existing moral code

- Does the individual have a generally intact moral sense about the rights and wrongs of their behaviour?

- How effective is this control normally, in this and other areas of their life?

- What has undermined their controls in this instance?

Intellectual understanding of issues

Is there any reason to believe that the individual genuinely did not perceive their actions to be harmful/illegal/serious? How able are they to learn from their mistake?

Cognitive distortion

Is any form of cognitive distortion (eg minimising cost, denigrating the victim, reframing the meaning of the behaviour) evident? Was this significant in the build-up to the behaviour, or was it largely a rationalisation afterwards?

Empathy with victim/s

- How accurate is the individual's perception of others' feelings?

- How much do they believe that this awareness should influence their actions?

- Is their in/sensitivity to the victim an exception, or the norm? Are they generally able to deny themselves gratification in response to others' needs, or not? What happened to overrule their empathy in this situation?

Impulsivity

Does the individual have difficulty in resisting immediate impulses, even in the face of clearly negative long-term consequences? If so, does it apply only to this type of behaviour, or more generally across a range of actions and situations?

Substance abuse

To what extent is substance use necessary for the behaviour to occur? As with mental illness, is it:

(a) necessary and sufficient by itself?

(b) necessary but requiring other factors to be present too?

(c) related but not causal (eg caused by the same factors as the behaviour itself)

(d) a reaction to the behaviour

(e) irrelevant?

Insight into past offending

While full insight (ie the same view as that of the assessor, with convincing extra detail) is certainly not essential in managing future behaviour safely, the following factors are likely to influence confidence in predictions about risk:

■ **Recognition of drive**

Does the individual recognise the strength of their motivational drive to behave in this way? Do they overestimate the role of external factors, including victim influence?

■ **Acceptance of risk cycle**

Is there an awareness of the High Risk Factors (HRFs) which tend to lead to harmful behaviour? These will include internal HRFs such as certain emotions, urges, trains of thought etc and external ones like particular situations, places, or interactions.

■ **Acknowledgement of future risk**

What evidence is there that the individual judges realistically the possibility of repeating the behaviour? This is a difficult issue to establish with accuracy, as most people will assert a quite unjustified confidence, because they need to convince either themselves, or the authorities, or both. It is important not to confuse desperate wishful thinking with 'denial' (another disastrously over-worked and misunderstood concept, too often the result of clumsy or hostile interviewing). Most people are capable of learning to make positive contingency plans without losing their fundamental optimism, given sensitive but firm guidance.

Motivational stage

It is not really surprising, given limited resources in the mental health field, that so many potential customers are turned away with the verdict of 'unmotivated'. Where only a proportion of those referred can be offered help, it makes more sense to reject the others on the basis of an expressed attitude to change, rather than some far more arbitrary factor such as ability to get up the clinic steps.

Where the cost of the harmful behaviour is high, however, professionals have less excuse for treating 'non-motivation' as if it were a simple all-or-nothing matter. From the least motivated (who claim to see no need for any change at all) to the nearly-motivated (who disagree with the professionals about what needs changing, or who fluctuate wildly), there are well established approaches and techniques most likely to help them move on to a position where greater change is possible. Where there is a great deal of resistance (for example, where the behaviour is bound up with lifestyle or self-image) periods of professional input will often need to be separated by intervals in which the person has the chance to absorb and consolidate what they have learned about themselves, before being ready to move on further.

There is no such thing as 'untreatability'. To describe someone in these terms means either:

(a) *'I don't have the skills to help this person change'*

(b) *'It would probably take longer than we've got'.*

Cost of the behaviour

- To the potential victim(s)

Is the likely result of the behaviour:

(i) life-threatening?

(ii) severe and irreversible?

(iii) significant?

(iv) tolerable, given a victim of average resilience?

- **To the assessed person**

How serious would it be for the perpetrator if they were discovered behaving in this way again?

- **To the assessor**

How well can the agency afford to have this behaviour happen again? This will be partly related to the costs to victim and perpetrator, but may also reflect the agency's values, its current standing in public opinion (local or national) and any media interest in certain types of cases at that time.

Assessment of applied risk

Emotional/social environment

Knowing everything there is to know about an individual, outside the context in which they have previously functioned, provides considerably less than half the information needed for a sound prediction. Trying to assess risk on the basis of the assessed person in isolation is as unreliable as marrying the subject of your holiday romance before you fly home. Having never known them in another environment, met their family and friends, learned how they cope in a crisis, or seen them when bored, angry, scared or hurt, all you really know is how attractive and plausible they can be when they put their mind to it.

Significant others

Reliable prediction depends heavily on corroborated evidence about how the person has responded to and been influenced by others in the past, across a wide variety of situations.

Intimate relationships

How does the individual relate to those closest to them? Whatever the expressed views of those others, what actual effect do they appear to have on the harmful behaviour?

Sub-cultural influences

The 'sub-culture' of an individual can be any group with which they identify, wider than the nuclear family but narrower than a national identity. It may be a religious congregation, council estate community, Hell's Angels gang, trade or profession, or a regional stereotype: the definitive features are attitudes or behaviours believed (by the individual) to be held by a group of people who are important in that person's sense of identity.

Most sub-cultures significant in harmful behaviour will themselves hold supporting deviant values, but others will exert a restraining or even paradoxical influence (eg family members whose presence is sufficient to prevent the behaviour occurring, or others who, while apparently opposing the behaviour, somehow manage to trigger it anyway.)

Situational triggers

Some harmful acts are powerfully influenced by external situations (eg a nightclub which stirs territorial aggression, Christmas evoking childhood fears of disappointment, or urban streets after midnight which automatically define all women present as promiscuous).

These will include ambient factors (background atmospheres) and precipitating factors (immediate triggers) which are known to have been influential in past behaviour. Don't assume that because the behaviour is negative, the triggering situation necessarily must be too; sometimes the drive to behave destructively is linked to good times.

Victim factors

The influence of the victim is one of the most powerful in the majority of serious offences. Contrary to popular stereotype, relatively few assaults occur between complete strangers; most perpetrators know their victims, often intimately.

Availability

- To what extent is the key behaviour aimed only at a limited number of people?

- How active will the perpetrator be in seeking them out?

- Will the potential victim need to behave in a certain way? How unusually? (For example, would a child need to say something highly offensive, or merely act in an age-appropriate way, in order to provoke an assault?) The victim's identity or presentation may be crucial; they may need to be the current partner, a parent, someone in authority, a blonde, or an obstacle in relation to a certain goal.

- How likely is the individual to meet the identified victim, or someone with the necessary qualities?

Capacity to resist

People who inflict harm range from those who will be deterred by, for example, assertive reactions in their victims, to those whose motivational drive is so strong as to ignore or overwhelm any resistance.

Is the victim, although usually assertive or even hostile by nature, less able to resist because of their dependence on the individual in question? Or is some other vulnerable type of person specifically targeted?

Power discrepancy

- Is the probable victim significantly less powerful than the individual in question?

- Is this imbalance the result of prescribed (inborn) or ascribed (learned) qualities? Remember that age, race and gender are not always the most relevant factors; intelligence, physical attractiveness, maturity and popularity are all highly influential in unequal relationships.

- Do the power discrepancies all tend to lean one way? (Is the perpetrator, for example, far more emotionally dependent than the victim?)

- Might the abuse be the only aspect of the relationship in which the perpetrator feels more powerful?

Influence and responsibility

While the responsibility for an act is always entirely that of the person who commits it, influence over the action may come from a variety of sources, including the victim.

What evidence is there that external influences have been important, or even necessary, in bringing about the harmful behaviour? How unusual does the influence (eg the behaviour of the victim) have to be in order for the harm to result? The necessary external triggers for an assault, for instance, may range from a deliberate insult, proactive sexual conduct by a child or the normal crying of a small baby.

Influence by others might be unnecessary for the behaviour to start, but significant in its continuing. What would the victim or others gain by further victimisation?

Applied cost

While the behaviour might be considered likely to cause a certain amount of harm in relation to a victim of average resilience, is there any indication that the most likely victim is particularly vulnerable? Someone who has already been abused, for example, or who has a fragile mental state may be far less able to tolerate further harm.

Is there a 'last chance' aspect which means that there is an especially high cost to the victim, perpetrator or others of the behaviour occurring again?

Reliability of detection

Acceptable risk does not always involve a low-probability and low-cost behaviour. Sometimes, where the environmental (applied) factors are favourable, and the behaviour likely to be detected before or shortly after it occurs, even serious or highly likely incidents may be considered manageable.

Urgency v cost

Does the seriousness of the anticipated behaviour mean that it must be prevented; ie that it is essential that increased risk is spotted immediately? Or would it be sufficient that it is detected as soon as it starts happening again? The higher the likely cost, the more urgent the need for reliable early feedback about risk indicators.

Presence of early warning signs

- To what extent are signs of increased risk (eg returning mental illness, rise in verbal hostility) noticeable to the individual concerned, members of the household or significant others?

- In the past, how quickly has the harmful behaviour followed such indicators?

- Is it likely that there will be sufficient time to identify the signs, and report and intervene effectively?

Openness to monitoring

Where there is a significant or high cost of the behaviour recurring, it will be necessary to back up 'in-house' vigilance with external monitoring by professionals. Even when the individual and/or those around them appear alert, informed and reliable, it is still important to establish a system of objective corroboration for at least a trial period. Ideally, this would continue until there has been clear demonstration that worrying changes are being reported promptly. (A period during which nothing changes and nothing has been reported is not sufficient evidence that the 'in-house' system is working!)

Are the early warning signs or minor episodes of the behaviour amenable to objective checking (eg blood testing to monitor compliance with medication, physical examinations for signs of injury, access to details of school attendance in cases of neglect etc)? Are those involved prepared to allow this monitoring to occur? Do the objective signs correspond with subjective reports?

Capacity of others to protect

If there is any doubt about the ability of significant others to protect the potential victim, it is essential to identify the obstacle/s. Often, the professional response itself can be undermining in an otherwise 'safe-enough' environment.

Acceptance of seriousness of past behaviour

Do those who need to offer protection:

(i)   accept that the perpetrator has acted in a harmful way in the past?

(ii) appreciate the responsibility/influence issues?

(iii) acknowledge the likely cost to the victim?

Acknowledgement of future risk

To what extent do they recognise the probable future risk? Many people underestimate the strength of deviant drive and over-play the effect of assumed unusual environmental factors, victim behaviour, stressors etc in the past. Another commonly misleading (though sincerely believed) argument is *'S/he has too much to lose by doing that again'*. Sadly, this applies to countless people who go on to behave in a risky fashion despite the enormous costs to themselves.

Recognition of need for protective strategy

Many people who pay lip-service to acknowledging the degree of future risk reveal their underlying, more worrying attitudes when pressed to impose new rules on themselves and others.

- Will it be possible for professionals to check that safe guidelines are being followed?

- Do all concerned appreciate that the perpetrator too is being protected by such a strategy?

Knowledge

Does everyone know what to look for? Are they armed with basic principles of risky behaviour as well as concrete examples?

Vigilance

- Everyone might be appropriately alert now, but how soon will they start to become complacent?

- How might vigilance best be maintained at a safe level? Sometimes (eg where professionals have overstated some element of the risk early on), those who need to be more cautious at later high-risk points may be over-confident when the time comes. (For example, someone who has been told that substance abuse would have a disastrous effect on their mental stability, but who has discovered that they can have a few pints without a problem, is more likely to experiment with greater quantities, or with drugs.)

Power to intercept/report

- How able are those doing the monitoring to report what concerns them, or to intervene to stop the behaviour if appropriate?

- Are there power or dependency issues which are likely to undermine their good intentions?

Perceived consequences of reporting

- How much would those involved have to lose by ending/reporting the behaviour?

- Do they understand the consequences of reporting low, significant and high risk signs?

- Has a clear contract been negotiated, describing what needs to be reported under each of these headings and what professional response they can expect to each? Too often, those trying to manage risk at home can feel that they are forever in danger of crossing some invisible line which only the professionals involved can see, and which will lead to a sudden and catastrophic reaction when they do cross it.

Writing it up

The final risk assessment report may well have a life far beyond the purpose for which it was produced, and is likely to re-emerge at key points in the assessed person's life, maybe for many years to come. Unsound assessments and poorly worded conclusions in particular have an uncanny tendency to haunt the unfortunate author for what seems like an eternity. It is always worth a few more moments, therefore, to check that nothing vital has been omitted nor carelessly expressed. Are you satisfied that:

- the purpose of the report, and its circulation limits, have been clearly explained?

- you have stated your areas of competence in carrying out the assessment, your limitations, what remains to be done and who should do it?

- that full use has been made of relevant theory and research?

- all sources have been acknowledged?

- you have distinguished between current risk status and the factors likely to increase/decrease it in the future?

And, most important of all:

- the evidence has clearly driven the conclusions?

The Risk Assessment Framework

Possible sources of error
- Related to the information available
- Related to the client/patient
- Related to the assessor
- Related to the agency/climate

Assessment of individual risk

Definition of the target behaviour

Probability of recurrence

Past behaviour
- *Type & frequency*
- *Actuarial prediction*

Motivational drive (theory-based formulation)
- *Mental illness*
- *Deviant v normal drive*
- *Influence of previous learning*
- *Necessary triggers/conditions*
- *Sources of reinforcement*

Controls & disinhibitors
- Existing moral code
- Empathy with victim/s
- Intellectual understanding of issues
- Cognitive distortion
- Impulsivity
- Substance abuse

Insight into past offending
- Recognition of drive
- Acceptance of risk cycle
- Acknowledgement of future risk
- Motivational stage

Cost of the behaviour
- To the potential victim(s)
- To the assessed
- To the assessor

Assessment of applied risk

Emotional/social environment

Significant others
- Intimate relationships
- Sub-cultural influences

Situational triggers
- Ambient factors
- Precipitating factors

Victim factors
- Availability
- Capacity to resist
  - Behavioural style
  - Type of victim
  - Relationship with aggressor
- Power discrepancy
  - Socially derived
  - Personally derived
- Influence and responsibility

Applied cost

Reliability of detection
- Urgency v cost
- Presence of early warning signs
- Openness to monitoring
- Capacity of others to protect
  - Acceptance of seriousness of past behaviour
  - Acknowledgement of future risk
  - Recognition of need for protective strategy
  - Vigilance
  - Power to intercept/report
  - Perceived consequences of reporting

Summary of risk

Probability of behaviour recurring	high/significant/low
Cost of behaviour recurring	high/significant/low
Sources of possible error	Towards over-/under-prediction of risk?

Early warning signs

High risk signs	Response
_____	_____
_____	_____
_____	_____
_____	_____
_____	_____

Significant risk signs	
_____	_____
_____	_____
_____	_____
_____	_____
_____	_____

Low risk signs	
_____	_____
_____	_____
_____	_____
_____	_____
_____	_____

Level of monitoring

Including:
- Anticipated frequency over time
- Objective corroboration required
- Criteria for relaxation of monitoring

References

The material in this chapter has been based on the framework originally presented in *Risk Assessment: A Practitioner's Guide to Predicting Harmful Behaviour* by Bryony Moore (1996). London: Whiting & Birch.

Department of Health (1990) HC (90)23/LASSL(90)11 – *The Care Programme Approach for People with a Mental Illness Referred to the Specialist Psychiatric Services*. London: DoH.

Chapter 10

Psychological Interventions for Mental Health Problems

Zaffer Iqbal & Max Birchwood

Introduction

Recent advancements in the area of mental health have provided clinicians with several innovative interventions that, as well as complementing established chemotherapy regimes, have provided effective maintenance of psychotic disorders and reductions in relapse. Two of these approaches will be considered in this chapter. Family-based interventions can target problem areas that may impinge upon the mental health of the client and his/her long-term recovery. A specific programme of assessment, education and therapeutic intervention will encourage the client and family to identify and manage such potential difficulties. Our attention will turn to exploring the framework for early intervention as a means of preventing relapse. In this chapter we will provide an overview of the approaches to the treatment of severe mental illness, in particular their efficacy and theoretical underpinning, and the implications of recent research for the provision of such services.

Family intervention

The Expressed Emotion concept

The potential for relapse in patients with a severe mental illness is well documented (Hogarty & Ulrich, 1977) and a stratagem reliant upon neuroleptic medication alone was not effective in curbing the high proportion of patients re-presenting within a year of a major psychotic episode. This problem encouraged the investigation of several possible causal factors during the 1970s, one of which was the concept of Expressed Emotion (EE) (Brown, *et al*, 1972). EE is a synthesis of the relative's attitudes to the patient and is composed of elements such as the frequency of critical remarks, significant emotional over-involvement, a lack of warmth, antagonistic behaviour and negative affect. Living with a high EE relative is argued to produce a high degree of stress and agitation in the patient, hence acting as a trigger for relapse. As such, patients who have regular contact and involvement with a high EE family member are significantly more likely to relapse (Birchwood, 1992; Kuipers & Bebbington, 1988).

Although this robust effect has been widely replicated, the development and characteristics of the high EE environment is less well defined. Brown *et al* (*ibid*) highlighted the link between maladaptive behaviour and criticism by relatives, and high EE has been linked with both social impairment and poor social functioning (Vaughn, 1986). Greenley (1986) suggests that these social deficits result in increased burden for the family and unpredictability in the behaviour of the patient.

A further problem with harnessing EE as a therapeutic device is the questionable nature of its stability. Relatives' levels of criticism have been reported as either increasing (Tarrier, *et al*, 1988) or decreasing (Hogarty, *et al*, 1991) following an acute psychotic episode. Birchwood and Smith (1987) argue that EE incorporates a 'state' element that fluctuates in accordance to the emerging relationship between the patient and family, and at the time when both parties are coming to terms with the emerging psychosis. Finally, and on a similar note, Kuipers and Bebbington (1988) suggest that EE stability is a composite of the relatives' current EE level and their ability to cope with the emerging schizophrenic illness. This apparent 'instability' of EE has been observed in a number of studies where up to a quarter of high EE families revert to low EE without any clinical input (Tarrier *et al*, 1988; Hogarty *et al*, 1991). Additionally, the former study also reports a minority of low EE families changing to high EE.

Assessment issues

A significant problem exists if assessment is to provide a stable measure of EE when such variations in EE level are reported over relatively short periods of time. Kuipers and Bebbington (1988) have suggested, based upon their findings, the existence of three disparate groups of relatives: a good coping group with a low EE that remains low; a poor coping group with high EE and a variety of psychosocial problems, and finally, a group of poor coping relatives (but with low EE) who will revert to high EE, dependent upon stressful circumstances. This third group of 'poor coping' families with low EE levels may be overlooked if a family intervention service is based solely upon a high EE inclusion criterion.

It is acknowledged that over 60% of high EE relatives report marked levels of stress, burden and coping difficulty (Leff & Vaughn, 1985) in comparison to low EE relatives. However, a sub-group of low EE relatives is identified as having high levels of stress coupled with impaired coping, sometimes identifiable in the family member afflicted with mental illness who also exhibits an 'impaired' social range. The lack of significant differences between this sub-group and the remainder of the low EE group suggest that other factors are also involved. Several studies have therefore suggested that regardless of levels of EE, the coping style of relatives faced with the problems and burdens prominent when caring for the person with a severe mental illness should also be examined (Hatfield, 1978; Barraclough & Tarrier, 1990).

A detailed outline of the types of coping style employed by relatives of patients who develop psychosis was provided by Birchwood and Cochrane (1990; **Figure 1**, below). Their results provided significant indications that styles of coping were associated with perceived control or burden, and that relatives making greater use of coercive, avoidant and disorganised coping styles experienced less perceived control, more stress and greater burden.

Figure 1 Examples of coping strategies (Birchwood & Cochrane)	
Coping strategy: Coercion	
Symptoms:	*'I would laugh at him to show him how stupid they are... I'd try to bring him to his senses and I'd say, "Just watch the TV, there's nothing going to happen!"'*
Withdrawal:	*'I'd tell him "buck yourself up" but he just ignored me so I'd say, "For crying out loud help yourself and buck yourself up, people are being kind..."'*
Slowness:	*'I'd say "for crying out loud, I'll do it myself... you're so slow you drive me up the wall"!'*
Coping strategy: Avoidance	
Symptoms:	*'I just leave him; whatever you say you won't convince him... if I try he only gets aggressive and I don't want that again.'*
Withdrawal:	*'I knew he was bad and did not want to force him to do things because I knew it would make him worse or even violent... I used to force him out but he would end up coming back because of some incident... I don't push him now because I don't want people to see him while he is ill.'*
Loss of independence:	*'I usually do everything for him to keep the peace... my husband tries but he (son) goes on at him until he ends up doing it.'*
Coping strategy: Ignore/accept	
Symptoms:	*'I was worried but thought it was a phase he was going through... I would ask him if he was all right then leave it at that... I didn't want to make a fuss about it.'*
Withdrawal:	*'With such a lot in the family we hardly noticed he wasn't doing very much and was quieter than usual... we ignored it really, left him to his own devices.'*
Loss of independence:	*'We saw it as part of his illness... we do as many things for him as he wants... we leave him time on his own.'*

Coping strategy: Collusion	
Symptoms:	'I sometimes pretended to hear the voices as well, to reassure him that he was not the only one.'
Withdrawal:	'I tell her who is coming to the door so if it's someone she doesn't want to see it gives her time to get upstairs.'
Loss of independence:	'I do most things she asks... I tell her that I don't mind... and I won't make her do things she doesn't want to... I don't want her to have this terrible illness again.'

Coping strategy: Constructive	
Symptoms:	'I'd say, "Just don't listen to them, try to forget them...". I'd try and distract her whenever I could.'
Withdrawal:	'I try to draw him into conversations all the time... I rattle on at him in the hope he will find something of interest... I suggest little jobs for him to do to get him going rather than sitting here moping.'
Loss of independence:	'I comment on it, tell her that she's doing wrong... it's a matter of 'restraining' her; by pointing out where she's going wrong in the hope that she will gradually improve.'

Coping strategy: Resignation	
Symptoms:	'I'd say, "Good God, there's nothing (poison) in the tea, I poured it myself" ...it made no difference so I just ignore him now.'
Withdrawal:	'I just ignored it and left him to it in the end... I used to call him again and again, he said he'd get up soon, he never did, so in the end I just left him to it.'
Loss of independence:	'I used to get annoyed and have a go at him... it's hopeless, there's nothing you can do about it... I'm resigned to it now, I just take each day as it comes.'

Coping strategy: Reassurance	
Symptoms:	'I tried to reassure him that there was too much love around him, nobody could get him... I always react in this way though I put it in different ways each time.'

In conclusion, the coping styles of family members can have strong implications for the level of EE observed (Smith, *et al*, 1993). Any service utilising the EE framework would require regular assessments if an intervention based on EE is to be provided. Such assessments would need to incorporate among others, measures of coping style, perceived stress and burden.

Evaluating the expressed emotion concept

The result of early EE research was the implementation of clinical trials in the 1980s testing the efficacy of offering a psycho-educational family-based intervention to the patient and his/her relatives. Due to the complex and dynamic nature of the EE concept and its associated difficulties as outlined above, it is suggested that, if employed as the 'gold' standard, EE would be a poor measure of treatment success (Goldstein & Kopeikin, 1981). Smith and Birchwood (1990) suggest that a broader focus than EE is required to measure success and that multiple outcome measures such as social functioning, relatives' burden, and patients'/relatives' satisfaction with the intervention be utilised in assessing the treatment's efficacy.

The problems of using EE levels as inclusion criteria have been discussed earlier in the chapter, and it has been suggested that psychosocial problems may exist in low as well as high EE families. An additional concern is the finding that some low EE families have attempted to cope with a challenging family member by using disengagement and distancing strategies (Vaughn, 1986; Smith & Birchwood, 1990). The danger in such cases is that the health professional, concentrating on reducing the risk of relapse, may overlook the needs of the family coping with the significant burden and stress of caring for a relative with psychosis.

Inasmuch as EE would be a poor indicator of the success of family intervention work, it is reasonable to suggest that, as a sole entry qualification, it would limit the availability of such a service to only those patients and relatives who are assessed as having a high EE score, usually at the point of hospital admission (Leff *et al*, 1982). There are distinct difficulties in recruiting patients during the acute stage of their psychotic episode. In addition, patients who have a history of poor contact with the services and/or are not regularly admitted upon relapse may have a similar level of need for family intervention (Smith & Birchwood, 1990).

There are clear pitfalls in evaluating the relationship between EE and relapse in studies where the measure of success is based solely upon the reduction of the patient's risk of relapse. In such cases, investigation of the links between EE and social outcome, or EE and the family's level of social skills are usually not possible. Evidence suggests that good patient outcome, in terms of relapse and social adjustment, is related to successful family coping strategies and a lack of family burden. Hence, expansion of the family intervention service's remit to enable relatives to cope by assessing the needs and wellbeing of the family may be a significant factor in the success of such an intervention.

Outcome studies

Overall, it can be confidently stated that the rates of relapse over 1–2 years produced by family intervention work are lower than those for standard treatment. The studies outlined show little difference between relapse and length of family intervention although it has been argued that a follow-up period of up to 12 months shows a less beneficial outcome for relapse than one of between 12 and 24 months (Penn & Meuser, 1996) (see **Table 1**, overleaf).

Table 1 Relapse rates from family intervention studies			
Study	n	Follow-up 9 or 12 months	24 months
Goldstein & Kopeikin			
■ family intervention	25	0*	–
■ routine treatment	28	16*	–
Leff *et al*			
■ family intervention	12	8	20
■ routine treatment	12	50	78
■ family therapy	12	8	–
■ relatives group	6	17	–
Kottgen *et al*			
■ family intervention	15	33	–
■ control (high EE)	14	43	–
■ control (low EE)	20	20	–
Falloon *et al*			
■ family intervention	18	6	17
■ individual intervention	18	44	83
Hogarty *et al*			
■ family intervention	21	19	–
■ social skills training	20	20	–
■ combined interventions	20	0	–
■ control	17	41	–
Tarrier *et al*			
■ family intervention	25	12	33
■ education only	14	43	57
■ routine treatment	15	53	60
Vaughn *et al*			
■ family intervention/education	18	41	–
■ routine treatment	18	65	–
Zhang *et al*			
■ family intervention	28	–	10
■ routine treatment	22	–	36
McFarlane *et al*			
■ multiple relative family intervention	83	–	16
■ single relative family intervention	89	–	27

*Study with 6 month follow-up period. (All subjects medicated unless stated).

A Family Intervention Service Model

In attempting to integrate family intervention with mainstream psychiatric treatment, careful consideration needs to be given to the issues we have outlined in this chapter. In particular, based upon the family centre 'model' established at All Saints Hospital in Birmingham, there are six specific aspects which are pertinent to developing such a resource.

The service does not use high EE status or acute admission as an entry point. Instead, the centre routinely initiates contact with individuals and their families at multiple entry points in the service including acute admission units, outpatient and maintenance medication clinics, day centres, and voluntary groups such as NSF and Mind. Service availability is not determined by referrals or specific individual requests for help but is offered routinely to families as one component of the psychiatric service.

Once an offer of help has been accepted, the specific characteristics and needs of the individual and family are assessed using various questionnaires and interview assessment measures. A needs/strengths profile is derived from the information, which is then used to plan a negotiated intervention. Services offered include: information and orientation to schizophrenia for patients and their families; helping the family and the individual cope and live with schizophrenia; training patients and families to recognise 'early warning signs' of relapse, and self-management of persisting symptoms.

Efforts are made to ensure that family needs are understood and responded to sympathetically within a framework of partnership (Hatfield, 1978). The approach with families is one that acknowledges the difficulties they may face in caring for a relative with schizophrenia, and sees the family as facing problems rather than as a 'problem family' in need of treatment. The emphasis is on helping the family to develop the necessary expertise, through the provision of expertise and skills to determine the most appropriate management strategies for the problem they face, rather than prescriptively providing solutions which families then follow. A crucial component is the negotiation of the goals of the intervention with the individual and the family; this not only defines needs and goals but also serves to overcome the 'adversarial set' between professional and family, which might be exacerbated when a therapy for the family is offered.

The family service has developed as a routine part of the total services offered to individuals with schizophrenia and their families. Close liaison is maintained with key professionals involved with a particular individual and through joint working and regular case reviews. Efforts are made to ensure that there is co-ordination and continuity in care and that the goals of the family intervention are in line with the overall treatment and rehabilitation plans for an individual.

The goal of maintaining patients in the community with their families requires the full use of community resources, both statutory and voluntary. The centre liaises closely with community agencies relevant to the particular needs of the individual and family. For example, in meeting the social and recreational needs for a given individual, use might be made of local community, recreation and adult education centres, social interest clubs or, if more specialised help is required, contact clubs and local day centres.

The availability of sufficient numbers of appropriately trained staff was identified as a key factor affecting the efficacy and continuity of family interventions within a routine psychiatric service. A crucial function of the family service is therefore one of dissemination, training and supervision. Three levels of training are routinely provided through in-service workshops and routine input to pre- and post-qualification training for all frontline professional staff: highlighting the needs of individuals with schizophrenia and their families; responding to the information and the emotional needs of individuals and their families following a diagnosis of schizophrenia, and helping families reduce the emotional and practical burden of schizophrenia.

A central resource of materials and expertise is maintained at the centre but, in addition, trained 'tutors' are identified as supervisors to whom staff can relate directly for information, support, and supervision. Back-up information materials are provided in the form of a teaching pack with a training manual, information booklets (Smith & Birchwood, 1985) and videos. The specific interventions are then offered routinely to families from staff trained in their use on the admission units, outpatient clinics, and in various community settings. This training and supervision structure thus promotes the long-term continuity of family interventions within the psychiatric service.

All aspects of the service are closely monitored and evaluated to ensure that the objectives of the intervention are being fulfilled, and that the quality of the service provision is maintained. Efforts to ensure that the dissemination of skills to frontline professionals does not dilute the intervention or prejudice quality are encouraged through the continued maintenance of the family centre as a central resource, together with the established system of 'in-house' supervision and training described above.

Early intervention for Relapse Prevention

Overview

Even an ideal combination of psychosocial interventions and drug therapy does not eliminate the potential for relapse (Hogarty *et al*, 1991). As such, the debilitating nature of relapse can result in the possibility of the individual developing residual symptoms and a greater probability of future regression (McGlashan, 1988), which in turn generally leads to greater social disablement (Birchwood, 1992).

Although the prediction of relapse may be only modestly effective, the focus of research upon the detection of early indicators to the loss of wellbeing does allow for early intervention. An investigation of the perceived wellbeing of patients attending for maintenance therapy (McCandless-Glincher *et al*, 1986) suggests that such indicators are useful in the formation of an early intervention strategy. Of the 62 subjects in this study, 61 said they could recognise early signs of relapse, and, as a result, the majority (50 out of 61) initiated some change in behaviour to combat this. These changes would include engaging in diversionary activity, seeking professional help, and resuming/increasing their medication. As these subjects had initiated symptom-monitoring and a range of resulting responses, it is possible that patterns of prodromal episodes, as precursors to relapse, may be identifiable.

This possibility was investigated in a large scale study where 145 subjects with a diagnosis of schizophrenia were recruited alongside 80 family members (Herz & Melville, 1980). The main question asked was: *'Could you tell that there were changes in your thoughts, feelings or behaviours that might have led you to believe that you were becoming sick and might have to go into hospital?'*. This was answered in the affirmative by 70% of patients and 93% of relatives. The results of this and a similar British study are detailed in **Table 2** opposite.

Both studies concur in finding dysphoric symptoms the most prevalent. There was agreement between patients in the Herz and Melville study that non-psychotic symptoms such as anxiety, tension and insomnia were part of the 'prodrome', and 50% of subjects felt that characteristic symptoms of the prodrome were repeated at each relapse. Finally, subjects reported the presence of many of the non-psychotic episodes during the non-acute periods of the illness.

Research has been conducted to investigate the effect of the putative prodromes, ie neurotic or dysphoric episodes, in a group of 54 schizophrenic patients (Hirsch & Jolley, 1989). In order to increase their ability to recognise dysphoric syndromes, patients and their keyworkers received a one-hour teaching session about schizophrenia that outlined the importance of dysphoric syndromes as a precursor to relapse. All subjects were symptom free at the commencement of the study, and received assessments using the SCL-90 (Derogatis *et al*, 1973), a self-report psychiatric measure developed for the assessment of psychiatric pathology, and Herz's Early Sign Questionnaire (ESQ)

Category	Birchwood *et al* (N=42) %	Rank [1]	Herz & Melville (N=80) %	Rank*[1]
Anxiety/agitation				
■ Irritable/quick tempered	62	2 (equal)	–	–
■ Sleep problems	67	1	69	7
■ Tense, afraid, anxious	62	2 (equal)	83	1
Depression/withdrawal				
■ Quiet, withdrawn	60	4	50	18
■ Depressed, low	57	5	76	3
■ Poor appetite	48	9	53	17
Disinhibition				
■ Aggression	50	7 (equal)	79	2
■ Restless	55	6	40	20
■ Stubborn	36	10 (equal)	–	–
Incipient psychosis				
■ Behaves as if hallucinating	50	7 (equal)	60	10
■ Being laughed at or talked about	36	10 (equal)	14	53.8
■ 'Odd behaviour'	36	10 (equal)	–	–

Table 2 Percentage of relatives reporting early signs

* There were many other symptoms assessed. Percentage reporting only shown for parallel data.

(Herz *et al*, 1982). All subjects received monthly assessments unless a dysphoric episode was evident. In such cases these questionnaires were administered at each such dysphoric episode and fortnightly thereafter. The requirement for relapse was defined as the emergence of florid symptoms, including hallucinations and delusions. Results showed that 73% of relapses were preceded by a prodromal period of dysphoric and neurotic symptoms within a month of relapse. These prodromes included symptoms such as depression, anxiety, interpersonal sensitivity and paranoid symptoms, and were confirmed by the SCL-90.

Although one half of the subjects in this study received maintenance medication and the other half received a placebo, all subjects were given additional medication upon the emergence of dysphoric

[1] The rank columns explain how confident relatives felt about certain early signs in predicting /detecting whether their family member with psychosis was relapsing. The rank will therefore show the most persistent indicators of relapse from the relatives point of view.

symptoms. Dysphoric episodes were far more common in the placebo group (76%) as opposed to the medicated group (27%). However, the prompt administration of medication does not provide clarification as to whether these dysphoric episodes were part of a reactivation of psychosis (true prodromes), and also whether such cases included 'false positives' possibly related to the use of a placebo. The use of the ESQ which is reproduced in **Table 2** (page 280) does underline the importance of symptoms of dysphoria/depression and the general blunting of drives and interest. Recorded experiences such as 'loss of control', 'fear of being alone' and 'puzzlement about objective experience' suggest the operation of psychological factors that we will discuss later in the chapter.

The results of the four major prospective studies of prodromal changes outlined by Birchwood (1992) suggest that psychotic relapse is preceded by non-psychotic dysphoric symptoms and low-level psychotic thinking, including ideas of reference and paranoid thoughts. However, the clarity of these results is clouded by the use of a targeted medication strategy (Hirsch & Jolley, 1989; Marder *et al*, 1984) in two of these studies which allows for potential confusion when attempting to decipher between putative prodromes and false positives. It is also suggested that the use of an early intervention strategy may have exaggerated the magnitude of the recorded prodromes. Subjects who do not relapse may develop fluctuations in levels of dysphoric symptoms, and fluctuations that are not part of a relapse (ie false positives), but which nevertheless may respond to medication if detected (highly likely) during the course of the study. Hence, such interventions may reduce the contrast between relapsed and non-relapsed groups.

A further potential complication is the finding that the pattern of prodromal symptoms suggests between-subject variability (Birchwood *et al*, 1989). Some patients may 'peak' on anxiety symptoms, others on disinhibition, and so on. Similarly, a small proportion may show no prodromal symptoms (Subotnik & Neuchterlain, *ibid*). The existence of prodromes of psychotic relapse is confirmed by the studies outlined above, although the limitation of group studies is evident from their inability to address the qualitative and quantitative between-subject variability in early signs and symptoms. This is supported by the finding that greater prediction was possible when patients were compared against their own baseline rather than that of others (Subotnik & Neuchterlain, *ibid*). Hence, it may be more useful to look at each patient's prodrome as a 'relapse signature', which contains core or common symptoms along with features unique to the patient. Identification of an individual's prodrome can, it is reasonable to assume, increase the overall predictive power of prodromal symptoms.

A Psychological Model of Prodromes

The research outlined above suggests **two stages in the relapse process**: **dysphoria**, including anxiety, restlessness and the blunting of drives, followed by **low-level psychotic pathology** such as suspiciousness, ideas of reference and so on. It is argued that strong features of the prodrome include 'loss of control', 'fear of going crazy' and 'puzzlement about objective experience' (Hirsch & Jolley, 1989). However, other studies suggest that a set of early symptoms is being overlooked. Some patients report a feeling of over-stimulation where external and internal events invade consciousness (Chapman, 1966). Visual and time distortions are commonplace and the resultant effect leads to feelings of derealization and depersonalisation (Donlon & Blacker, 1975). Patients often consult physicians with vague and diffuse somatic symptoms which suggest an overactivation of biological systems (Offenkrantz, 1962).

We argue that the patient faced with the myriad of symptoms intrinsic to psychosis attempts to rationalise and search for meaning in these experiences in order to provide him/herself with meaning and control. Those with little experience of relapse may be puzzled by these perceptual changes that occur and may respond to them with fear and confusion. Patients with greater experience will be aware of the 'danger' represented by the emergence of such symptoms and respond with a sense of foreboding, as they realise that something is about to happen over which they have little or no control, ie relapse. Dysphoria may therefore be regarded as a response to the emergence of a threatening or ominous event (the relapse), or a response to the failure to control what may be regarded as a highly dangerous and alarming event. The stress and ominous feelings this may create could accelerate the relapse process (see **Table 1,** p276).

Critical periods

Although little prospective research exists investigating the long-term effects of severe mental illness from first episode onwards, the available findings suggest that positive and negative symptoms stabilise within 24 months and that no further deterioration affects about 25% of the sample (Thara *et al*, 1994). This suggestion that deterioration reaches a plateau within the first two years of illness was suggested during the earliest days of mental health research (Bleuler, 1978), and has been reinforced by later studies (Carpenter & Strauss, 1991).

It would appear that for many individuals afflicted with severe mental illness, the initial period following the first episode may provide the best possibility for successful secondary prevention. Furthermore, the role of psychosocial adjustment within this framework, although not a well-researched topic, provides evidence which suggests that it may play a key role in the relapse prevention (Birchwood *et al*, 1997). Research indicates that nearly two-thirds of subjects, followed-up at an early or first-episode stage of illness, can have attempted suicide over a six year period since onset (Westermeyer *et al*, 1991). The necessity to focus upon the critical period of early psychosis is, we feel, the next step for intervention trials.

Implementation in a service context

As with the development of a family intervention provision, the necessity for close co-operation between patient, carer and professionals is of paramount concern in the early detection and treatment of relapse. The notion of an **'informed partnership'** between all parties suggests a clear set of initial stages where education and engagement can be undertaken. Information provided about early intervention and prodromes needs to be incorporated alongside general information about serious mental illness. The responsibility that is being placed upon the individual and relative to recognise components which may constitute a potential relapse and the need for treatment requires succinct explanation. The stability of the relationship provided by the professional will be reflected in the successful engagement and compliance of the patient to the early intervention treatment.

Individuals with a history of repeated relapse or who are at high risk due to factors – such as high EE, recovery from a recent relapse or low-dose maintenance medication – may be suitable for early intervention regimes. Patients who receive high doses of maintenance medication may not be suitable for a regime which relies upon increasing drug dosage to combat potential relapse, but may benefit from early intervention procedures based upon psychosocial designs (Penn & Meuser, 1996). In the case of clients receiving very high doses of medication or with severe drug-related symptoms, the likelihood of discriminating a prodrome against such a background would appear to be very difficult. Similarly, the absence of insight may hinder the potential usefulness of an early intervention strategy.

Four potential problem areas have to be addressed if an effective early intervention service is to develop. Firstly, the identification of 'early signs' would require intensive regular monitoring of mental state at least fortnightly, which is rarely possible in clinical practice. Secondly, some patients may choose to conceal their symptoms as relapse approaches and insight declines (Heinrichs *et al*, 1985).

Thirdly, many patients experience residual or persisting symptoms, cognitive deficits or drug side-effects which may obscure the validity of the prodromes. Finally, the characteristics of prodromes may vary from individual to individual and this information may be lost in the use of generalised scales for pathology and group design in research studies. This particular problem may be overcome by the use of precise interviewing techniques when obtaining information from the client, his/her family and close associates. A correlation between the accounts from such individuals may lead to greater accuracy in discriminating a future prodrome.

The use of the Early Signs Interview and Early Signs Scale (Birchwood, 1992) provides an ongoing system of monitoring with observations taken on a fortnightly basis, although the frequency of observations can be increased if there is any cause for concern. A sense of ownership over the collected data is to be encouraged and patients can be provided with regularly updated information at each interview in the form of printouts and graphs.

Upon the emergence of a prodrome both the patient and their family will require intensive support and counselling in order to combat the strain that may be associated with the possibility of relapse. The use of stress management techniques, diversionary activities and general support will help alleviate these concerns (Brier & Strauss, 1983), although quick access to such services would be a crucial component of any such intervention. Weekly, daily or even inpatient care – a powerful tool in the repertoire of early intervention work – can be offered not only to alleviate anxiety but also to emphasise the 'shared burden' which needs to be projected for the success of any such service.

Summary

In this chapter we have briefly reviewed the rationale, intervention and service implications of two new approaches to the psychological treatment of psychosis.

The argument for employing EE research within a clinical framework is strengthened by family intervention treatments, which indicate that targeting this particular factor will reduce the risk of potential relapse. However, it is important for the clinician to be aware of the burden and stress which families may also experience in such situations, and to associate good patient outcome with successful family coping and decreased family burden. In developing a family intervention service it is important to engage clients and their families if the risk of non-compliance is to be lowered. It is important that the service integrates effectively with existing treatment resources and crucial that it is reinforced by a training system available to all staff, which would provide the specialist skills required for such a service provision.

The usefulness of early intervention for relapse prevention lies in the accurate detection of indicators to the loss of wellbeing and, as such, requires a system of symptom monitoring and prodrome detection. The overall predictive power of early intervention is further enhanced by the identification of the individual client's prodrome and specific 'relapse signature'. The development of an early intervention service would require intensive and regular symptom monitoring, but also precise interviewing techniques in order to avoid client-specific information being lost. Upon the identification of a prodrome, the client and family will require intensive support and counselling, as well as rapid access to services.

In conclusion, we have suggested that recent research in the psychosocial approaches to serious mental illness provides robust evidence that, of the underlying abnormal processes and functioning experienced by clients and families, many are 'normal' and can be addressed therapeutically through the use of the cognitive-behavioural strategies. Each requires a collaborative partnership between client, carer and service provider which must be implemented in the context of a structure of care in which the client's needs are managed on a long-term basis in conjunction with other treatment modalities.

References

Barraclough, C. & Tarrier, N. (1990) Social functioning in schizophrenic patients I. The effects of expressed emotion and family intervention. *Social Psychiatry and Psychiatric Epidemiology* **25** 125–129.

Birchwood, M. J. (1986) The control of auditory hallucinations through the use of monoaural auditory input. *British Journal of Psychiatry* **149** 104–107.

Birchwood, M. J. (1992) Early intervention in schizophrenia: theoretical background and clinical strategies. *British Journal of Clinical Psychology* **31** 257–278.

Birchwood, M. J. & Cochrane, R. (1990) Families coping with schizophrenia: coping styles, their origins and correlates. *Psychological Medicine* **20** 857–865.

Birchwood, M. J., McGorry, P. & Jackson, H. (1997) Early intervention in schizophrenia. *British Journal of Psychiatry* **170** 2–5.

Birchwood, M. J. & Smith, J. (1987) Expressed emotion and first episodes of schizophrenia. *British Journal of Psychiatry* **152** 859–860.

Birchwood, M. J. & Smith, J. (1987) Schizophrenia and the Family. In: J. Orford (Ed) *Coping with Disorder in the Family*. Beckenham: Croom Helm.

Birchwood, M. J., Smith, J., MacMillan, J. F., Hogg, B., Prasad, R., Harvey, C. & Bering, S. (1989) Predicting relapse in schizophrenia: the development of an 'early signs' monitoring system using patients and families as observers. *Psychological Medicine* **19** 649–656.

Bleuler, M. (1978) *The Schizophrenic Disorders: Long-Term Patient and Family Studies* (trans. C. Clements). New Haven: Yale University Press.

Brier, A. & Strauss, J. S. (1983) Self control in psychiatric disorder. *Archives of General Psychiatry* **40** 1141–1145.

Brown, G. W., Birley, J. L. T. & Wing, J. K. (1972) Influence of family life on the course of schizophrenic disorders: a replication. *British Journal of Psychiatry* **121** 241–258.

Carpenter, W. & Strauss, J. (1991) The prediction of outcome in schizophrenia V: eleven year follow-up of the IPSS cohort. *Journal of Nervous and Mental Disease* **179** 517–525.

Chapman, J. (1966) The early symptoms of schizophrenia. *British Journal of Psychiatry* **112** 25–251.

Derogatis, L., Lipman, R. & Covi, L. (1973) SCL-90: an outpatient psychiatric rating scale – preliminary report. *Psychopharmacology Bulletin* **9** 13–17.

Donlon, P. T. & Blacker, K. H. (1975) Clinical recognition of early schizophrenic decompensation. *Disorders of the Nervous System* **36** 323–330.

Falloon, I. R. H. (1988) Expressed emotion: current status. *Psychological Medicine* **18** 269–274.

Goldstein, M. J. & Kopeikin, H. S. (1981) Short and long-term effects of combining drug and family therapy. In: M. J. Goldstein (Ed) *New Developments in Interventions with Families of Schizophrenics*. San Francisco: Jossey-Bass.

Greenley, J. R. (1986) Social control and expressed emotion. *Journal of Nervous and Mental Disease* **174** 24–36.

Hatfield, A. B. (1978) Psychological costs of schizophrenia to the family. *Social Work* **25** 355–359.

Heinrichs, D., Cohen, B. P. & Carpenter, W. T. (1985) Early insight and the management of schizophrenic decompensation. *Journal of Nervous and Mental Disease* **173** (133).

Herz, M. I. & Melville, C. (1980) Relapse in schizophrenia. *American Journal of Psychiatry* **137** 801–812.

Herz, M. I., Szymonski, H. V. & Simon, J. (1982) Intermittent medication for stable schizophrenic outpatients. *American Journal of Psychiatry* **139** 918–922.

Hirsch, S. R. & Jolley, A. G. (1989) The dysphoric syndrome in schizophrenia and its implications for relapse. *British Journal of Psychiatry* **suppl. 5** 46–50.

Hogarty, X. & Ulrich, X. (1977) Temporal effects of drug and placebo in delaying relapse in schizophrenic outpatients. *Archives of General Psychiatry,* **34** 297–301.

Hogarty, G. E., Anderson, C., Reiss, D., Kornblith, S., Greenwald, D., Ulrich, R. & Carter, M. (1991) Family psycho-education, social skills training, and maintenance chemotherapy in the aftercare treatment of schizophrenia, II: two year effects of a controlled study on relapse and adjustment. *Archives of General Psychiatry* **48** 340–347.

Koenigsberg, H. N. & Handley, R. (1986) Expressed emotion: from predictive index to clinical construct. *American Journal of Psychiatry* **143** 1361–1373.

Kuipers, L. & Bebbington, P. (1988) Expressed emotion research in schizophrenia: theoretical and clinical implications. *Psychological Medicine* **18** 893–909.

Leff, J. (1989) Controversial issues and growing points in research in relatives' expressed emotion. *International Journal of Social Psychiatry* **35** 133–145.

Leff, J. P. & Vaughn, C. E. (1985) *Expressed Emotion in Families.* New York: Guildford.

Leff, J., Kuipers, L., Berkowitz, R., Eberlein-Vries, R. & Sturgeon, D. (1982) A controlled trial of social intervention in the families of schizophrenic patients. *British Journal of Psychiatry* **141** 121–134.

Marder, S. R., Van Putten, T., Mintz, J., McKenzie, J., Labell, M., Faltico, G. & May, R. P. (1984) Costs and benefits of two doses of fluphenazine. *Archives of General Psychiatry* **41** 1025–1029.

McCandless-Glincher, L., McKnight, S., Hamera, E., Smith, B. L., Peterson, K. & Plumlee, A. A. (1986) Use of symptoms by schizophrenics to monitor and regulate illness. *Hospital and Community Psychiatry* **37** 929–933.

McGlashan, T. H. (1988) A selective review of recent North American follow-up studies of schizophrenia. *Schizophrenia Bulletin* **14** 515–542.

Offenkrantz, W. C. (1962) Multiple somatic complaints as a precursor of schizophrenia. *American Journal of Psychiatry* **119** 258–259.

Penn, L. P. & Mueser, K. T. (1996) Research update on the psychosocial treatment of schizophrenia. *American Journal of Psychiatry* **153** 607–617.

Smith, J. & Birchwood, M. J. (1990) Relatives and patients as partners in the management of schizophrenia. *British Journal of Psychiatry* **156** 654–660.

Smith, J. & Birchwood, M. J. (1987) Specific and non-specific effects of an educational intervention with families living with a schizophrenic relative. *British Journal of Psychiatry* **150** 645–652.

Smith, J. & Birchwood, M. J. (1985) *Understanding schizophrenia (vols. I-IV).* West Birmingham Health Authority: Health Promotion Unit.

Smith, J., Birchwood, M. J., Cochrane, C. & George, S. (1993) The needs of high and low expressed emotion families: a normative approach. *Social Psychiatry and Psychiatric Epidemiology* **28** 11–16.

Subotnik, K. L. & Nuechterlain, K. H. (1988) Prodromal signs and symptoms of schizophrenia relapse. *Journal of Abnormal Psychology* **97** 405–412.

At the Core of Mental Health © Pavilion 2000

Tarrier, N. (1989) The effect of treating the family to reduce relapse in schizophrenia. *Journal of the Royal Society of Medicine* **82** 423–424.

Tarrier, N., Barraclough, C. D., Vaughn, C., Bamrah, J. D., Porceddu, K., Watts, S. & Freeman, H. (1988) The community management of schizophrenia: a controlled trial of a behavioural intervention with families to reduce relapse. *British Journal of Psychiatry* **153** 532–542.

Thara, R., Henrietta, M. & Joseph, A. (1994) Ten year course of schizophrenia – the Madras longitudinal study. *Acta Psychiatrica Scandanavica* **90** 329–336.

Vaughn, C. (1986) Patterns of Emotional Response in Families of Schizophrenic Patients. In: M. J. Goldstein, I. Hand and K. Halweg (Eds) *Treatment of Schizophrenia: Family Assessment and Intervention*. Berlin: Springer.

Westermeyer, J. F., Harrow, M. & Marengo, J. T. (1991) Risk for suicide in schizophrenia and other psychotic and non-psychotic disorders. *Journal of Nervous and Mental Disease* **179** 259–266.

Chapter 11

Healing and Curing: Deinstitutionalising Psychiatry

Michael Radford

Introduction: from revolving doors to revolving services

Nuts and bolts

'Getting the nuts and the bolts together' can describe the objectives of recovery-oriented, community-based practice. This draws attention to the changes of attitude needed to counter the marginalising description of people with mental health problems as 'nuts' from whom others, inwardly or outwardly, have been socialised to bolt. It also serves to emphasise the wide range of practical measures required to support each other in everyday meaningful life. Caring is not enough: attention needs to be focused on the attitudes and the practical measures aimed not only at 'curing' but also at 'healing' and 'recovery'. Community psychiatry can also be dubbed *'psychiatry with the blinkers off'*. Shedding institutional blinkers involves more than working away from hospital. Though for many this change of setting is challenging enough to make some of the changes necessary to getting the nuts and bolts together, it is quite possible for the increase in uncertainty to make us transpose defensive attitudes or invent new

ones. Shedding blinkers, genuinely deinstitutionalising psychiatry, involves perception of other perspectives, readjustment of power relations and less damaging ways of containing uncertainty.

Revisiting Kathleen Jones' history of the mental health services is a good way to grasp the agenda of change there has been over the last generation. Jones (1972) described three 'revolutions' that were happening in the mental health system between the passing of the *National Health Service Act* in 1946 and the publication of *Better Services for the Mentally Ill* (Department of Health,1971). The Act required local authorities to pass control of the mental hospitals to the newly formed health authorities, and hospital care was separated from primary care.

> *'The first major change after 1948 was the entry of statutory authorities into the field of community work, and the consequent shift in the role of voluntary organizations. Local authority mental health departments began to shoulder the burden of care in the community... After 1948, local authority care, day and night hospitals, sheltered workshops and other experimental forms of care did much to break down the old distinction between being totally well (at home) and totally sick (in hospital). Britain began to attempt the provision of a flexible range of services to meet the varying needs of individuals.'*
> (Jones,1972)

The pharmaceutical revolution

Jones describes *'the pharmaceutical revolution'*, which started with the trials of Chlorpromazine in the early 1950s at All Saints Hospital in Birmingham, and were conducted by the pychopharmacologist who can claim to be the city's first professor of psychiatry. There were then to be found rows of people in catatonic states who were brought out of their frozen state when given the drug and who reverted when it was stopped (Cy Elkins, personal communication). Later in the decade, after the drug was licensed, such people were able to work in the new factory started by the Birmingham Industrial Therapy Association. In similar projects across Britain, people who were patients and ex-patients of the mental hospitals were 'getting nuts and bolts together' – counting them and putting them into plastic bags! This was an unfamiliar activity for people who had been lining the walls of the hospital, which allowed them to be perceived differently; but it did not fulfil the more ambitious projects of social inclusion and 'recovery' because there was little effect on power relations. It was a start, but more was needed for services to become community-based and recovery-oriented.

Jones stated that the development of psychopharmacology allowed for extramural treatment and a shift from talk of 'aftercare' to talk of 'alternative care'. She acknowledged the limits of medication *'as it was gradually realised that the psychotropic drugs alleviated, but did not cure'.* The following years have seen the recognition of the potential for permanent damage from anti-psychotic medication in the form of tardive dyskinesia and of reversible yet disabling damage to social and sexual function. Despite the development of drugs with fewer side-effects, Jones' conclusion as to their limits still stands for most people with major mental illness (in particular, chronic schizophrenia and resistant depression).

Thornicroft and Tansella (1999) quote the conclusion of one of the leading psychiatrists of the day:

> *'Certainly if we had to choose between abandoning the use of all the new psychotropic drugs and abandoning the industrial Therapy Units and other social facilities available to us, there would be no hesitation about the choice: the drugs would go.' (Lewis 1959)*

The administrative revolution

'The administrative revolution' was Jones' term for such things as the development of open door policies, the recognition that mental hospitals *'catered for a range of residential and occupational needs that could be re-provided outside the walls, the experimentation with "therapeutic communities" in the hospital and the growth of outpatient clinics, hostels, therapeutic social clubs, psychiatric units in general hospitals and mental health social work in the community'.* It is important to remember that this process started before the introduction of the new medications (Shepherd, 1957) and was initiated by concern for human rights and the recognition of unacceptable levels of abuse. It is easy for some nostalgic critics of care in the community to forget the damning mental hospital inquiries of the 1950s, '60s and '70s.

To Jones' lists can now be added the continued pace of mental hospital closures and the replacement of revolving door admissions with the possibility of provision of significant amounts of care and treatment centred outside hospitals in people's own homes and workplaces (Radford,1992). This Copernican revolution is both logical and logistically feasible: services can be made to revolve around a person and their family, instead of requiring the person to move around the service facilities. The person and their situation become the hub, not the water tower or the acute hospital bed.

When properly resourced and supported, such components of the spectrum of care allow professionals to avoid the potential of *'Radford's special law of psychiatric perversity'* under which we can sometimes seem to spend half our time persuading people to come into hospital and the other half persuading them to leave. (The general law, which was conceptualised only to make mental health trainees watch out for our propensities to perversity, is that if a service user finds the courage to express an opinion, mental health professionals will try to convince him of the opposite.)

Both short-term *'acute crisis resolution'* and long-term *'assertive continuing care'* can be provided and, when properly organised, can reduce the need for hospital services, making them affordable. This has been shown in randomised controlled trials, which although not blind, *are* more representative of regular service populations than most drug trials, and which have shown outcomes as good as, or better than, more traditional services as well as being preferred by users and carers (Stein & Test, 1980; Radford, 1992). Despite being against the then-current ideology of 'normalisation' of mental illness by moving its centre of treatment from mental to general hospitals (Hoenig & Hamilton, 1969) this innovation has been spreading (Stein, 1992). There was really no evidence of any benefit to service users and their families of the move to general hospitals, but there was much less resistance from psychiatrists.

Doctors are not the only ones to be suspicious of the move to comprehensive community-based treatment. A key element is seen to be the **'assertive continuing care team'** (or **'assertive outreach team'**), and the practices of the new teams have been regarded with suspicion by some patients who see them as moves to re-colonise their lives as much as did the staff in the old long-stay wards. There is also recognition among some professionals that, unless there is an emphasis on TCL (Training in Community Living), patterns of dependency can be recreated and maintained (TLC – tender loving care, is not enough). Thus new patterns of delivery can turn out to be anti-recovery (see below). More positively, Sashidharan (1999) makes the point that there is a good chance of avoiding the abuse that can occur in hospital, and providing better anti-racist and culturally competent services, when these are carried out in people's own territory. From my own experience in the multi-racial Sparkhill community mental health team, I agree with his argument, but there is no guarantee that new service patterns alone will deliver these crucial agendas, because personal and institutional racism are so deeply ingrained and pervasively portable.

The NHS plan published in July 2000, calls for 335 home treatment teams to be established in the UK by 2004 (DoH, 2000) and expects a saving of 30% acute beds. The chief reason to support this initiative is that it increases choice for staff and service users and when properly operated is usually preferred by them and their families and carers. Developing manpower (person power) is a key problem also addressed in the plan.

The legislative revolution

The third of Jones' revolutions in mental health services was 'the legislative'. She refers to changes that followed the 1957 Royal Commission. The terms of reference set in 1954 were as follows:

> *'To inquire, as regards England and Wales, into the existing law and administrative machinery governing the certification, dentition, care (other than hospital care or treatment under the* National Health Service Acts 1946–52)*, absence on trial or licence, discharge and supervision of persons who are, or are alleged to, be suffering from mental illness or mental defect, other than Broadmoor patients; to consider, as regards England and Wales, the extent to which it is now, or should be made, statutorily possible for such persons to be treated as voluntary patients, without certification; and to make recommendations.'*

The reference to dentition is not only a reminder of the now discredited theory of focal sepsis as a cause of disease, including mental illnesses which lead to the (often involuntary) removal of the teeth of many confined to institutions, but also a reminder of the same intervention as a sad and desperate remedy for managing the behaviour of people who came to be biting themselves or others. It should remind us of the damaging results of false theories on the one hand and of lack of useful theory on the other. One such theory, widely held at the time, was that there was no recovery from schizophrenia. Good progress notes at the time used to read 'well institutionalised'. The aim was to provide safe and uncontroversial exclusion.

The *1959 Mental Health Act* in England and Wales allowed for widespread voluntary and informal treatment in state mental hospitals for the first time. The *1983 Act* also incorporated liberal civil rights concerns. More recently, however, the *Mental Health Patients in the Community Act of 1995* which introduced the *Supervised Discharge*

Act of 1996, was concerned to increase legal control. Discussions in 1998–9 of a new *Mental Health Act* seemed to reflect a political agenda of shifting responsibility for social control even more strongly to mental health professionals. This is in contrast to the Italian *Law 180* that followed the reforms in Trieste. These were much later than those in Britain but more radical in tone. *Law 180*, passed in 1978, placed responsibility for suicide on the individual and for threats of harm to others on the police. Doctors are responsible for compulsory treatment in respect of people's health and not for social control. Dilemmas similar to those in England and Wales exist for those exercising this responsibility, but the atmosphere is different (Pino Pini, personal communication). The same is true for Belgium, Spain and Germany where the courts decide if someone needs compulsory treatment, as used to be the case in the UK. In these countries, *'psychiatrists treat people, but it is not their job to be responsible for individual citizens' behaviour in the community'* (Turner *et al*, 1999).

The control or containment of uncertainty in both intra-psychic and inter-personal areas has always been a central issue in mental health theory and practice. It is probably the main role of mental health professionals as defined by the expectations of others. A minority seem to relish this role of controlling other people's lives, but most psychiatrists, as doctors, want to be in the role of treating individuals without being agents of social control. The same is just as true of other mental health practitioners.

The need for a philosophical revolution?

The role of psychiatry in mental health and the role of mental health in society are problems confronting all mental health practitioners. Struggling with the dilemmas presented by negotiating these often conflicting roles reveals the possible need for a fourth revolution: what in Jones' vein could be called *'the philosophical revolution'*. Delays in publishing the UK *National Service Framework for Mental Health* were variously put down to the problems in finding an acceptable solution to the confinement of people with *'dangerous severe personality disorder'* and to cost problems with the Treasury. But there are philosophical differences. The key difference from the *National Service Framework for Coronary Heart Disease* and the model for breast cancer is that an attempt is being made to negotiate, through mental health, an agenda for social care and control and not just for the medical treatment of illness. The aim of this chapter is to draw attention to some of the philosophical debates involved. Space allows only a sketch, but teachers, practitioners and service users may value some awareness in order to make sense of some of what is going on in current debates.

Healing, curing and recovery

A re-examination of the underlying theoretical bases of mental health activity is demanded, not only because of the continuing dilemmas between the wishes to ameliorate the distress caused by complaints seen as symptoms of mental illness ('cure'), the demands to limit related behaviours ('containment') and the pressure to keep situations stable ('maintenance'). It is also necessary because of the shifting ideologies underpinning the rapidly changing contexts and practices, described above as Jones' three revolutions. Mental health services are different from other health and social welfare systems because they carry a greater symbolic load in the handling of various anxieties about rational control in Western society. They are set in a number of conflicting philosophical, moral and ethical discourses.

Instead of the previous practices aimed at the exclusion of irrationality (see Bracken's analysis, page 308), present 'modernised' services emphasise the twin projects of 'recovery' and 'social inclusion'. The draft strategy, published in 1999 by the largest of the regional health authorities in England, stresses these projects. It is backed up by four papers which explore the concepts commissioned by the West Midlands Regional Office from the International Mental Health Network, which is a loose alliance of service users, carers and professionals, and both clinicians and managers (Carling & Allott,

1999a, b and c; Carling *et al*, 999). Recovery and social inclusion are also emphasised in the pan-Birmingham Mental Health Strategy document (jointly produced by the social services department and the health authority) and are restated in the *National Service Framework* (Department of Health, 1999).

Within current discourse about recovery-oriented, community-based mental health, there is a pivotal, but inconsistently conceptualised, distinction between 'curing' and 'healing' (and recovery). Two sets of activities often overlap and may interact, either positively or negatively, but should not be confused. The former is aimed at fixing disorders of a physical (and, perhaps, psychological) mechanism. The latter is aimed at restoring 'full' human functioning (and meaning) after a breakdown. I do not mean to indicate a predetermined endpoint, but rather a process in which we are all involved. Some psychotherapies and most physical therapies aim to cure and make claims to be 'empirical' or 'scientific'. Curing in this sense is something done *to* a patient. The term 'patient' was introduced as a general term by the British empiricist philosopher and physician, John Locke (1632–1704), who used it to distinguish between an active 'agent', which was the (mechanical) cause of an effect in a passive 'patient', which was acted upon by such an agent. Later it was used in medical discourse to refer to those upon whom doctors practise.

By contrast, healing, in the sense above, is something undertaken together with fellow human beings. Inasmuch as the activities of 'curing' are allowed to produce habits of passivity, they are liable to be a handicap to the 'healing', which can lead to 'recovery'. This idea is quite familiar to the practice of psychiatric rehabilitation. It is perhaps less familiar when discussed in the discourse on complementary medicine. It could be argued that some Shamanistic practices were done to the recipients, but most traditional or complementary practices require full participation in a validation process, the end point of which is reaffirmation of the person and reintegration to the processes of social groups and valid social roles. Chinese medical practices, such as acupuncture, are based on the

At the Core of Mental Health © Pavilion 2000

principle of balancing the flow of energy in the whole person. Perhaps this is why mental health service-user groups are keen to advocate complementary practices as alternatives to the psychiatric practice that is being offered to them. Complementary practice is generally seen as holistic and psychiatric practice is often experienced as reductionist. There may be some curing, but complementary medicine should probably be seen as contributing to healing and be evaluated in terms of reintegration and not primarily of symptom relief (see **Chapter 12**).

The process of recovery is not initiated until both mechanism and meaning are being restored, until both curing and healing have begun (Hill, 1970).

'Recovery' is a term used in the 1990s in a new sense in discourses about mental health practice. In their review, Tooth, Kalyanansundarum and Glover (1997) find the term being used with two meanings. The first is in the questioning of an assumption of universally poor prognosis for conditions arising, for example, from the schizophrenias. This strand seeks to separate the effects of the disorder itself from the effects of how those diagnosed have been treated. When the social and psychological factors in the consequent disability are ameliorated, it is claimed that as many as 26% of people with chronic conditions previously thought irrecoverable, can be rehabilitated and stay independent of the services. This is about the same as the encouraging outcomes in 'early intervention' studies, when these aims and measures are applied near the onset.

The other meaning of 'recovery' is that, even when their illness cannot be cured, in the sense of total symptom remission, people can 'get on with their lives', finding purpose and meaning independent of the mental health system. The study by Tooth *et al (op cit.)* questioned service users with a DSM IV diagnosis of schizophrenia who were functioning well, about who and what had been most helpful in their recovery. Some acknowledged medication, but most put as the key factor the quality of the relationships they had had with particular people, which included some service professionals (those who were experienced as committed to their recovery as people), as well as some friends and family members.

In an accessible feature article, Mike Smith (1998a) repeated that *'the core of our message is that professionals must start to see the route to recovery being with the person not with the professional. There may be many things we can do to help a person on the road'* and we should find out what these are and do them. The participatory workbooks on *Working with Voices* and *Working with Self-Harm* exemplify this (Coleman & Smith, 1997; Smith, 1998b).

The recovery literature exposes the need for rethinking service planning and professional training, in order to offer more competent engagement with people suffering with mental health problems. Williams and Lindley (1996) have reviewed the recent theory and experience of working with service users in the UK to do this. These authors have had a long commitment to the process and conclude that the fashionable strategy of market consumerism is not enough to correct the problems in the mental health system. This is because of the reluctance to link structural inequalities with their profound psychological consequences and thus not to recognise sufficiently the power imbalance and the effects of internalised oppression. Service users as consumers do not have free choice and have been trained not to expect it. Protest, or lack of it, are equally liable to be pathologised.

> *'When the social context is ignored it is easy to view psychological distress and disturbance as individual aberration. By locating the problem within the victim, mental health services protect the interests of those who are privileged rather than meet the needs of those who seek help.'*

This has resulted in provision which is *'irrelevant, risky and stigmatising, within contexts that are unsafe. There is an appreciable risk that those using services will be sexually and/or physically abused'*. Service users are angry.

Williams and Lindley (*ibid*)conclude that *'in the final analysis it is neither just, nor realistic, to expect mental health services to be transformed by those who have least power. It is vital that service users, professionals and carers find better ways of struggling for change together.'*

In a piece entitled 'The myth of recovery', Whitwell (1999) described the beginning of a study that would have paralleled that of Tooth *et al.* He pointed out that 'recovery' cannot be understood in the usual sense of getting back to the state of being before the illness (or mental health problem) started, because people identifying themselves to him as 'recovered' nevertheless reported continuing symptoms, reduced tolerance of stress, restricted lifestyle, unemployment, stigma and poverty. Whitwell revisits and recommends the term 'survivor' which many, who have had experiences of having mental health services applied coercively, have borrowed from those rebuilding their lives after physical or sexual abuse, or from experiences in prison and of racism. In a chapter on recovery from racism, 'Healing our Wounds: liberatory mental health care', bell hooks (1996) writes of the need to link individual work for self-recovery with progressive action for political change. She emphasises the importance of fighting the internalised oppression which has allowed behaviours, used adaptively to survive coercion, to be confirmed as racist stereotypes. I think that similar things have been allowed to happen to those in the mental health system.

According to Whitwell (*ibid*) the term 'survivor' *'is generally unpopular with psychiatrists because of its negative implications'*, (identifying not only mental illness but also psychiatric services as assaults on personhood), *'surviving the damage and coping with disability and disadvantage are alternatives to the medical model'*. I disagree that they are alternatives: both are needed as I will argue below. But it is important to challenge the ethical domination of some versions of 'the medical model'. There are a number of definitions of the medical model (Clare, 1986) and Parsons' description of 'the sick role' is complementary. A key aspect of this is that patients should follow the advice of doctors (Parsons, 1951) in order to legitimise exemptions from social duties.

Parsons' definition is particularly problematic when applied to the dilemmas arising from dealing with chronic conditions, when people cannot get cured. For people with long-term conditions, alternatives are needed to the sick role.

Mere survival, however, is not enough. Whitwell refers back to traditional healing for a different frame of reference: *'the strength to carry on and survive personal damage is one of the perennial themes of art and literature'.* Healers, and others through contact with them, *'derive strength from the damage they have sustained and overcome'.* Recovering service users can help others towards recovery. When a stage is achieved beyond bleeding into each other's wounds, the authenticity and role modelling can be more important to the healing process than medical, or any other, advice-giving.

The same is true of mental health professionals. Those entering mental health professions often do so following traumas in earlier life and the effect of this deserves more attention. Psychiatric nurses, for example, have been shown to have had more such experiences than a comparison group of general nurses, and they both have had more than a group of workers in the computer industry (Virdi, 1993). Such factors in motivation should be distinguished from effectiveness, but healing qualities resulting from growth stimulated by such personal experiences are important in mental health work. Without such abilities there cannot even be adequate engagement with service users, and without human engagement there can only be coercive service delivery. This is a source of protest by service users against the 'assertive outreach' strategies now in the *National Service Framework*. I suggested we should be using the term 'available outreach' (Radford, 1992) – this is more in line with what people want. The necessary attitudes were examined by Professor Sir Denis Hill 20 years ago. Writing about the qualities of a good psychiatrist, Hill (1978) warned that the worst kind of clinician is one capable only of routinely applying the current fashion of treatment according to the latest fad of diagnosis. This picture of 'the medical model' is behind some of the attacks on psychiatrists and is not defensible.

Ron Coleman (1999) identifies himself as a 'survivor' and distinguishes between symptomatic recovery, social recovery and personal recovery. For him, only the last has satisfactory value and it consists first in reclaiming power through building self-confidence, self-esteem, self-awareness and self-acceptance and second in reclaiming ownership of one's life and experience. Also, it depends on the external existence of real choices and, through all of this, on having allies and personal relationships with friends, neighbours, family, lovers and those mental health workers who are committed to recovery. He describes the COPS (Choice, Ownership, People and Self) Recovery Programme and provides a model care plan to aid recovery. This sets out a structure for the person to consider and write down their personal development wishes, their strengths, coping abilities and problems, and the help they would like to have. It focuses on aims-led instead of needs-led assessment. There are three prerequisites:

> *'If you cannot do the following three things, then you are not ready to use the plan:*
>
> *1 Be honest with yourself.*
>
> *2 Take responsibility for your own recovery.*
>
> *3 Be committed to your own recovery.'*

A pay off for the effort is that:

> *'It may help professionals to base their services upon what YOU REALLY WANT, and not what THEY THINK YOU NEED. It may help them to identify their own training needs and plan appropriately for the future of mental health services'*
> (Coleman, 1999)

Coleman's important book, *Recovery: an alien concept*, challenges all parties in the mental health system. Coleman was diagnosed as having schizophrenia at a major London teaching hospital when he was in a severe personal crisis and hearing voices. It took him ten years to recover and to get off neuroleptics. Psychiatrists are still under the kind of time pressure that makes it difficult to listen and understand such experiences. At the time, there was not the present recognition that hearing voices can be a normal experience (Romme, 1996). Part of Coleman's recovery came from working with Marius Romme, Sandra Escher and others in establishing the UK (and later, the international) Voice Hearers Network. In passing, it is worth noting his and other service users' accounts of the difficulties in coming off medication that is widely regarded as non-addictive. The voices became more distressing and the usual advice is then to continue taking the medication. What he needed and arranged for himself, was more personal support. Recent UK government statements are that non-compliance should no longer be a legal option for people with the diagnosis who have a history of difficult behaviours. In the future it is possible that Coleman would not be allowed to recover.

Another point made by Whitwell (*op cit.*) is that an over-optimistic attitude can lead to insufficient recognition of damage done to people by mental illness; this can result in (false) transactions with service users and carers, in which service professionals offer the hope of recovery in the sense of cure, and thus deny the reality of such damage and the depth of the struggles that ensue. This is a form of denial that makes it ever more important to separate the potential and actual effects of the illness from the potential and actual effects of the treatment. False optimism, as well as false pessimism, will impede recovery processes.

Another aspect of therapeutic optimism is the danger of the many psychological theories which continue (falsely) to pathologise and to offer 'cures' to people encountering problems of life which are not mental illnesses. Stokes (1994) made the same point when he wrote that *'therapist and client may remain endlessly "glued" together as if generation of hope about the future were by itself a cure'.* Although beyond the scope of this chapter, it is important to be aware of the debates that have ranged from Lewis (1953) through Scheff (1966) and Fulford (1989) to Bolton and Hill (1996) on the possible interactions of social, psychological and physical processes, and to avoid simplistic reductionist theory and practice. True cures would be greatly welcomed, and the search goes on. However, when none are available, it is the healing agendas that lie at the centre of the approach to mental health, based on recovery and social inclusion.

Aspects of enlightenment: freedom and rationality

Certainty through exclusion

Foucault (1965) provides a genealogy of the actions and attitudes directed at people with severe mental health problems following the Western Enlightenment. He makes key distinctions between the activities of mental health service providers as a practical mental health system and a wider, more generalised, political mental health system. The former, in his account, acts more or less to keep in place psychosocial processes by which irrationality in social and personal life generally is controlled and uncertainty reduced.

This distinction is of the greatest importance because conflation between the irrationality of persons with mental illness and irrationality in cultural, political and other group processes hides the true social and political causes of human violence, by identifying them with mental illness. This was not Foucault's point, but it is important because failure to make this distinction allows for the idea that it is some kind of individual pathology that leads to violence. Except in rare cases, violence perpetrated by people with mental illness has the same causes as in anybody else. It is this that makes impossible and unfair the role that psychiatrists have had as agents of social control whether willingly or otherwise.

Table 1 Modernist divides in European and American psychiatry

1 Western Enlightenment projects to increase certainty by exclusion

(The System)	(The Self)	(Science and Scientism)
Segregating mad people	Suppressing madness within	Applying rational thought
The asylums project	The rational individual	The university clinics
	(and the Freudian project)	

2 Enlightenment values paradoxically confronting such projects:

liberté	fraternité	égalité

3 Some resulting new practices:

De-institutionalisation	Club-house movement	Advocacy
Normalisation	Social Firms	Pick and mix/Smorgasbord
(Move to General Hospitals)	The search for a new	(Educational models)
Open employment	psycho-social-dynamics	mutual learning processes

4 How can we contain the re-emergence of uncertainty?

Please write here how we might together avoid a new Napoleonic solution ....

....

....

5 Eastern Enlightenment: factors to increase wisdom by inclusion

Faith	Energy	Mindfulness	Equanimity	Wisdom

Foucault's thesis, echoed by Bracken (1995) and summarised in **Table 1**, above, was that the activities of mental health workers could be understood as subservient to the mental health system and that, inspired by the Western Enlightenment, this lead to the:

■ segregation of mad people via the asylum project

■ suppression of madness within, via the myth of the rational individual

■ the application of rational thought in treating mentally ill patients via the university clinics project. It is necessary to note that there are historical inaccuracies in Foucault's account (Fish, 1999). This does not mean, however, that his theories do not provide insight into the political functions that the mental health system has come to serve.

Pat Bracken – a psychiatrist currently working in a home treatment team in Bradford which employs service users in recovery – has provided an analysis of the influence of Western Enlightenment on the theory and practice of mental health services and, in his practice, a practical confrontation (Bracken, 1995; Bracken & Cohen, 1999). His thesis is summarised in the columns of the upper part of **Table 1**, to which I have added a section suggesting that the enlightenment values exemplified in the French Revolution confront the consequences of an uncritical rationalism that was transmitted by Descartes from Aristotle (see discussion of **Science and scientism**, p311). Bracken goes further than Foucault in problematising the psychoanalytical project (see The self, below). As an appendix in the table, I have also added some contrasting ideas from Eastern Enlightenment traditions to show that there are older and broader ideas available and current in the world.

The system

Foucault sees significance in the fact that the Western Asylums Project designed to subject 'pauper lunatics' to moral treatment and which came to protect communities from mad people, took place against a background of the Western colonisation of large parts of the world's population. White racist stereotypes were invented and served, for a while, to insulate humanitarian protest. Dehumanising practices were accompanied by dehumanising theories. Judged to fall short of the ideal of the rational man, Black, Asian and Irish people were thought of as less than fully human and the same attitudes were applied to women, children and later to the inhabitants of lunatic asylums. The persistence of these attitudes leads to the recognition that the non-White populations nowadays found in European inner cities are placed in (at least) 'double jeopardy' when faced with mental health problems (Fanon, 1952).

The self

In the second of Bracken's themes (**Table 1**, second column), there is a similar point to be made about the assumption that White patriarchy equates to the rational individual ideal of Western enlightenment. There is an enormous quantity of literature and debate on the self, from enlightenment ideas to what are now being called post-modernist. The context here is that the enlightenment thinkers invented and propounded a new notion of the self, that was derived from the 'I' in Descartes' answer to ontological doubt (*'I think, therefore I am'*). This 'Enlightenment Self' was the essence of the individual. It included only conscious thoughts and feelings and excluded aspects that were foreign to its identity. It was conceived as a fixed constituent of the person, separate from other people, autonomous, coherent and in control of its domain. As it became free of the 'tutelage' of others (Kant, 1784), it needed a boundary of what was 'me' and 'not-me'. Aspects of the self that did not fit were excluded, disowned. On this account, those aspects were identified as the 'Excluded Other': characteristics of the self that resembled those of other (denigrated) groups were denied. Jung called it 'the shadow' (Martin, 1955/'76).

These political descriptions had great influence and underpinned the marginalisation of people who were separated from power over themselves. Madness within was suppressed: the consequence of being publicly categorised as 'mad' became very frightening because it would lead to social exclusion. This is still the case, even if in a less extreme way.

At the level of life history, an example of the opposite temporal order of self-development is suggested by Tolstoi's assertion that Anna Karenina should by read at three stages of a person's life: first for the romance, second for the politics and last (the most mature) for the spiritual philosophy.

As an iterative method of self-development, a person may embrace, explore and celebrate, by themselves or in groups, each of their affinity group identities – old, middle-aged or young; White or Black; male or female; owning, middle or working class; village of residence and country of birth; Animist, Atheist, Bhuddist, Christian, Hindu, Humanist, Islamic, Jain, Jewish, Pagan, Sikh, Stoicist, Zoroastrian, or many more; in this context especially helper or helpee, and so on. Then we might work to become conscious of the characteristics of the excluded others, of the groups whose differences help maintain our restricted identities, because we have been trained to suppress and deny characteristics of ours that are like theirs. Finally, we may seek to enlarge ourselves by becoming conscious of, and embracing a wider and deeper humanity: one which is inclusive and not exclusive in its identification.

Another exercise can be described as 'holding the third corner'. One triangle in mental health politics is that with professional, service user and community (or it may be carer) on each of the corners. Collusion is often seen between the three possible parings, each of which exclude a third. Professional and service user may join up to blame, or denigrate the concerns of families or public opinions. Families and service users may blame professional for poor service performance, or even for the creation of mental illness. Professionals, families (and public watchdogs) may conspire to remove the practical expression of rights and endanger the freedom of service users. Holding the third corner does not allow such pseudo-mutualities: it is less comfortable, but it is more likely to result in healing and recovery for all.

Science and scientism and the re-emergency of uncertainty

The third column in **Table 1** – Bracken's third theme – represents the application of scientific method to the phenomena of mental illness through the practice of university clinic professorship. Most of the theory that informs psychiatric practice comes from this application of rational-scientific thought to mental health problems.

As stated above, a key doctrine of the Enlightenment was that *'the truth is manifest'* to any individual and does not depend on interpretation from the church or an expert body (Popper, 1960). It could be recognised by an authority within each person, either through clear thought or clear perception. There is a body of specialist common sense in psychiatry, but it is not necessarily true. It may well change quite radically, and cannot be put forward as the truth. Instead, in my view, the place of science is not as a replacement of common sense, but as a method of application of the current common sense, which may include various well tried recipes for treatment and formulae to contain our own and others' uncertainties. MacIntyre and Popper (1983) describe a *'new medical ethics'* that corresponds to the clinical method of evaluating intended effects, and monitoring for both expected side-effects and for unexpected, unintended effects. They advocate the liberal conceptualisation of what is now seen as audit and evidence-based practice. In order to be free of false and oppressive Western knowledge claims, Popper (1998) suggests that we should go back before Aristotle to Xenophenes for the basis of a new and responsible professional attitude. We could also go outside Western philosophy and study the practice of Eastern enlightenment.

This means that patient and doctor, recipient and clinician, must be partners in the application of current knowledge. Even if we are to regard scientific knowledge as *'common-sense writ large'* (Popper, 1959) and as having no guarantee of truth, it is still true that we do have shared experience derived from professional activity. *We do know something* and we know that this should be made available to service users in an appropriate manner. What we know is the result of shared practice – common sense. This means that in its application, there should be shared information, informed choice and scientific monitoring. All of this is set out by Thornicroft and Tansella (1999) in an accessible and well structured way; this book and the *National Service Framework for Mental Health* could usefully be read in conjunction with this chapter.

Social inclusion

The theory and practice of recovery-oriented, community-based mental health services thus differs radically from 'traditional' (cure or containment) hospital-based practice. New approaches to old problems are being searched for in the light of current conceptualisation of the changes of practice that were often informed more by condemnation of past scandals than by coherent theory. An example is the introduction of 'activation' programmes in the mental hospitals because it appeared that doing nothing was bad for residents. According to Franca Basaglia (1998), when her late husband was leading the liberalising reforms in Grosjne and Trieste (Basaglia, 1981), he was *'metaphysically lazy'*. By this she meant that the point was to change that world, not to understand it; or, at least, not to spend so much time agonising over the theory as to do nothing in practice.

A table listing some of the differences in the two approaches was recently provided by Marius Romme (1999). It is a typical and useful summary and I thank him for permission to reproduce it here.

The development of 'social psychiatry' has blurred the distinction between traditional psychiatric theory and practice and (community) mental health theory and practice. There is, however, still a tension to be found between three strands of the psychiatric enterprise. This is echoed in other mental health practitioners and provides another example of where it is healthy to hold the third corner. There is not only a political struggle between 'organic', 'psychological'/'psychodynamic' and 'social' psychiatrists respectively, there are also philosophical problems in finding a common framework in which their respective contributions can be discussed, and in agreeing the criteria by which their claims to knowledge can be evaluated. The first is a metaphysical issue which I once called 'Hill's problem' (Radford, 1983). The second is the epistemological one discussed in the previous section, which has been at the centre of critical debate since the beginning of the Western Enlightenment and is concerned with the search for certainty and the place of 'Science' in filling the need.

A striking and repeated finding is that the prevalence of schizophrenia goes down when national unemployment figures go down in the USA and the UK alike (Warner, 1985; Thomas, 1997). Analysis of this fact demonstrates the importance of external choices in society and the role of open employment in particular in the recovery from schizophrenia. Social inclusion is also predicated on supplies of good housing and of support to enable people to make use of training, employment and leisure resources.

Other cultural conditions also change the prognosis of schizophrenia. The good prognosis for schizophrenia reported in rural India (WHO, 1979; Jablenski, 1989) appears even better in the traditional

Table 2 Community care and traditional care	
Community care	**Traditional care**
1. Based on existentialism	Based on positivism
2. Focused on reintegration (by restoring a balance between individual and society)	Focused on cure (by banishment of symptoms)
3. Social function oriented (focused on the interactions with society) pathology)	Illness oriented (focused on individual
4. Process-oriented (working towards a personal journey of self-discovery and making choices)	Intervention-oriented (working with methods and protocols in a prescribed way)
5. Based on negotiation and emancipation	Based on social control
6. Made to measure personal needs	Standardisation
	(Romme,1999)

community, at least for social inclusion and probably also for symptoms. Respect for the value of such culture is being demonstrated by Chaterjee, a psychiatrist currently working in a tribal area of India. He reports (Conferences in Birmingham and Trieste, 1998) that external influences are seen to be responsible for both physical and psychiatric afflictions. The sufferer is supported by the group against misfortune which is seen neither as his deficiency nor his fault. There are aspects of the social attitudes in this example of tribal India that can be seen as more advanced that those in modern city life.

Confronting the excluded other: relating to the bizarre

A crisis of representation is an aspect of postmodern discourse (Bertens, 1995). Psychiatric diagnosis is one such representation. Myths about clinical records are others.

'Nuts' and 'bolts' are representations: they have real effects which expose basic processes in the response to the fear of collapse, death, dissolution and disintegration that we all carry. They also refer to real people who stand independent of any representation, even if no representation can fully capture reality. Real people can get hurt and/or can get helped. It is irresponsible to lose sight of this and lapse into solipsism. In his recent and revealing book on the representation(s) of disease(s), Gilman (1988) suggests that:

> '...we project our fear onto the world in order to localise it and, indeed, to domesticate it. For once we locate it, the fear of our own dissolution is removed. Then it is not we who totter on the brink of collapse, but rather the Other. And it is an-Other who has already shown his or her vulnerability by having collapsed.'

The point that Gilman wants to show is that the representations of, for example, people with schizophrenia that are invented and passed on between psychiatrists have aspects that are derived from our personal existential fear, as well as our shared observations. These influence our behaviour towards such other persons. He takes the use of the concept 'bizarre' and of the 'praecox experience' to bring this out. This is commonly used to define thought or behaviour as 'schizophrenic', and at bottom is a subjective judgement between what Karl Jaspers called 'the understandable' and the 'non-understandable' (1913/1963).

> *'The 'bizarre' sense in the observer of the schizophrenic has been seen as resulting from what has come to be labelled as the 'praecox feeling', a term coined by H. C. Rumke, who observed that as a diagnostician he was 'guided by the "praecox feeling"' which arises in the examiner. Only highly experienced psychiatrists can employ this compass. In his study of transference and counter-transference, U. H. Peters has emphasised that the praecox feeling is not an emotional reaction to the patient but rather is rooted in the 'non-rational' memory of the psychiatrist. These views of the praecox feeling stress that it is the application of a diagnostic label based on cumulative experience in observing schizophrenics. That this feeling is the result of the interpretation of phenomenological clues may be the source of Peters' observation that the more one knows the patient, the less reliable is the praecox feeling as an indicator of schizophrenia, for the accumulation of other data will tend to mask the initial impression of psychopathology' (Gilman, op cit.).*

If I had been diagnosed as having schizophrenia and could not escape the mental health system, I would want Peters to be my psychiatrist. As Gilman put it:

> *For whether we distance ourselves from it, or whether we adopt it as our mask, we use the bizarre as our sign of our own completeness. In the first case we demarcate our sense*

of self from the Other; in the second, we consciously adopt the external label of difference as a means of showing our control over the world. In both cases we know we are not different. We play a role, and that role defines difference as that which lies outside of ourselves. Thus we use the stereotype of the bizarre language of the schizophrenic as a means of defining our own sanity.'

There is also much to say about the nuts and bolts of meeting and treating people with severe disruptions of personality development. Many have suffered traumatic stress as children. Until the indefinite ages of between 16 and 18 such children are seen as victims and their disturbed behaviour is excused. After this, or before if they perpetrate severe crimes, they are seen as unco-operative, difficult or dangerous.

Douglas Bennett used to say that helping people with personality disorder was the next challenge for those working on the theory and practice of psychiatric rehabilitation. Watts and Bennett (1983) put up an argument that a rehabilitation approach may have more to offer than a curative one. Other psychiatrists are seeking to distance themselves politically as well as emotionally from any responsibility for this group of people. This is a key current issue in British psychiatry. It is about resources, scapegoating, roles and responsibilities. We cannot always avoid engagement when harm to self or others is threatened or when this has occurred.

The persisting paradox of paternalism: user empowerment and the place of psychiatry in mental health

The death of certainty presents a great challenge to psychiatry. This issue is discussed in the conclusions of a postmodern analysis of the politics of schizophrenia by Philip Thomas (1997):

'My colleague Pat Bracken (personal communication) argues that one of the most important tasks facing psychiatry, indeed the whole of medicine, is that facing up to the loss of certainty means that it must redefine ethics. To this, I would add that psychiatry needs an ethics of intersubjectivity. This is because psychiatrists must recognise their own perspective and the way this affects and colours their relationships with their patients... Only then can the conflict between professional and personal languages be made explicit.'

The role of science in the definition of what it is to be professional in the light of the discussion in this chapter needs to be changed from the commonly accepted one. Instead of applying 'scientifically established knowledge' with common sense and a code of ethics, we should be applying common sense and our ethical codes with 'scientific method' (Radford, 1983). This means that we do not have to (pretend to or struggle to) separate the impact of ourselves from our practice by being professionally disengaged. What does follow is that, as responsible clinical professionals, we should learn to be aware of the impact on both 'curing' and 'recovery' outcomes of what we do and how we are; and to take responsibility for this.

Figure 3 is drawn to bring out the complementary processes in which secondary care mental health services are engaged. On the left is represented what can be called 'the cure model'. As with coronary heart and cancer problems, the task is to screen, refer, diagnose, treat and cure (by removing the pathology). People with such conditions should get timely access to the appropriate levels of technical expertise. People with mental health problems need the same in order to be cured of any treatable underlying conditions, such as a brain tumour or a metabolic disorder, that may have been unrecognised. Thereafter, the main diagnostic role of psychiatrists is to recognise functional psychosis (the schizophrenias or manic and depressive illnesses) and negotiate the application of medical treatment as far as it is useful and to take responsibility for it.

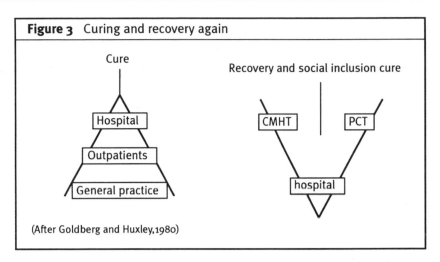

Figure 3 Curing and recovery again

Cure

Recovery and social inclusion cure

Hospital

Outpatients

General practice

CMHT   PCT

hospital

(After Goldberg and Huxley, 1980)

However, when illnesses are not curable by present knowledge, the task is to improve symptoms and help the person to live as fully as possible. In the 'recovery' model, community mental health teams and primary care teams have a shared role in supporting the processes of personal development and social inclusion. By virtue of their medical training, psychiatrists in mental health teams are well placed for the first task, part of which is to transmit knowledge of the limits of medical intervention. They may have some training in the processes of recovery and social inclusion, but can claim no supervening expertise. This sounds very obvious, but the different processes can be confused. The use of hospital beds in the recovery and social inclusion process, for example, can be seen as very different from their use in the diagnosis and cure process. Some services are trying to create separate residential facilities for respite care.

This confusion has led to uncertainty about the psychiatrist's role in community mental health teams. The extent to which 'the cure model' should dominate is controversial when there is no real cure for many of their patients. Psychiatrists' resistance to recovery-oriented, community-based practice is important because of the persisting levels of hegemony over the mental health system retained by doctors since the profession took over control of the county asylums in the nineteenth century turning them into 'mental hospitals'. This was the move that changed the regimen from moral treatment to medical treatment. Inasmuch as there was attention paid to treatment of physical diseases and attention to study of outcome, this was not totally negative. The trouble is that hegemony implies more than taking over people's lives and purpose: it also colonises the foundations of their personal meaning (Williams, 1983). This is why it is so hard to shake off. The less these systems are challenged, the more they will be unwittingly espoused by new generations of doctors and other powerful professionals. Nurses are the largest professional group in mental health services, but have not been able to provide any effective challenge because, according to Hopton (1997), reform in mental health nursing has concentrated on person-centred psychology which softens but does not alter the social and political relations; and because under the current UK *Mental Health Act,* '*all the real power in the relationship between mental health services and service users resides with the consultant psychiatrist*'.

In establishing dialogue with service users, therefore, it is useful to be aware of the impact of the behaviour of those with more power on those with less.

Psychiatrists have key roles in the management of inpatient beds and in the use of the *Mental Health Act,* which allows for compulsory admission and treatment. Decisions about the use of the *Mental Health Act* are occasions when the psychiatrist and approved social worker override the autonomy of a service user. Training for both has been increased as the ethics have been more conscious. The Code of Practice emphasises the importance of respect. Here, the professional's duty of beneficence becomes paternalistic. Positive beneficence (the duty to do good) and negative beneficence (the duty to avoid harm) are both problematic here. The amount of persuasion that should be applied at other times is also difficult to judge, but the final decision can be the service user, until the capacity to form informed consent is impaired.

This is, however, a central problem in mental health practice, indeed in all medical practice. Even in something as routine as the competence of voluntary inpatients to give fully informed consent to neuroleptic medication, strict tests have shown that only few (five per cent) are so competent when assessed in a sophisticated way (Paul & Oyebode, 1999). This study was described by the authors as 'very modest', but it is very important. They show that in the real world, patients' consent is actually based on desire for symptom relief and their trust in their doctors.

Not to act paternalistically at times would be negligent. Indeed, it is also paternalistic to push a person towards autonomy and out of dependency. Perhaps the only clear thing to say is that these processes should be as open as possible.

The restoration of full humanity: can we find less damaging ways to contain uncertainty?

Whether and how people could cope and adapt to the ever increasing rate of social change was the subject of *Future Shock* (Toffler, 1970) and was being widely discussed at the time Jones published her account of the revolutions in mental health services. Toffler addresses the escalating uncertainties in Western society over a similar historical period to that reviewed by Jones (1972), mainly in the United States, since the Industrial Revolution and the growth of capitalism. He documented the consequent and accelerating rate of social change, the impact of scientific discovery and technological invention, the break-up of traditional arrangements (based on European feudalism), and the impact of diversity on individual identities. He writes:

> *'When diversity converges with transience and novelty, we rocket society towards an historical crisis of adaptation. We create an environment so ephemeral, unfamiliar and complex as to threaten millions with*

*adaptive breakdown. This breakdown is future shock...
To survive, [the individual]... must search out totally
new ways to anchor himself, for all the old roots –
religion, nation, community, family, or profession – are
now shaking under the hurricane impact of the
accelerative thrust.'*

Popper (1946) wrote of '*the strain of civilisation*' and his political philosophy was devoted to defining the structures that would be needed to bring into being an open society and to preserve it from its enemies. Because we have such an important impact on making our own environment which in turn has such an important effect on making us, Popper (1994) suggested that '*it is our duty to remain optimists*'. This is not to deny present difficulties or the need for honesty in facing them. In one of his Kantian moments he asserted that, although honesty was demonstrably not always the best policy, honesty was better than policy. The attitude of optimism is a way of relating to the world and to death.

In his analysis of human existential anxiety and ontological insecurity, Paul Tillich (1952) wrote of the fear of loss of being through death, of relatedness to others through isolation and of the loss of personal meaning. I found my copy in a second-hand bookshop in Madison on a visit as the guest of Len and Karen Stein, and it left me with a very strong impression of how whole-hearted were the community mental health services pioneered there, and how important it was to implement them to escape the pretences for caring involved in 9 to 5 provision. Such time limits have been part of the staff security structure – we can cut off and go home, and we need to do this. Working in a team which is organised to provide continuity through crises makes this much easier: we do not have to say 'I've got to go home now, come back in the morning' and then carry the anxiety. We can say '*I've got to go home now, but my colleague is here*'.

A necessary and urgent task to achieve this type of approach is the deconstruction of many aspects of contemporary psychiatry, and of false certainties; and the creation of a new frame of reference for professional activity in the light of the destruction of certainty. Without the full participation of the recipients of mental health care in a dialogue that really confronts the 'excluded other', mental health practitioners cannot succeed in reincorporating mutual projections and entering into the process of reclaiming our full humanity.

Acknowledgements

This chapter has been influenced by discussions at the Birmingham Philosophy and Psychiatry group with Femi Oyebode, Pat Bracken, Moli Paul and others. Some of the ideas on the genealogy of ethics in mental health were presented at the South Birmingham User Forum early in 1998 and were developed as a paper for the First International Conference on De-institutionalising Psychiatry in Trieste, October 1998.

I am indebted to many discussions with Razia Yaqoob; she is an intellectual companion and one of the 'friends of my mind'; to Sue Turner, for showing me the importance of holding the third corner; to Brian Deakin, a fellow Sparkle Award winner, who made the space to discuss an earlier draft of this chapter and to validate me; to Pam Virdi and Jenny Bywaters, also friends of my mind, who read the penultimate draft; to members and clients of the Sparkhill Community Mental Health Team over the last fourteen years; to Keith Munnings, who is teaching and encouraging me in Samatha meditation practice; and to Bill Fulford, Paul Sturdee, and other teachers on the Warwick University postgraduate course on the Philosophy and Ethics of Mental Health.

Most of all I am grateful for the support and insight given to me by the writings of Sir Karl Popper, a man described in his Guardian obituary by Jonathon Rea as *'the first and the greatest of the post-modern philosophers'*, to his representation of intellectual life as an unended quest, to his concern with practical matters and for the encouragement of a letter in which he praised my paper on psychoanalysis and the science of problem-solvingman, saying it was a very good contribution to the discussion, '*a discussion in which I have taken no part*'.

References

Adorno, T. & Horkheimer, M. (1947; 1986) *Dialectic of Enlightenment*. London: Verso.

Bakhtin, M. M. (1981) *The Dialogic Imagination*. Austin: University of Texas.

Basaglia, Franca (1998) Address to 'The First International Conference on De–institutionalising Psychiatry', Trieste, 1998.

Basaglia, F. (1981) Breaking the Circuit of Control. In: D. Ingleby (1981) (Ed) *Critical Psychiatry: The Politics of Mental Health*. London: Harmondsworth.

Bennett, D.H. & Freeman, H. L. (1991) *Community Psychiatry*. London: Churchill Livingstone.

Bennett, D. H. & Watts, F. N. (1983) *Theory and Practice of Psychiatric Rehabilitation*. Chichester: John Wiley.

Berlin, I. (1999) *The Roots of Romanticism*. London: Chatto and Windus.

Bertens, H. (1995) *The Idea of the Postmodern: A history*. London: Routledge.

Bolton, D. & Hill, J. (1996) *Mind, Meaning and Mental Disorder: The nature of causal explanation in psychology and psychiatry*. Oxford: Oxford University Press.

Bracken, P. (1995) Beyond liberation: Michael Foucault and the notion of a critical psychiatry. *Philosophy, Psychology and Psychiatry* **12** 139–150.

Bracken, P. & Cohen, B. (1999) Home treatment in Bradford. *Psychiatrist Bulletin* **23** 349–352.

Castel, R. (1985) Moral Treatment: Mental Therapy and Social Control. In: P. Cohen and A. Scull (Eds) *Social Control and the State*. Oxford: Blackwell.

Carling, P. J. & Allott, P. (1999a) *Core Vision and Values for a Modern Mental Health System Developing Services Together Directional Paper 1*. Birmingham: West Midland Partnership for Mental Health.

Carling, P. J. & Allott, P. (1999b) *Beyond Mental Health Services: Integrating resources and supports in the local community developing services together directional paper 2*. Birmingham: West Midland Partnership for Mental Health.

Carling, P. J. & Allott, P. (1999c) *User-Based Outcomes in a Modern Mental Health System Developing Services Together Directional Paper 4.* Birmingham: West Midland Partnership for Mental Health.

Carling, P. J., Allott, P., Smith, M. & Coleman, R. (1999) *Principles of Recovery for a Modern Community Mental Health System Developing Services Together Directional Paper 3.* Birmingham: West Midland Partnership for Mental Health.

Clare, A. W. (1986) The Disease Concept. In: P. Hill, R. Murray and A. Thorley (Eds) *Essentials of Postgraduate Psychiatry.* London: Grune and Stratton.

Clarkson, P. (1995) *The Therapeutic Relationship in Psychoanalysis, Counselling, Psychology and Psychotherapy.* London: Whurr Publishers.

Coleman, R. (1999) *Recovery: An alien concept.* Gloucester: Handsell.

Coleman, R. & Smith, M. (1997) *Working with Voices: Victim to Victor.* Stockport: Handsell.

Dalai Lama (1995) *The Power of Compassion.* London: Thorsons.

Deegan, P. (1996) Recovery as a journey of the heart. *Psychiatric Rehabilitation Journal* **19** 74–83.

Department of Health (1999) *National Service Framework for Mental Health.* London: DoH.

Department of Health (1971) *Better Services for the Mentally Ill.* London: HMSO.

Department of Health (2000) *The NHS Plan: A Plan for Investment, a Plan for Reform.* London: DoH.

de Swaan, A. (1990) *The Management of Normality: Critical essays in health and welfare.* London: Routledge.

Durrell, L. (1969) *Spirit of Place: Letters and essays on travel.* London: Faber and Faber.

Fanon, F. (1952/67) *Peau Noire, Masques Blancs* (trans. C. L. Markmann, 1967). New York: Grove Press.

Fish, V. (1999) Clementis's Hat: Foucault and the Politics of Psychotherapy In: I. Parker (Ed) *Deconstructing Psychotherapy.* London: Sage.

Foster, A. & Roberts, V. Z. 1998) *Managing Mental Health in the Community: Chaos and containment.* London: Routledge.

Foucault, M. (1965) *Madness and Civilisation: A history of insanity in the age of reason.* New York: Random House.

Foucault, M. (1984) What is Enlightenment? In: *The Foucault Reader* (Edited by P. Rabinow; trans C. Porter). London: Harmondsworth.

Fowles, J. (1977) *Daniel Martin*. London: Cape.

Freire, P. (1978) *Pedagogy in Process: The Letters to Guinea-Bissau London: Writers and Readers*.

Fulford, K. W. M. (1989) *Moral Theory and Medical Practice*. Cambridge: Cambridge University Press.

Gaukroger, S. (1995) *Descartes: An intellectual biography*. Oxford: Clarendon Press.

Giddens, A. (1991) *Modernity and Self-Identity: Self and society in the late modern age*. Oxford: Polity Press.

Gilman, S. (1988) *Disease and Representation*. New York: Cornell University Press.

Goldburg, D. P. & Huxley, P. (1980) *Mental Illness in the Community*. London: Tavistock.

Hall, C. (1992) *White, Male and Middle Class: Explorations in feminism and history*. Oxford: Blackwell.

Hill, D. (1970) On the contributions of psychoanalysis to psychiatry: mechanism and meaning. *British Journal of Psychiatry* **117** 609–615.

Hill, D. (1978) The qualities of a good psychiatrist. *British Journal of Psychiatry* **113** 97–105.

Hobson, R. F. (1989) *Forms of Feeling: The heart of psychotherapy*. London: Routledge.

Hoenig, J. & Hamilton, M.W. (1969) *The Desegregation of the Mentally Ill*. London: Routledge and Kegan Paul.

Hopton, J. (1997) Towards a critical theory of mental health nursing. *Journal of Advanced Nursing* **25** 492–500.

hooks, b. (1996) *Killing Rage: Ending Racism*. London: Harmondsworth.

Illich, I. (1973) *Deschooling Society*. London: Harmondsworth.

Illich, I. (1975) *Tools for Conviviality*. Glasgow: Fontana.

Jablenski, A. (1989) An Overview of the World Health Organisation Multi-centre Studies of Schizophrenia. In: P. Williams, G. Wilkinson and K. Rawnsley (Eds) *The Scope of Epidemiological Psychiatry*. London: Routledge.

Jaspers, K. (1913/1963) *General Psychopathology*. Translated by J. Hoenig and M. W. Hamilton Manchester: Manchester University Press.

Jones, K. (1972) *A History of the Mental Health Services*. London: Routledge and Kegan Paul.

Jumble, J. (1999) *The Light Side Survivors*. Birmingham: Footprint.

Kant, I. (1784) An Answer to the Question: What is Enlightenment? In: P. Waugh (Ed) (1992) *Postmodernism: A Reader.* London: Edward Arnold.

Laugharne, R. (1999) Evidence-based medicine, user involvement and the post modern paradigm. *Psychiatric Bulletin* **23** 641–643.

Leggett, J. (1997) Medical scientism: good practice or fatal error? *Journal of the Royal Society of Medicine* **90** 97–101.

Lewis, A. (1953) Health as a social concept. *British Journal of Sociology* **4** 109–124.

Lewis, A. (1967) Empirical or rational? The nature and basis of psychiatry. *Lancet* **2** 1–9.

Lewis, A. (1991) Dilemmas in psychiatry. *Psychological Medicine* **21** 581–585.

Lewis, A. (1959) The Impact of Psychotropic drugs on the structure, function and future of psychiatric services in hospitals. In: P. Bradley, P. Deniker & C. Radonco-Thomas. (Eds) *Neuropsychopharmacology.* Amsterdam: Elsevier.

Luhrmann, B. (1997) *The Sunscreen Song* (class of '99) E.M.I. Music Australia Pty. Ltd.

Lyotard, J. F. (1984) *The Post-modern Condition: A report on knowledge* (trans. by G.Bennington and B. Massumi). Manchester: Manchester University Press.

MacIntyre, N. & Popper, K. R. (1983) The critical attitude in medicine: the need for a new medical ethics. *British Medical Journal* **287** 1919–1923.

Main, T. F. (1953) The ailment. *British Journal of Medical Psychology* **30** 129–145.

Martin, P. W. (1955/76) *Experiment in Depth: A study of the work of Jung, Eliot and Toynbee.* London: Routledge and Kegan Paul.

May, J. (1993) *World as Lover, World as Self.* London: Rider.

Milcinski, M. (1999) Zen and the art of death. *Journal of the History of Ideas* **60** 385–397.

Morrison, T. (1987) *Beloved.* London: Chatto and Windus.

Mosher, L. & Burti, P. (1994) *Community Mental Health: A practical guide.* New York: Norton.

Mulhall, S. & Swift, A. (1992) *Liberals and Communitarians.* Oxford: Blackwell.

Mullen, P.E. (1996) Jealousy and the emergence of violent and intimidating behaviour. *Criminal Behaviour and Mental Health* **6** 199–205.

Mullen, P. E. & Martin, J. L. (1994) Jealousy: a community study. *British Journal of Psychiatry* **164** 35–43.

National Health Service Act 1946

Nietzsche, F. (1874) Untimely Meditations. (Trans by R. J. Hollingdale, 1983). Cambridge: Cambridge University Press.

Osbourne, T. (1998) *Aspects of Enlightenment: Social theory and the ethics of truth.* London: UCL Press.

Oyebode, F., Brown, N. & Parry, L. (1999) Clinical governance in practice. *Advances in Psychiatric Treatment* **5** 399–404.

Parsons, T. (1951) *The Social System.* lllinois: Free Press.

Paul, M. & Oyebode, F. (1999) Competence of voluntary psychiatric patients to give valid consent to neuroleptic medication. *Psychiatric Bulletin* **23** 463–466.

Phillips, A. & Rakusen, J. (1989) *The New Our Bodies, Our Selves.* London: Harmondsworth.

Popper, K. R. (1960) On the Sources of Knowledge and of Ignorance. In: K. R. Popper (Ed) (1963) *Conjectures and Refutations.* London: Routledge and Kegan Paul.

Popper, K. R. (1982) The Open Universe: An Argument for Indeterminism. In: W. W. Bartley III (1982) *Logic of Scientific Discovery (postscript).* (Ed). London: Hutchinson.

Popper, K. R. (1992) *Unended Quest: An intellectual Autobiography.* London: Routledge.

Popper, K. R. (1994) *The Myth of the Framework: In defence of science and rationality.* London: Routledge.

Popper, K. R. (1998) *The World of Parmenides: Essays on the Pre-Socratic Enlightenment.* (Edited by A. F. Peterson.) London: Routledge.

Queredo, A. (1968) *The Development of Socio-medical Care in the Netherlands.* London: Routledge and Kegan Paul.

Radford, M. D. (1983) Psychoanalysis and the science of problem-solving man: an appreciation of Popper's philosophy and a response to Will (1980). *British Journal of Medical Psychology* **56** 9–26.

Radford, M. D. (1992) The Copernican revolution in mental health services: replacing the revolving door. *Journal of Mental Health* **1** 229–239.

Reeves, A. (1998) *Recovery: An holistic approach.* Gloucester: Handsell.

Reiff, P. (1966) *The Triumph of the Therapeutic.* London: Chatto and Windus.

Romme, M. A. J. (1996) *Understanding Voices: Coping with auditory hallucinations and confusing realities.* Maastricht: Rijksuniversiteit.

Romme, M. A. J. (1999) Inaugural Lecture, University of Central England.

Rose, N. (1990) *Governing the Soul: The shaping of the private self.* London: Routledge.

Rose, N. (1996) *Inventing Ourselves: Psychology, power and personhood.* Cambridge: Cambridge University Press.

Russell, B. (1948) *The History of Western Philosophy and its Connection with Political and Social Circumstances from the Earlier Times to the Present Day.* London: Allen and Unwin.

Sashidharan, S. P. (1999) Alternatives to Institutional Psychiatry. In: D. Bhugra and V. Bahl (Eds) *Ethnicity: An Agenda for Mental Health.* London: Gaskell.

Scheff, T. (1966) *Being Mentally Ill: A sociological theory.* London: Wiedenfeld and Nicholson.

Shepherd, M. (1957) *A Study of Major Psychosis in an English County.* London: Chapman and Hall.

Smith, M. (1998a) The road to recovery. *Mental Health Practice* **2** 26–27.

Smith, M. (1998b) *Working with Self-harm: Victim to victor.* Stockport: Handsell.

Stein, L. I. (1992) Innovating Against the Current. In: L. I. Stein (Ed) *New Directions for Mental Health Services.* San Francisco: Dass.

Steiner, G. (1968) *In Bluebeard's Castle: Some notes towards the re-definition of culture.* London: Faber and Faber.

Stein, L. I. & Test, M. A. (1980) Alternative to Mental Hospital Treatment, 1: Conceptual model, treatment program and clinical evaluation. *Archives of General Psychiatry* **37** 292–397.

Stokes, J. (1994) The Unconscious at Work in Groups and Teams – Contributions from the work of Wilfred Bion. In: Anton Obholzer and Vega Zagier Roberts (Eds) *The Unconscious at Work: Individual and Organisational Stress in the Human Services.* London: Routledge.

Szasz, T. S. (1961) *The Myth of Mental Illness.* New York: Hoeber-Harper.

Tagore, R. (1913) *Sadhara: The Realisation of Life.* London: MacMillan.

Tart, C. (1996) *Neurophysiology and philosophy* – conference talk.

Taylor, C. (1989) *Sources of the Self: The making of the modern identity.* Cambridge: Cambridge University Press.

Thomas, P. (1997) *The Dialectics of Schizophrenia.* London: Free Association Books.

Thornicroft, G. & Tansella, M.(1997) *The Mental Health Matrix: A Manual to Improve Services.* Cambridge: Cambridge University Press.

Tillich, P. (1952) *The Courage To Be.* New York: Yale University Press.

Toffler, A. (1970) *Future Shock*. Ontario: Bantam Books.

Tooth, B., Kalyanansundaram, V. & Glover, H. (1997) *Recovery from Schizophrenia: A consumer perspective*. Centre for Mental Health Nursing Research. Queensland University of Technology Locked Bag No 2, Red Hill, Q 4064.

Turner, B. S. (Ed) (1990) *Theories of Modernity and Postmodernity*. London: Sage.

Turner, T., Salter, M. & Deahl, M. (1999) *Mental Health Act* Reform: should psychiatrists go on being responsible? *Psychiatric Bulletin* **23** 578–581.

Virdi, P. (1993) *Driven to Heal: Factors influencing the career choices of mental health professionals*. Birmingham University Thesis (MEd. Counselling).

Wall, C. & Gannon-Leary, P. (1999) A sentence made by men: muted group theory revisited. *European Journal of Women's Studies* **6** 21–29.

Warner, R. (1985) *Recovery from Schizophrenia: Psychiatry and political economy*. London: Routledge and Kegan Paul.

Watts, F. N. & Bennett, D. (1983) Neurotic, Affective, and Conduct Disorders. In: F. Watts and D. Bennett (Eds) *Theory and Practice of Psychiatric Rehabilitation*. Chichester: Wiley.

Wetphal, M. (1999) Soron Kiekegaard. In: R. H. Popkin (Ed) *The Pimlico History of Western Philosophy* . London: Pimlico.

Whitwell, D. (1999) The myth of recovery from mental illness. *Psychiatric Bulletin* **23** 621–622.

WHO (1979) *Schizophrenia: an initial follow-up*. Chichester: Wiley.

Williams, J. & Lindley, P. (1996) Working with mental health service users to change mental health services. *Journal of Community and Applied Social Psychology* **6** 1–14.

Williams, R. (1983) *Keywords: A vocabulary of culture and society*. London: Fontana.

Wing, J. K. & Brown, G. W. (1970) *Institutionalism and Schizophrenia*. Cambridge: Cambridge University Press.

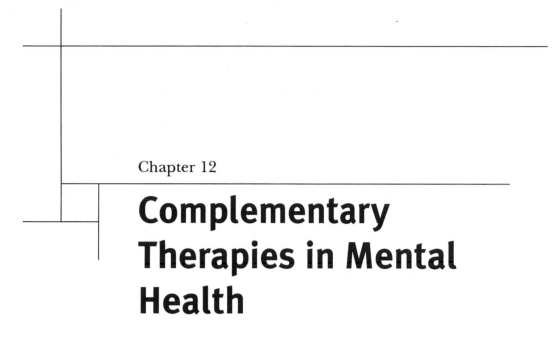

Chapter 12

Complementary Therapies in Mental Health

Annie Mitchell

Introduction

Over the next few years, it seems likely that ideas and practices from complementary medicine will be increasingly influential in the mental health field, as we struggle to facilitate community care within which people can lead meaningful lives, with services they want and which are relevant to their needs, rather than those others think they ought to have. The provision of complementary healthcare for people experiencing mental health difficulties (being so far at an early stage of development) is patchy, little documented and hardly researched. Certainly one of the most striking features of the currently changing pattern of health provision overall is the large increase in numbers of people choosing to consult with complementary practitioners, along with a growing interest in self and mutual help approaches. People who go to complementary practitioners apparently do so initially for pragmatic reasons, usually wanting help with chronic, intractable problems (which often involve pain, both physical and emotional). Those who continue their use of complementary approaches mainly do so alongside, or in parallel with, their use of orthodox medicines (Sharma, 1992).

The reasons for the shift towards greater use of complementary therapies are complex and varied. Their appeal seems to extend far beyond any simplistic notions of narrowly defined effectiveness of treatment. The attraction seems to lie in a mixture of their more egalitarian approach to the therapeutic relationship, their recognition of links between lifestyle and illness, the individual nature of the treatments offered and the success of treatments for symptom management, along with a perceived relative lack of noxious side effects. A central and crucial factor is their potential to bring meaning to the experience of suffering by making connections between physical, mental and spiritual circumstances and aspects of people's lives. In Western healthcare we urgently need to find ways of bridging the Cartesian divide referred to by Radford in **Chapter 11**, which has so often led to fragmented and fragmenting treatment, and which has exacerbated the splitting and disconnection so often experienced by those in distress: the complementary therapies seem to offer a promise of healing this mind – body split.

Their potential for bringing order to the chaotic experience of illness and distress might indicate that complementary therapies could have much to offer in mental health care, yet until recently, they have been little used or discussed within Western mental health settings. Individual practitioners have perhaps been unsure about how to provide treatment to people with severe mental health difficulties, and in any case most people with such difficulties are not in a position to pay for private treatment, yet complementary therapies have only rarely been made available within the public sector. There is now a growing demand for complementary treatment in mental health care, coming from the grass roots, fuelled by the concerns of people in the user movement to have services which are less dominated by the psychiatric medical model: more cohesive, more humane and more personally empowering (Breggin, 1993; Rogers & Pilgrim, 1996). At its best, complementary therapy offers the user an opportunity to work with a practitioner with whom he or she can form a mutually respecting relationship, who can take the time and trouble to learn about the person's life and concerns and who will offer therapeutic techniques modified to the individual's particular circumstances, along with specific advice about links between life-style and wellbeing. Such a personally tailored approach must be attractive to those who are dissatisfied and disaffected by the shortcomings of orthodox approaches in which even those who want to listen and understand sometimes seem constrained by the limitations of their professionalism and conceptual models.

Many complementary therapies have their origins in lay and folk knowledge so are strongly rooted in a self, and mutual help, non-expert, approach to healing. There is much use of the traditional healing powers of magic, symbolism and ritual in many complementary approaches – the power of which have been neglected and diminished within the rationalism of science but which, used wisely and with care, may have much to offer those who need help in the creative use of irrationality and intuition.

The Mental Health Foundation conducted a user-led study which investigated the strategies used by people in emotional distress to attempt to take control of their lives. People were found to develop their own individual ways of coping, which brought a whole range of everyday activities, therapies and treatments into an overall strategy for living with mental health problems. People particularly appreciated having someone to talk to, who listened and took them seriously, although this did not necessarily involve an 'expert treatment'. Many people used and valued alternative and complementary therapies (these findings will be enlarged below) and the report concluded:

> *'We believe that access to all forms of treatment or therapy should be equal and that alternative and complementary therapies and talking treatments should be available to all who want them. Information about, and access to, the many different treatments and therapies described in our survey is very limited for most people. This is mainly due to the lack of availability of alternative and complementary therapies within the mental health services.'*
> (Mental Health Foundation, 1997)

In this chapter we will look at some common features of complementary therapies, consider their possible benefits for users in mental health, examine the issue of evidence of effectiveness, identify some of the issues and challenges in providing complementary therapies in mental health care and, finally, conclude by considering possible ways forward.

What are the complementary therapies?

In some ways it is misleading to write of 'complementary therapies' as if they were a homogenous set of approaches, which they certainly are not, coming as they do from a huge range of social and cultural conditions and systems of knowledge and belief. Despite their diversity, however, complementary therapies can be thought of as having certain defining features, at least from a culturally relative perspective. In a negative sense, complementary therapies have been defined as those approaches to therapy and diagnosis which lie outside current Western medicine or outside the institutions where conventional healthcare is taught and provided (Pietroni, 1992; Zollman & Vickers, 1999), thus appealing to those users and providers who are disenchanted with orthodox medicine – or psychiatry in particular, in the case of mental health treatment. Complementary therapists do not, on the whole, use the diagnostic system of bio-medicine in which clusters of symptoms are grouped together as disease entities, which are then used not only as the basis for treatment decisions, but also to categorise **people**. The problem of labelling, with all its stigmatic and stereotyping consequences, may be side-stepped in complementary approaches in which treatment decisions are (ideally) based on a consideration of the individual **pattern of functioning** of the person, including their particular physical, mental and social conditions and dispositions. The person's temperament, spirituality, lifestyle and relationships, are considered to be at least as important as specific symptoms. In theory, at least, such approaches should avoid pathologising the individual, although

At the Core of Mental Health © Pavilion 2000

as we will see below, complementary therapies are not without their own risks of victim blaming.

Positive approaches to defining complementary therapies consider their commonalities. Complementary therapies can be defined as those approaches with certain core features, including, in particular, an attempt to **recruit the person's own self-healing capacity**. They are generally considered to aspire to:

- emphasise **the interconnection of mind, body and spirit**

- use (relatively) **non-invasive techniques**

- have **few side effects**

- make much use of **time, touch and talk**

- involve the **individual as active participant** in treatment

- **treat the individual rather than the disease**

- incorporate **beliefs** which may not accord with those of western science

- work **with** rather than against **symptoms**

- attempt to understand **what symptoms mean in the context of the individual's life, lifestyle and social context.**

(Adapted from Fulder, 1996 and Vickers, 1996a)

Are the therapies alternative or complementary to orthodox medicine?

The therapies may be seen as either alternative or complementary to orthodox medicine in two respects: the pattern of their use and their underlying system of beliefs. Most people who use the therapies do so in the complementary sense of moving between and within different systems of treatment according to their particular need at the time, basing their choice on personal preference, on word of mouth recommendations from other users and on lay beliefs about what therapies are relevant for which difficulties (Vincent &

Furnham, 1994). The Mental Health Foundation Study (1997) found that only 10% of their sample of mental health users regarded their choice of complementary therapies as completely alternative to orthodox health care.

Many of the therapies might more aptly be considered as alternatives to orthodox medicine in terms of the system of beliefs underpinning their understanding of illness. Complementary therapies are derived from a variety of traditions, many of which are very different from that of biologically based Western medicine, and often involve understandings which are at odds with medical science. The therapies may be considered to be alternative in so far as their holistic underpinning, with a recognition of the interconnection of the social, personal, physical and spiritual realms, provides a counterpoint to the reductionist approaches of biological medicine.

There is debate about the value, or otherwise, of the integration of complementary healthcare into more orthodox health systems with a fear that, in practice, **incorporation** (with biomedicine retaining its supremacy) is a more likely outcome than **true integration** (as promoted by the Foundation for Integrated Medicine, 1997) with an equal valuing of conceptual frameworks and methods. Many practitioners will choose to remain outside orthodox healthcare systems so as to maintain their conceptual and methodological integrity, while others may wish to join the system so as to influence it from within, to make their treatment more readily available and, perhaps, to gain greater public acknowledgement and recognition of their role in healing. In summary, while many of the therapies *are* alternatives (in the sense of being *different* to biomedicine), so too are other currently available approaches to mental health work, such as psychology, psychotherapy, counselling, social work, and community intervention, many of which share many of the defining features of complementary therapies. In terms of service provision and patterns of use, different approaches should perhaps best be regarded as complementary parts of a coherent and holistic mental health system.

Complementary therapies in practice – what do they involve?

There are various ways of describing and differentiating the complementary therapies. There are so many different therapies and they are interpreted so differently according to the particular practitioner, that it is not possible to describe them within the constraints of this chapter. Useful sources include Stephen Fulder's *Handbook of Complementary Medicine* (1996) which gives an overview of the principles and practice of most of the therapies most commonly encountered in Britain. A series of articles written for the *British Medical Journal* as an 'ABC of complementary therapies' (Zollman & Vickers, 1999) reviews the claims and evidence of effectiveness across therapies and presenting problems and is due to be published as a book in Spring 2000. In a more succinct form, for mental health users, Mind have produced a helpful *A–Z of Complementary and Alternative Therapies*, including a guide to choosing a therapist (Mind, 1995). Jan Wallcraft (1998) has provided an essential source book on research, policy and practice for the use of complementary therapies for a wide range of mental health problems, which was produced for the Mental Health Foundation. This detailed report describes and reviews approaches currently used by complementary practitioners in mental health work, giving many clearly described clinical and case examples.

One useful way of considering the relevance and applicability of different complementary approaches is to find out how they deal in practice with four central components of the treatment act: the therapeutic relationship, understanding and explanation, application of technique and practical advice (Mitchell & Cormack, 1998). These headings provide a useful framework for thinking with users about which therapies may suit them as individuals, taking into account their particular preferences and needs.

Therapeutic relationship

It is often said the complementary therapies offer more equal therapeutic relationships, with more time for warmth, empathy, compassion and understanding. While this may often be the case, it is not necessarily so, and seems to depend more on the interpretation of the particular practitioner than on the specific therapy.

Understanding and explanation

The therapies and therapists have a range of views about causes, cures and maintaining factors for illness and distress, and will differ in the degree to which these understandings and explanations are made explicit. In particular, some approaches deal with spiritual issues, which are commonly neglected in Western medical approaches and about which users may have strong views. It is worth considering the extent to which the particular system of beliefs may resonate with, or constructively challenge, that of the person considering their use.

Application of technique

Therapeutic modalities vary tremendously across several dimensions, and it is useful to consider the extent to which the approach involves the following aspects of treatment:

- **Use of touch.** Touch is central to many treatments (such as massage, reflexology, osteopathy, chiropractic, cranial osteopathy) but not to all. Homeopathy and herbal medicine, for example, rarely involve touch in treatment.

- **Use of creativity and visualisation.** The creative therapies (art, music, drama) and many shamanistic traditions use imaginative techniques.

- **Invasive techniques.** Acupuncture is most commonly quoted as using an invasive technique involving the use of needles or moxibustion, but massage, chiropractic and osteopathy may also be described as invasive in the sense of involving physical manipulation.

- **Use of talk.** Talk is central in many disciplines, both as a means of assessment and as a therapeutic intervention in its own right, but different treatments will be differentially talk-focused: massage, meditation, aromatherapy, reflexology and healing, for example, require relatively little talking whereas talk is central in homeopathy and in some aspects of Chinese medicine.

- **Instruction giving.** Alexander technique and the Feldenkrais method give direct instruction in posture and movement and their practitioners consider themselves to be teachers rather than therapists.

- **Prescription of medication or remedies.** Herbal medicine (Western and Chinese) and homeopathy can seem, in some ways, quite parallel to Western medicine in their reliance on the use of herbs and remedies (albeit not drugs as currently understood), aromatherapy involves the use of oils not taken internally, whereas other approaches such as massage, reflexology, yoga, do not involve any sort of substances.

Practical advice

Therapists and therapies differ in the extent to which they promote self-help strategies around the practicalities of life (sleep, exercise, rest, relaxation, diet and nutrition), but many will offer clear advice in these areas. In particular Chinese medicine, naturopathy, herbalism and exercise therapies such as T'ai Chi and Shiatsu all emphasise practical action on the part of the user. It is arguably the case that it is particularly in this area of developing confidence around self-help that many complementary therapies have most to offer mental health users.

There is certainly scope for giving people more information and opportunity to talk through what different complementary therapies may offer. It is, however, important to bear in mind that in the absence of systematic evidence about the relative value of different treatments, it is most important to find a therapy and practitioner with whom the person can feel comfortable, safe and realistically hopeful.

Research evidence on complementary treatment in mental health

There has so far been little systematic investigation of the effectiveness of complementary approaches in mental health, as, indeed in health care more broadly – Zollman and Vickers (1999) noted that in 1995 only 0.08% of NHS research funds were spent on complementary medicine. It is important however to recognise that absence of evidence of effectiveness is not the same as evidence of absence of effectiveness. Rather, it means that we just don't know yet. There are problems about establishing evaluation research in complementary medicine: dominance of the pharmaceutical industry, lack of funding for research and for developmental pilot work, disagreement about appropriate methodologies for evaluation of holistic treatment, lack of agreement about meaningful, relevant and measurable outcomes, as well as a need for clarification about the aims of treatment, and about whose criteria for success should pertain.

Establishing appropriate research remains problematic for several reasons. First is a seemingly intractable *Catch 22* situation. It is difficult to get funding for research other than large scale clinical trials, and such trials are difficult to implement until basic developmental pilot work has been done, which first requires some funding for service provision on which to base the pilot work. But the funding for the service provision is first dependent on evidence of effectiveness. Moreover, many researchers and practitioners disagree about whether the methodology of double blind clinical trials, which requires controlling all the variables, is appropriate for evaluating holistic approaches where the various components of treatment are considered to act together synergistically (Yamey, 2000). Users and carers themselves need a greater voice in making research more relevant to their own concerns. Research such as the already quoted work by the Mental Health Foundation (1997) may inspire inclusion of more broadly based, user-centred criteria for success, which may be more difficult to operationalise than traditional measures, such as symptom change or treatment satisfaction, but which would be more meaningful and valid to those undergoing treatment. User-valued outcomes, particularly pertaining to complementary care, may include increased sense of meaning, improved sense of wellbeing, feeling able to cope, having explanations which make sense, being in control of treatment and being respected as a significant individual.

Notwithstanding the difficulties in establishing research, there are some relevant empirical findings. Specifically, there is evidence from clinical trials to support the use of the herbal remedy hypericum in the treatment of mild to moderate depression (Linde *et al*, 1996); massage for anxiety and acupuncture for substance dependence (Vickers, 1996b); hypnosis for anxiety, panic disorder, and sleeplessness and to enhance the effects of cognitive behavioural therapy for some conditions (Vickers & Zollman, 1999). There are no systematic trials yet available investigating the impact of complementary therapies on people with psychosis or severe mental illness.

Wallcraft (1998) went beyond clinical trials and meta-analyses to incorporate clinical accounts, case studies and anecdotal claims in her overview of evidence of effectiveness of complementary approaches across a range of mental health problems. She cautiously concluded that while very many unanswered questions remain, evidence is emerging that at least some complementary approaches may be of value in treating some mental health problems. So far, there seems to be demonstrable potential for promoting mental health and relieving the symptoms of anxiety, depression and insomnia with the following approaches: transcendental medicine (though not Ayurvedic medicine as a whole); acupuncture (though not other aspects of traditional Chinese medicine such as herbal remedies); nutritional medicine (especially amino acids and some other supplements); herbal medicine (especially hypericum); homeopathy; massage; aromatherapy; reflexology. Although there are relatively few descriptive reports of the use of treatments with people with psychosis or severe mental illness, the tentative information so far available is generally encouraging.

Importantly, complementary therapies are *'well accepted and often much appreciated by patients and do not appear to have many adverse effects'* (Wallcraft, 1998). People with anxiety and depression accounted for between a quarter and a third of all referrals to complementary practitioners in two integrated general practices, and the patients, many of whom had longstanding problems of five years or more, overwhelmingly felt that they had benefited from therapies which had often provided hope, where other treatments had failed (Hooper *et al*, 1996; Hotchkiss, 1995). In summary, there is now sufficient research, clinical evidence and personal testimony to justify the further development, investigation and evaluation of complementary approaches for people with mental health difficulties.

What are the different stakeholder perspectives on complementary therapies in mental health?

Users

Health service users in general, as well as desiring cure or control of their symptoms, want to be treated as real people and to be given explanations to help make sense of illness and treatment which will then lead to the possibility of personal control (McIver, 1993). Mental health service users in particular want:

- their needs for housing, income, social life and employment to be met

- help and support

- respect and trust

- choice and consultation.

(Mental Health Foundation, 1994)

Complementary approaches may be well suited to contributing to attempts to satisfy the latter three points while the first point puts the potential role of treatment into context. User rights, put forward by the NHS Executive's Mental Health Task Force Users Group (1994) form a backdrop against which it again seems clear that, from the user's perspective, complementary approaches have a part to play in overall mental health care provision. Users are considered to have the right to:

- receive the least restrictive, least harmful treatment that is suitable for their needs

- be informed of harmful, or potentially harmful, effective medical treatment

- treatment that is compatible with their beliefs

- be informed of alternatives to medical treatment

- be treated or cared for by a trained, supervised, competent person.

The study of users' views, mentioned earlier, by the Mental Health Foundation (1997) reported on over 400 people's experience of mental health services and treatments and provided strong evidence of the value placed by many users on approaches which promote personal coping. Those surveyed (many of whom responded through their own concern about treatment, therefore, is a largely self-selected sample) indicated strong appreciation for talking treatments (counselling and psychotherapy) and for a range of alternative and complementary therapies, finding them much more helpful than psychiatric approaches. Between 85% and 97% of those who used complementary and alternative therapies and 88% of people with talking therapies found them helpful, compared with 67% of people using anti-depressants, just over 50% of those using major tranquillisers and only 30% of those who had ECT. Art and creative therapies had been experienced by nearly half of the sample and were found to help in expressing feelings, to focus the mind, to distract, to relax and through the provision of support and empathy.

Physical therapies (including osteopathy, aromatherapy, acupuncture, massage, reflexology) and exercise and postural therapies (such as yoga, Alexander technique and physical exercise) had both been experienced by about one third of those surveyed. Benefits mentioned included relaxation, being treated as a whole person, gaining a sense of being able to take control over their own treatment and promoting a sense of wellbeing. Treatment involving diet, natural supplements or remedies (naturopathy, herbalism, homeopathy) had been used by about one quarter of the people. Benefits here were more uncertain. It was noted that these treatments involved a more passive acceptance of treatment as compared with the more active engagement of mind and body in other treatments, and this may have led people to have similar expectations of them to those often held of conventional medical treatments.

Overall, the positive benefits of complementary therapies and alternative treatments for users was seen to be compatible with those of other active self-help actions (including hobbies and leisure activities, as well as spiritual support), and focused around promotion of a sense of structure and meaning in life. Up to half of the people sampled would like to try more and other complementary and alternative therapies; this demand for a greater range of provision seems likely to be still growing.

Purchasers

A study by the National Association of Health Authorities and Trusts (Mouncer, 1993) found that around 70% of purchasing authorities were, at that time, in favour of complementary therapies being available on the NHS. Being in favour in principle does not, however, necessarily translate into actual purchasing, especially in these days of financial constraint and competing demands for resources. A particular challenge of complementary therapy is the increased emphasis on evidence-based purchasing, which means that purchasing authorities are reluctant to buy treatment whose effectiveness has not been demonstrated in clinical trials.

The particular views of purchasers of mental health services about complementary therapies have yet to be ascertained, but given the current crisis in mental health services, along with the supposed attention to user views (Rogers & Pilgrim, 1996), there is certainly the case for the purchase of more complementary health provision, at least on the grounds of popular demand. Purchasers need information based on a range of sources, including the results of innovative research strategies encompassing broad views on what constitutes effectiveness. These should take into account, for example, the new emphasis on prevention, supposedly targeted by the shift of resources from secondary to primary care, and to which complementary medicine should be well placed to contribute, insofar as the holistic approach seeks to tackle causes as much as symptoms.

Providers

Many orthodox practitioners, including nurses, GPs, occupational therapists and psychologists are extending their skills and conceptual frameworks through learning complementary techniques. Indeed, much complementary treatment may already be implicitly purchased in this way. Complementary therapies may mesh particularly well with social and psychological approaches. They share an emphasis on the meaning of symptoms and on the therapeutic relationship as a vehicle for change, but complementary practitioners also bring in an acknowledgement of the bodily aspects of distress which are largely neglected by psychologists and social workers.

On the other hand, the challenge of alternative world views, incompatible treatment approaches and competition for resources may lead to rivalry, envy and mutual suspicion between some orthodox and non-orthodox practitioners. Users may be aware of this suspicion, as evidenced for example in a study which found that over half of those patients with cancer who were using alternative treatment did not reveal this to their medical practitioner (Downer *et al* 1994).

The ambivalence of psychiatrists is shown in their response to the NAHAT survey of views about complementary medicine in which the Royal College of Psychiatrists stated that, while recognising the value of those therapies whose efficacy had been proven and vindicated by research, *'they would not recommend that these be widely available on the NHS, at a time when existing services are funded inadequately'* (Mouncer, 1993).

At a political level, professional vested interests run deep and complementary practice will have to run the gauntlet of challenge from the medical profession if it is to make serious inroads into service provision. Nevertheless, the earlier antagonistic medical attitude to complementary practice has softened considerably, at least, in its official stance as conveyed in the BMA Report (1993).

How might complementary therapy be made available to users?

There are several possible routes for the provision of complementary treatment for people with mental health difficulties.

Private treatment with individual practitioners

It has sometimes been assumed that people with psychological distress are over-represented amongst patients of complementary practitioners, but this does not seem to be the case. In their 1995 study, Furnham and Beard found no difference in mental health status between three groups of people: regular users of complementary medicine, those who exclusively use orthodox medicine and a mixed group who use both. It seems extremely unlikely that people with severe mental health difficulties in particular, will be able to afford to buy private complementary treatment to any significant extent. This route, then, is unlikely to make a major impact on service provision, unless, as discussed overleaf, individual users receive the means to control their own healthcare budget.

Treatment purchased through primary health care

The implications for complementary health provision of the much heralded locality-based purchasing through primary care trusts are as yet uncertain. Given that the lead figures in locality purchasing will be GPs, there is scope both for optimism and uncertainty. GPs are known to be increasingly favourable to complementary medicine and are more favourable towards it than are hospital doctors (Whelan, 1995). They are open for several reasons, including being overwhelmed with those chronic conditions which conventional medicine often finds it difficult to alleviate, let alone cure, and sometimes even makes worse, amongst which mental health difficulties must be at the forefront.

A national survey of access to complementary health care via general practice (Thomas *et al*, 1995) showed that an estimated 40% of GP partnerships in England and Wales were willing to provide access to complementary treatment. Many of the pilot developmental schemes for the integration of complementary and orthodox medicine have been based in primary health care settings, and have demonstrated the value of complementary approaches for people experiencing anxiety and depression (Hooper *et al*, 1996; Hotchkiss, 1995; Welford & Hills, 1996).

However, GPs have little experience and expertise in working with people with severe and enduring mental health problems; the numbers of such people in any one practice are quite low and often GPs lack confidence in meeting their needs locally. There is no evidence available, so far, of complementary treatments being offered for people with severe and enduring mental health problems within primary health care, although this is a route that some practices, or groups of practices, may wish to pursue.

Treatment purchased through health authorities/ commissions or through joint funding with social services

There are three possible mechanisms here. First is through the purchase of complementary therapies as part of the package of services provided within a specialist NHS provider unit, such as community or mental health trusts. In this model, complementary therapists would be employed to work alongside the whole range of other practitioners, such as occupational therapists, community psychiatric nurses and psychologists, within the orthodox system. This is the integrated model of service provision with its own particular advantages and disadvantages. It offers complementary medicine the potential to influence the system from within but at the risk of being swallowed up by the prevailing ethos.

The second mechanism would be through the purchase of complementary therapies from separately contracted independent providers. This model, advocated by Whelan (1995) would require practitioners to group together to develop comprehensive services as clinics and holistic centres and to market their services to purchasers in a business-like way. The potential advantage of this approach is that it may harness the entrepreneurial spirit of many practitioners and provide the means of developing a real robust alternative to the medical model. It also requires practitioners to find convincing methods to demonstrate their cost effectiveness and to contribute a broader and deeper debate about relevant outcomes.

The third and most direct mechanism for purchasing would be individually, for example, through the care manager via the Care Programme Assessment process. There is no documentation on the extent to which this is happening already – with few resources available, the scope for creative purchasing of this type is small, yet it is possible to speculate that if the financial resources did reach the individual user (if people were given real power), they would choose to buy complementary approaches in preference to conventional treatments. As things stand, commentators have recognised that users and their families have insufficient money within their own control to make choices about how they wish to be helped (Blom-Cooper & Murphy, 1991).

Voluntary sector provision

Traditionally the most exciting, innovative and user-centred approaches have been through the voluntary sector who have the freedom and licence to create imaginative services. It seems likely that many new developments in offering complementary therapy to long term users will be through day centres and drop-in centres within organisations such as Mind. In such settings, users themselves can be involved in finding out what therapies and therapists suit them, and in making decisions about how best to involve them in their lives.

In summary, visionary joint commissioning or purchasing of mental health care should facilitate the provision of a co-ordinated but not monolithic range of services, which together meet a whole range of preventative, social and health needs. Complementary therapies may form part of this range of services. Sometimes this may be through the enrichment of current practice of NHS care providers who adopt new ideas and techniques from other traditions. Sometimes it will be through the direct public sector purchase of alternative practice as individual practitioners or sometimes as collaborative partnerships between practitioners or in partnership with voluntary sector provision.

Examples of practice

Projects in which complementary treatments are made available to mental health users are quietly mushrooming across the country, but none have yet been formally documented. Two national conferences have facilitated some networking between those who are interested in further developments: the first was organised by the King's Fund in 1995 (Jennings, 1995) and the second by Pavilion in 1997 (the proceedings of which are unpublished). Wallcraft's report (1998), already mentioned, summarises the information currently available.

Two examples give a flavour of how complementary therapies may be provided in practice. The stress project in Islington developed originally within the voluntary sector via a group of neighbourhood charitable projects (Biznieks, 1997, personal communication). The project became funded through a mixture of direct commissioning by the local health authority and local authority (social services), a grant from the Department of Health and independent fundraising. The project was based on medical referrals with clearly specified criteria for acceptance for treatment. A therapy programme was offered over a period of about a year for any individual user, consisting of one talking therapy (from a range of various cognitive and counselling approaches), along with up to two complementary therapies (including treatment such as massage, reflexology, homeopathy, acupuncture). The aim of the work was crisis prevention targeted at those in greatest need, and over half the users were identified as having severe and enduring mental health problems. Users were debriefed at the end of their treatment: further funding would be needed to secure ongoing supportive therapy for vulnerable people. The value of the service to users and referrers seemed to lie in its firm base in the community, its separateness from the mental health service (thereby avoiding stigmatisation) and its apparently beneficial therapeutic impact on clients' quality of life, self-esteem and ability to cope.

Another project was the complementary therapy project in Leeds (Bergin, 1997, personal communication 1997), which grew out of a stress management group within a social services day centre, where user interest stimulated the establishment of a multidisciplinary and user steering group with initial funding from the Mental Health Task Force. Users self-referred to the project, although requiring agreement from their GP or psychiatrist. A range of therapies were offered, including hypnotherapy, Shiatsu, osteopathy and acupuncture. Practitioners with professional qualifications and insurance were initially interviewed by a member of the steering group and had regular supervision with the co-ordinator of the day centre and through social services. Informal evaluation indicated that users valued receiving a service offered by people who have time to listen and who gave physical and emotional care in a tangible form. Challenges included establishing secure financial support and gaining the consent of those medical practitioners who are suspicious of a new approach which has not yet been formally evaluated.

General issues in the provision of complementary therapies in mental health

Medico-legal responsibility

Guidelines for the employment of therapists in the NHS include specifications that therapists give evidence of Professional Body membership (with Codes of Conduct) insurance cover and appropriate qualifications in their therapy (Hooper *et al*, 1996). There is an increasing push for statutory registration of the therapies; this has already been achieved by osteopathy and chiropractic.

However, Stone and Matthews (1996) have warned that while increasing regulation may appear to be in the interest of consumer protection, the consequent increase in the professional power and authority of the therapist may diminish the egalitarian popularity of complementary medicine. They question whether, to the extent that the therapeutic relationship is based on mutual responsibilities and sharing of information and power, holistic medicine is actually capable of being formally regulated in a meaningful sense. They argue instead for a patient-centred non-statutory regulatory framework with clear systems for registration, a strong code of ethics and effective and accessible grievance procedures.

Complementary practitioners in any case, along with other health professionals, are bound by their 'duty of care' towards their clients which requires them to take 'reasonable care in all circumstances', including recognising the limits to their professional training and competence. Wallcraft (1998) gives a helpful set of criteria for the practice of complementary therapies within the NHS, based on a set of guidelines for using a complementary therapy within an NHS Trust, which considers issues including authorisation, consent, supervision and insurance.

Practice issues

Challenges for complementary and orthodox practitioners working together within mental health settings may include the following:

- Complementary practitioners dealing with a very different client population from that encountered in private practice. The experiences of people who are homeless, poor, from a range of ethnic origin and social background may be unfamiliar for many practitioners.

- Becoming aware of, and overcoming, prejudices about people with mental health difficulties. Practitioners may need to develop complex understandings about the multi-factorial nature of mental health problems and about how to facilitate people's own choices about treatment decisions. Most complementary therapy training does not specifically deal with mental health issues and practitioners have not traditionally viewed themselves as particularly competent in dealing with severe mental health difficulties.

- Dealing with demands of teamwork. Many complementary practitioners enjoy the independent nature of private practice and may find the complexity of inter-professional relationships in teamwork to be of mixed benefit – in some ways it diminishes their autonomy while in others it gives greater support and new understandings.

- Dealing with professionals' prejudices about one another's work. People will need to cope with envy and competitiveness, as well as finding ways of enriching one another's practice through learning about different world views and approaches.

- Developing confidence in one another's therapeutic approaches. Complementary practitioners may need and want help and supervision, for example in finding out how to deal safely, confidently and sympathetically with disclosure by users of sensitive material. Equally, orthodox practitioners may need to remember that for users, ordinary human attention, listening and being taken seriously are often experienced as at least as helpful as more expert treatment including counselling and psychotherapy.

- Acknowledging and respecting one another's contribution and promoting appropriate but not intrusive communication with patients and between practitioners when more than one approach is being used.

- Clarifying medico-legal issues around recommendation, referral and delegation of treatment.

Questions of harm

Can complementary therapies cause harm? Any therapeutic discipline which has the potential for benefit must also have the capacity to cause damage if inappropriately applied. Four possible areas of difficulty are:

- misapplication of technique

- emotional or physical exploitation

- wrong application of a therapeutic modality when another treatment could be more helpful

- victim blaming.

In order to avoid technical failure or exploitation of patients, complementary therapists, just as much as orthodox practitioners, need to maintain effective systems for regular supervision and personal support, along with continued post-training education. Orthodox practitioners often raise the concern that people who use complementary treatments may thereby forego the benefits of more orthodox approaches. In practice this seems unlikely to happen to any significant degree since most people do not shift completely to complementary medicine and, in any case, usually turn in that direction only when orthodox approaches have already been found to be ineffective. The emphasis on gentle restoration of health, rather than removal of disease, implies a recognition of the significance of growth, development and empowerment, but also holds the seed of a potentially harmful tendency to over-emphasise the individual's own responsibility for their wellbeing, while taking less regard of the contextual factors which constrain individuals' choices and opportunities. Many traditional complementary approaches *do* recognise the role of community and social factors in promoting or preventing distress and disorder, but the way such approaches have been applied in Western culture has tended to emphasise the individual's role in managing his or her own circumstances. Our current awareness of the role of the structural inequalities in society which underpin ill health (Wilkinson, 1996) must alert us to the value of searching for alternative ways of tackling social, as well as individual sources of distress. Traditional medical systems such as Ayurvedic and Chinese medicine, coming from cultures which value dependence and inter-connectedness relatively more than in the West, with its emphasis on independence and autonomy, may have much to offer in this respect. Currently however, the focus is on the new insights which complementary therapies may bring to individual treatment.

Summary

The potential role of complementary therapies in mental health may include:

- the use of specific techniques for managing particular symptoms

- alleviation of stress, particularly at times of crisis, for users and carers

- providing an alternative source of pleasure or relaxation

- helping users to find an increased sense of meaning in life

- primary and secondary prevention through focusing on positive health

- providing therapies which may be more in tune with the belief systems of people from a wide range of cultures

- facilitating personal empowerment through encouraging active participation in treatment and offering self-help advice

- promoting self-esteem and enhancing morale through offering care and concern along with time and touch

- offering hope in seemingly intractible situations.

We need more publications in the area of complementary therapy in mental health, including descriptive studies of service innovations, single case studies, critical reviews of already published work, audit of current practice, qualitative studies of users' motivations and experiences in using the therapies, as well as clinical trials. Finally, the potential impact of any therapy in mental health work (complementary and orthodox) must be seen in a context of awareness of the crucial importance of economic factors in influencing people's physical and psychological wellbeing. Complementary therapies, or indeed expert treatment of any kind, will not be a panacea but may play a modest role in improving people's mental health along with improved social support, income, accommodation and opportunities for meaningful leisure and occupation.

References

Bergin, S. (1997) Personal Communication, Complementary Therapy Project, Roundhay Road Day Centre, Leeds.

Biznieks, I. (1997) Personal Communication, Stress Project, Shelburne Road, Islington.

Blom-Cooper, L. & Murphy, E. (1991) Mental health services and resources. *Psychiatric Bulletin* 15 65–68.

BMA (1993) *Complementary Medicine: New approaches and good practice.* Oxford: Oxford University Press.

Breggin, P. (1993) *Toxic psychiatry.* London: Harper Collins.

Downer, S. M., Cody, M. M., McCluskey, P., Wilson, P. D., Arnott, S. J., Lister, T. A., Sleuin, M. L. (1994) Pursuit and practice of complementary therapies by cancer patients receiving conventional treatment. *British Medical Journal* 309 86–89.

Foundation for Integrated Medicine (1997) *Integrated Healthcare – a way forward for the next five years? A discussion document.* London: FIM.

Fulder, S. (1996) *Handbook of Alternative and Complementary Medicine.* Oxford: Oxford University Press.

Furnham, A. & Beard, R. (1995) Health, just world beliefs and coping style preferences in patients of complementary and orthodox medicine. *Social Science and Medicine* **40** 1425–1432.

Hooper, J., Ruddlesden, J., Heyes, A., Ash, S. & Styan, S. (1996) *Introducing Complementary Therapists into GP Practices in Huddersfield and Dewsbury: Evaluation Report.* Huddersfield: West Yorkshire Health Authority.

Hotchkiss, J. (1995) *The First Year of a Service Offering Complementary Therapies in the NHS.* University of Liverpool: Liverpool Centre for Health, Department of Public Health.

Jennings, S. (1995) *Complementary Therapies in Mental Health Treatment.* London: King's Fund.

Linde, K., Ramirez, G., Mulrow, C. D. & Pauls, A. (1996) St John's Wort for depression: an overview and meta-analysis of randomised clinical trials. *British Medical Journal* **313** 253–258.

McIver, S. (1993) *Obtaining the Views of Users of Primary and Community Care Services.* London: King's Fund.

Mental Health Foundation (1994) *Creating Community Care.* London: Mental Health Foundation.

Mental Health Foundation (1997) *Knowing Our Own Minds.* London: MHF.

Mental Health Task Force User Group (1994) *Guidelines for a Local Charter for Users of Mental Health Services.* London: NHS Executive.

Mind (1995) *A–Z of Complementary and Alternative Therapies.* London: Mind Publications.

Mitchell, A. & Cormack, C. (1998) *The Therapeutic Relationship in Complementary Healthcare.* Edinburgh: Churchill Livingstone.

Mouncer, Y. (1993) *Complementary Therapies in the NHS.* Birmingham: NAHAT.

Pietroni, P. C. (1992) Alternative medicine: methinks the doctor protests too much and incidentally befuddles the debate. *Journal of Medical Ethics* **18** (1) 23–25.

Pietroni, P. C. (1990) *The Greening of Medicine.* London: Gollancz.

Rogers, A. & Pilgrim, D. (1996) *Mental Health Policy in Britain.* Basingstoke: MacMillan.

Sharma, U. (1992) *Complementary Medicine Today: Practitioners and patients.* London: Routledge.

Stone, J. & Matthews, J. (1996) *Complementary Medicine and the Law.* Oxford: Oxford University Press.

Thomas, K., Fall, M., Parry, G., Nicholl, J. (1995) *National Survey of Access to Complementary Health Care Via General Practice.* University of Sheffield: Medical Care Research Unit, Sheffield Centre for Health and Related Research.

Vickers, A. (1996a) *Massage and Aromatherapy: A guide for professionals.* London: Chapman and Hall.

Vickers, A. (1996b) Complementary medicine in mental health care. *Psychiatry in Practice* 11–14

Vickers, A. & Zollman, C. (1999) ABC of complementary medicine: hypnosis and relaxation therapies. *British Medical Journal* **319** 1346–1349.

Vincent, C. & Furnham, A. (1994) The perceived efficacy of complementary and orthodox medicine: preliminary findings and the development of a questionnaire. *Complementary Therapies in Medicine* **2** 128–134.

Wallcraft , J. (1998) *Healing Minds.* London: Mental Health Foundation.

Welford, R. & Hills, D. (1996) *Glastonbury complementary health service.* Unpublished report by the Glastonbury Health Centre.

Whelan, J. (1995) Complementary therapies and the changing NHS: a development officer's view. *Complementary Therapies in Medicine* **3** 79-83.

Wilkinson, R. G. (1996) *Unhealthy Societies: The afflictions of inequality.* London: Routledge.

Yamey, G. (2000) Can complementary medicine be evidence based? *Western Journal of Medicine* **173** 4–5.

Zollman, C. & Vickers, A. (1999) ABC of Complementary medicine: what is complementary medicine? *British Medical Journal* **319** 693–696.

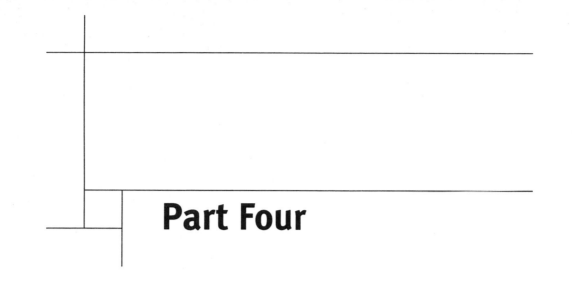

Part Four

Chapter 13

Users' Views of Mental Health Services

Marian Barnes

Introduction

This chapter explores what those who receive mental health services think about them. I am not writing this chapter as a user of mental health services and this fact needs some discussion. Elsewhere I have written:

> *'One of the most fundamental objectives of user groups is to claim the right to self definition for people whose identity and 'problems' have been defined by professionals. Reclaiming the right to define themselves and their problems is a prerequisite for attaining other objectives.'*
>
> (Barnes & Shardlow, 1996)

Why then did I agree to write this chapter?

My interest and involvement in this subject derives initially from my identity as a researcher working first in social services departments and then in university departments. In developing my practice as a researcher I have been challenged by people who use services claiming that I use their experiences for my own purposes, observing them as objects of research and acting in a similar way to service providers who regard them as objects of professional intervention. I have sought to respond to this by developing ways of conducting research which involve people as participants or 'active subjects' within the research process. That is not only a statement of values, but also a belief that to know and understand the world requires us to look at it from the perspectives of those who do not have the power to define it through, for example, determining the substance of professional education or what is considered to constitute 'knowledge' in formal terms. My understanding has been developed by working with people who use mental health services in research and other contexts.

But my interest in this subject is not just that of a researcher. It is also a personal and a political interest. Approximately one third of the population will experience mental health problems at some stage in their lives. Mental distress is a normal part of human experience. Whilst my personal experience is limited to discovering that I had once been recorded by my GP as suffering from an 'anxiety state', family members have had more extensive experience of mental distress and of mental health services. Just as those who have used mental health services may never be confident that they have reached the point of being an 'ex-user', all of us are *potential* users of mental health services. That is not to deny the qualitative difference of experience of those who have been diagnosed as mentally ill, but to recognise that people who use mental health services are not 'other', but are fellow citizens and could be us.

The political dimension of my interest concerns ways in which it might be possible to create an inclusive society. Self-organisation on the part of mental health service users and others who have been subject to exclusionary policies is vital if stigmatising policies and practices are to be overcome. But the achievement of those objectives also requires the creation of alliances which recognise that inclusion benefits all, not just those who have been excluded. Thus my contribution here is not intended to usurp the direct expressions of those who have experienced mental health services, nor is it intended to suggest that those experiences only achieve legitimacy if they are filtered through the lens of research. It is intended to reflect a shared ownership and responsibility for action, and to contribute to the creation of welfare services which enable social inclusion and social justice.

In this chapter I will be drawing on user-led research as well as my own research and that conducted by others who have also sought to research *with*, rather than *on*, users of mental health services. Quotes which are not referenced come from my own research and have not been published elsewhere. But first, I want to reflect on some of the reasons why users' views of mental health services may not be heard or taken seriously.

Finding a voice

In *Keeping in Touch with the Talking* (Ritchie *et al*, 1988) a man who had been a 'patient' in a psychiatric hospital for ten years was quoted as saying: *'if you don't keep your hand in with the talking, you get not to talk at all'.* He was reflecting on the isolation often experienced by people with long-term mental health problems, which can make it difficult for people to find a voice to express their views. One of the conclusions of the above report was that *'...individuals simply need people to talk to, someone who will have a conversation, listen to what they have to say and, most importantly, show some interest in them'* (*ibid*).

Social isolation, both within psychiatric hospitals and amongst people with mental health problems living 'in the community' can make it difficult for people to find a voice. However, when they do express their views, the validity of what they have to say may be discredited. They may be considered to 'lack insight' into their condition, or the nature of their illness may be cited as reason for disbelieving what they have to say. At times they may be legally denied the right to make their own decisions about whether or not to receive treatment.

People who have experienced severe mental disorder may accept that there are times when decisions about their care and treatment need to be taken by others. However, that does not mean that they should be regarded as permanently 'incompetent', nor that mental illness is necessarily associated with lack of capacity to take decisions. An activist in a mental health user group described one function of the group:

> *'One of the major roles that we can play is actually to say, "We are users, we can participate at this level, we can articulate, we can challenge, we can negotiate, we can write papers, we can do this", instead of [being] some bumbling idiot that doesn't know what they are doing.'*
> (Barnes & Shardlow, 1996)

Elsewhere, a young man involved in a newly formed user group talked to me of the way in which being part of that group was a way of 'practising to participate' in other forums. Finding a voice and then being able to express that voice to service commissioners or providers can be very difficult for people who have experienced having little say over their treatment and, in some instances, of being told that they are not competent to make decisions for themselves. User groups provide an important source of support for people to develop skills and confidence in expressing their views, taking control of their own lives, and in contributing to shaping services for others (Barnes & Shardlow, 1996, 1997; Harrison, 1993).

At the same time, the voices of mental health service users can be experienced as threatening by professional service providers. When users have had the opportunity to express their views they have often been very critical of service providers. Those messages can be difficult to hear. A manager in Birmingham interviewed about a user council project there said:

> *'Users' voices are angry and unreasonable... and [are] seen in those kinds of terms.'*

He went on to suggest why it may be more difficult to hear the views of users of mental health services than of users of other services:

> *'Perhaps it's expressed in more extreme terms within this service and there are two possible explanations. One is users of these services have as characteristics of their problem, features of their behaviour which lead them to express themselves in those kind of terms: they may be paranoid for example. The alternative explanation is equally valid...they genuinely are more oppressed (because they can be subject to compulsory detention)'*
> (Quoted in Barnes & Wistow, 1994)

Whilst some service managers talked about the need for support and encouragement if people were to express their views in a way which had previously been denied to them, there was a view that the user councils had provided an opportunity for an angry and extreme voice to be unleashed against service providers (*ibid*). Professional defensiveness in the face of views expressed within users' councils was considered to be particularly evident in the responses of some medical staff. Users who had been hospital inpatients were clearly very angry about both the attitude of psychiatrists and about users' lack of involvement in treatment decisions. Many of them did not experience benefits from the medical treatment they were given and felt that they were not offered any other choices. In fact, the three psychiatrists interviewed responded very differently to the challenges offered by users. One regarded the views expressed as stupid and ill-informed, but one of his colleagues reflected a different view, recognising that the users were forcing doctors to face up to uncomfortable questions about the efficacy of the treatments they were providing, as well as making positive contributions to the development of alternative service models.

It has not just been in Birmingham that the expression of views by mental health service users has caused difficulties for service providers. Mind, East Sussex County Council and Brighton Health Authority co-organised 'Common Concerns', a conference which brought together users and mental health professionals. It was described by Ros HeppleWhite, then-Director of Mind, as *'a turbulent three days, as people's roles and sensitivities and aspirations were to some extent subject to uncomfortable analysis'.* (HeppleWhite, 1988). Whilst health and social care professionals are being increasingly encouraged to involve users individually and collectively in decision-making about services, many still find this challenging and many users find it hard to express their views to those who have considerable power over them.

Experiencing mental health problems

It is not possible to consider users' experiences of mental health services without also considering the experience of mental illness, or indeed 'madness' as some would prefer. Both fictional and autobiographical accounts are testimony to the way in which a diagnosis of mental illness has far reaching and long-term impacts on the way in which it is possible to live one's life. It has a fundamental impact on an individual's sense of self, on the way others view them, and on the objective opportunities people have for pursuing personal objectives. The experience of mental illness and of receiving mental health services are bound up together. In her preface to *The Loony Bin Trip*, Kate Millett (1991) writes:

> *'This is an account of a journey into that nightmare state ascribed to "madness" that social condition, that experience of being cast out and confined... It is a journey many of us take. Some of us survive it intact, others only partially survive, debilitated by the harm done to us: the temptations of complicity, of the career of "patient", the pressures towards capitulation. I am telling this too in the hope that it may help all those who have been or are about to be in the same boat, those captured and shaken by this bizarre system of beliefs: the general superstition of "mental disease", the physical fact of incarceration and compulsory drugs, finally the*

threat of being put away and locked up forever, or if released, stigmatised throughout the rest of one's life.'

Mental health problems can in themselves undermine confidence, self-esteem and a coherent sense of self. Such difficulties can be exacerbated by lay views of mental illness and by policies and practices within mental health services which deny the capacity of people to be involved in determining their needs and how these might best be met.

> *'On two occasions, about eight years apart, I experienced the intense distress, depersonalisation, and sense of unreality that is often described as the onset of acute psychosis. During the first experience, believing that I needed medical help, I voluntarily admitted myself to a mental hospital. For six months I was in and out of hospitals (several times involuntarily), was given large doses of tranquillising drugs, and was generally made into a mental patient. I was told, and I believed, that my feelings of unhappiness were indications of mental illness. At one point, a hospital psychiatrist told me that I would never be able to live outside a mental institution. By the time of my final discharge I was convinced of my own inferiority, a feeling that lasted for years.'*
> (Chamberlin, 1988)

Mental illness is associated with abnormality and deviance and the disputed nature of many diagnoses of mental disorder has been the cause of abuse perpetrated by the mental health system on those who are regarded as deviant. That has been the case not only in the Soviet Union where political dissidents were labelled mentally ill and incarcerated, but also in this country where women giving birth to children outside marriage have, in the past, been admitted to long stay psychiatric hospitals. Women in particular have found that madness and lack of conformity to gender roles are closely associated in the minds of lay people and of mental health professionals (Matthews, 1984; Ussher,

1991). In view of this it is not surprising that one of the objectives of user groups is to emphasise the normality of mental distress:

> *...a vicar's wife once said, "What if I invite these people into my home? How would they be?" And I said, "Well they'll be like you, they'll have two eyes, a nose and a mouth and two ears." You know, they think they're going to see something weird and they don't know that perhaps they'll have a nervous breakdown and start with a mental illness'.*
> (Quoted in Barnes & Shardlow, 1996)

At an individual level 'becoming ordinary' has been identified as an objective of people leaving psychiatric hospitals and seeking to reclaim their ability to function effectively in the community (Lorencz, 1991). However, this may involve recognising how 'normality' or 'ordinariness' are understood by those with power to prevent discharge and pretending an intention to go along with this. Lorencz's research describes a range of behaviours, including controlling anger and denying hearing voices or hallucinating, intended to convince professionals of the person's readiness for discharge, whilst Judi Chamberlin (1988) quotes examples of women pretending plans to return to college, get a job or get married.

'Ordinary life' is not always protective of people's mental health. Many women who become long-term users of mental health services have been sexually abused, and the diagnosis of borderline personality disorder – which often attaches to women who have been traumatised by abuse – can feel like a punishment of the victim, and not the perpetrator, of that abuse for others' abusive behaviour (eg Briere, 1984; Bryer *et al*, 1987). The experience of mental distress is tied up with the experience of abuse, and the disbelief or silencing with which descriptions of abuse are often received by mental health professionals can be experienced as further abuse within the mental health system (Sayce, 1996).

Black people's experience can be similar. Racism can contribute not only to the experience of mental distress, but also to the treatment received within the system (Fernando, 1991). Fernando suggests that schizophrenia is over-diagnosed amongst Black people who are seen to be both 'alien' and 'inferior'. A perception of the 'dangerousness' of Black people may account for evidence that Black people of African or Caribbean origin are more likely to be subject to the controlling powers of mental health legislation (Bowl & Barnes, 1990) and receive higher doses of medication and more frequent physical restraint (Lipsedge, 1994; Moodley & Thornicroft, 1988)

Mental distress and mental illness can be experienced throughout life. There are few personal accounts of the experience of mental distress in old age, but it is important also to recognise the way in which depression in old age can be associated with loss of physical health, of roles, of partners or families, and how experience of mental health services may exacerbate that sense of loss (Murphy, 1982). Depression is the most widespread mental health problem in old age (Copeland *et al*, 1987), but dementia is perhaps the most feared disorder of age. There are some powerful fictional accounts which provide sensitive attempts to enter into the worlds of those with dementia or at least to provide some understanding of what the experience of dementia may mean. Michael Ignatieff's autobiographical novel, *Scar Tissue* (1993), recounts a son's experience of his mother's dementia and explores the way in which awareness is considered to fragment:

> '*By this stage, I was all in pieces inside her; name, face, texture of skin, shape of my eyes, all tumbling over and over in the darkness of her mind. Upon occasion, she would catch a piece of the broken mirror and hold it long enough to know who I was. That shard would slip loose and sink back into the shadows and she wouldn't give a flicker of recognition.*'

For many people the experience of mental distress is also an experience of stigma and discrimination (Read & Baker, 1996; Ritchie *et al*, 1988). Amongst the findings from a Mind survey of experiences of the impact of mental illness on everyday lives, were the following:

- 34% of those responding said they had been dismissed or forced to resign from their jobs

- 47% said they had been abused or harassed in public

- 26% were forced to move home as a result of harassment

- 25% had been turned down by insurance or finance companies.

The Ritchie *et al* study (*ibid*) reported people talking of losing not only their jobs, but of family breakdowns, and of young people who had left home being forced back into their parental homes because of poverty. Even those who become active in mental health user groups can find it difficult to admit to being mental health service users because of the stigma associated with this:

> '...*everybody accepts their mental health problems in different ways because some of our members – one especially comes to mind – he feels terribly ashamed. Now I've said to him time and time again, "Why? It's an illness." But we can't get through to him.*'

This is why mental health user groups are not only involved in action intended to improve the nature of mental health services, but on a broader front to raise public awareness and overcome stigma (Barnes & Shardlow, 1996 and 1997; Rogers & Pilgrim, 1991).

As well as exclusion resulting from stigma, people who experience mental health problems for lengthy periods are also likely to be living in difficult financial circumstances and often extreme poverty. Personal accounts of the impact of mental illness are supported by research such as that reviewed by Warner (1994) which provides evidence of the links between economic circumstances and schizophrenia. Recovery from mental illness is made more difficult if people are also worrying about getting welfare benefits sorted out and having enough money to pay their bills (Davis & Betteridge, 1990).

Another aspect of the experience of mental illness can be the constraints on the formal rights of citizenship. People considered incapable of managing their own financial affairs may have to apply to the Court of Protection before they can spend money belonging to them. Those in psychiatric hospitals may be effectively prevented from voting, and compulsory hospital admission and medical treatment runs counter to usual expectations that decisions whether or not to accept health care are freely entered into. These constraints apply only to a small proportion of those diagnosed as mentally ill, but nevertheless represent a significant aspect of the experience of long-term mental illness for that minority, and a source of concern for many more.

Thus, when people who use mental health services reflect on their experiences of using services, it is neither possible nor helpful to ignore their wider experiences of mental illness and the effect this has on their lives. Mental health services are judged not only on the day-to-day experience of service use, but on their capacity to contribute to overcoming social exclusion and to facilitate people's opportunities to live as citizens within their communities.

Even when help is sought directly in relation to the symptoms of mental illness, this will often be only part of the reason for approaching service providers. Rogers *et al* (1993) found that only 10.7% of those they surveyed gave 'mental illness' as the reason for their first contact with mental health services. Amongst the other reasons people sought help were: marital problems, work stress, bereavement and physical illness. Rogers *et al* (*ibid*) also give examples of the way in which the process through which certain types of experiences or behaviours come to be defined as mental illness involves a series of negotiations which often start in the lay world of encounters between family, friends or strangers. Such negotiations can involve both voluntary and coercive contact with mental health services. It is at this point that experiences of mental distress become tied up with experiences of mental health services. This is why it is important to address the issue of whether or not people are able to negotiate their own perspectives on the nature of their problems, or whether they find themselves subject to definitions which do not equate with their own perceptions of their needs or problems.

Experiencing services

Hospitals

Whilst many users recognise that there are times when admission to hospital is necessary to provide protection, treatment, or asylum (Rogers *et al*, 1993), the reality for many is that the experience of being in hospital is one of isolation, powerlessness and fear. Poor, overcrowded physical environments provide little opportunity for healing.

Reports produced by user council project workers in mental health services in one part of Birmingham reflected considerable criticism of hospital services. Users were unhappy with the physical environment in which services were provided; they were concerned about high levels of medication and a lack of choice over the treatments they were given; and about the attitudes of staff, in particular doctors, who were widely perceived to be *'impolite, arrogant, disrespectful, dismissive of users' wishes'* (quoted in Barnes & Wistow, 1994). Perring (1992) reports users' experiences of routined and impersonal treatment regimes, with little opportunity for ordinary activity and little preparation for the time when they would leave the hospital environment. Perkins (1996) reports the experiences of women who had been using mental health services and being admitted to hospital for at least a decade. They talked of lack of privacy, of not being treated as an adult, of the need for women-only spaces and to be able to choose their keyworker or doctor. Underlying many of their observations was the experience of not being listened to and not being believed – both by friends and by mental health workers.

Being admitted to hospital, particularly under a section of the *Mental Health Act*, can feel like being completely cut off from ordinary life (Hutchings, 1989). As the number of hospital beds has decreased, hospital wards have become full, if not overcrowded, and admission can be a frightening experience because levels of disturbance can be high. Admitting someone to hospital because they are at risk of harming themselves or others does not necessarily represent a move to a 'place of safety'. There is often a lack of privacy and women have been subject to unwanted sexual advances and active abuse by both patients and staff whilst in hospital (Wood & Copperman, 1996). Suicide attempts or self-harming will lead to 'specialing' – constant observation to prevent a repeat of such action. Whilst intended as protection against further harm, this intrudes fundamentally on privacy and on any sense of being in control of your own situation. Linda Hart, herself a psychiatric nurse who was admitted to the same hospital in which she worked, has described this experience:

> *'Let me out, let me out. The voice is laughing at me, the keys jingle like wind chimes; the staff are walking musical xylophones with only the upper keys in use. I'm rooted to the chair because I dare not get up in case I come up against a locked door and lose my determinedly held control. Keep the lid on. Be subject to all the indignities of powerlessness. Play the game, be the model patient to get the specialing lifted and perhaps a long desired walk outside. Present as "normal".'*
> (Hart, 1995)

The loss of autonomy and of separation from the world outside is particularly extreme for those admitted to high secure 'special' hospitals. Special hospital patients are utterly dependent on the staff of the hospital and on others detained with them to meet every need: for shelter, food, entertainment, for social and emotional contact, for care and treatment, and for respect and rehabilitation. This dependence exists in an environment in which conflict between the provision of care and the protection of society is usually resolved in favour of security. For women in particular, the experience of detention in a special hospital can be highly damaging. The incidence of self-harm amongst women in special hospitals is very high. But women also report verbal, physical and sexual abuse by members of staff, as well as an absence of opportunity for physical exercise and for creative activity (Eaton & Humphries, 1996; Hemingway, 1996; Barnes & Stephenson, 1996).

The notion of 'asylum' as a place of safety is largely absent from many accounts of users' experiences of psychiatric hospitals. Nevertheless there are attempts to reclaim the positive meaning of the term from the pejorative ways in which it has been applied to 'madhouses'. Wallcraft (1996) notes the range of practical meanings the term can have for those who regard themselves as survivors of psychiatric services, including the possibility of self-referral to an acute unit on the understanding that there will be no forced treatment and that personal preferences will be respected. But crisis houses away from the hospital setting, run by professional staff but with substantial user input, and less formal safe houses provided by friends and by other service users, are also seen as important elements of a system of support in times of crisis.

Wallcraft's inclusion of hospital admission as providing a potential for asylum reflects a range of views and experiences which identify positive as well as negative features of periods of separation from 'ordinary life'. Even Eaton and Humphries (*ibid*) found that women in special hospitals developed friendships which could provide a form of asylum for each other. In a rather different context, Prior (1995) discusses an example of a man who was a long-stay patient in a psychiatric hospital in Northern Ireland who *'refused to leave hospital, on the grounds that he was quite happy with his life'* he had *'a job, somewhere to sleep, and a place to keep the bicycle'* (Case notes, 1969). Mental health user groups are rarely campaigning for complete abolition of hospital or other types of residentially based mental health services. Rather, they are seeking to ensure that the quality of such service can offer genuine asylum and specialist help over which users have control, and which acknowledges and respects their individual needs.

Experiencing community services

One of the main objectives of community care is to replace the warehousing of large scale institutions with more individually responsive services. The development of the Care Programme Approach (CPA) and the introduction of community care assessments were both intended to base service responses around the needs of individuals and to enable service users to play a more active part on the process of determining their own care package. So what do users think about this approach to services? Beeforth *et al* (1994) conducted an evaluation based on users' views of case management in four health districts. The key positive themes emerging from this study were:

- what people valued most was their relationship with their case manager

- people felt they were listened to and allowed to make choices

- practical help with housing and benefits was valued

- case managers were seen to help people make better use of their time

- case managers were also able to help with sorting out family relationships.

But users expressed dissatisfaction as well. Care management itself cannot resolve problems relating to the shortage of community facilities and the difficulties of findings jobs. Nor can it resolve dissatisfaction with hospital admission and medication. But overall, this study indicated a positive response to case management and a wish that this would continue. An earlier report produced by users working with staff at what was then RDP (now the Sainsbury Centre for Mental Health) was rather less positive about case management:

'The central issue in improving systems of care is not case management, with all its implications of users

> *being "managed"' by professionals, but quality, with*
> *quality defined in terms of what users want and need.'*
> (Beeforth *et al*, 1990)

Nevertheless, 'care workers' were considered to be important in helping users find their way through the service system. Choice of care worker and access to an independent advocate were considered to be rights which should be enjoyed by all users and the report called for statutory funding of advocacy services.

The potential of user involvement in the process of assessment has been recognised in Avon where users and professionals have jointly developed an approach intended to support users in conducting their own self-assessments as a preliminary to discussing their needs with care managers (Avon Mental Health Measure, n.d.).

The Centre for Mental Health Services Development at the King's Fund has developed an approach to the strategic planning of mental health services based on stakeholder conferences which have focused on achievements or outcomes for users (Smith, n.d). They list the characteristics of a service which users have suggested would meet their needs. Such a service would provide help to users:

- with emotional problems
- in getting through a crisis
- in finding somewhere to live
- to have a full life during the day
- in making and keeping friendships
- by providing care which is rooted in an understanding of their culture or background
- in getting a reasonable income
- in finding someone to speak on their behalf if necessary
- in getting and holding down a job

■ in linking with others of the same race/culture and/or gender

■ in learning new skills.

This largely reflects the earlier work by Ritchie and her colleagues in Birmingham and emphasises the significance of help with the ordinary activities of life, rather than that of specialist mental health services. It is the way in which mental illness affects people's lives as a whole which causes people to seek help as much as (if not more than) the symptoms of mental illness *per se.*

Users of community mental health services tend to be less critical than those using hospital services. Indeed, one day centre manager in Birmingham said she had encouraged users of the centre to be more critical – but with limited success. Similarly, users who received home visits from their psychiatrist, or who met him at a drop-in centre felt little motivation to become involved in a user council because there was no sense of compulsion in the way in which services were provided (Barnes & Wistow, 1994). It is the experience of compulsion, whether as a result of action under the *Mental Health Act* or the result of lack of information, choice or the exercise of professional power, which underpins many of the dissatisfactions expressed by users of mental health services. This is why there has been widespread opposition from users to extensions of compulsory powers into community settings (Neeter, 1993).

Rogers *et al* (1993) reported a majority of users in their survey having a more positive response to the help received from their GP than from their psychiatrist. This was often associated with the GP's distance from hospital-based psychiatry and with what was perceived to be a more open and sympathetic manner of relating to the user. On the other hand, some users viewed their GP's lack of specialist mental health expertise in a negative light. One particular criticism of GPs is that they are too ready to prescribe medication and spend too little time talking to their patients. The inadequacy of community-based counselling services was a concern raised by users with me in an unpublished study of mental health needs in Shropshire. Whilst help with the ordinary activities of life is fundamental to any community-based service to meet the needs of those with mental health problems, users are also concerned that a reduction in hospital-based services should not been a reduction in services overall. They are seeking a range of services and treatments which are accessible at times of need without necessitating hospital admission.

Innovations in primary care services in some parts of the country are leading to more attention being given to mental health in this context. In Birmingham, a project exploring users' views of primary care services has led to the establishment of criteria to be used in assessing the quality of mental health services in primary care (Bailey, 1994). These include criteria relating to information provision, to the availability of shared care programmes with community mental health teams, and access to specialist counselling services.

Finding somewhere to live and some opportunity for creative activity are often particularly difficult for those experiencing severe mental health problems. Accommodation needs are varied and changing, and lack of appropriate accommodation can lead to re-admission to hospital. Ritchie *et al* (1988) report experiences of a number of people for whom difficulties – obtaining permanent accommodation, being placed in unfamiliar environments away from friends and family, being left without support at critical times and so on – were contributing to their mental distress. Rogers *et al* (1993) report high levels of satisfaction with residential accommodation (group homes, hostels etc), although there were varying levels of autonomy experienced by those living in such accommodation. The rigidity of the regimes was more likely to be as reason for a negative evaluation than was the quality of the physical environment.

Innovative projects which provide supported opportunities to work are generally well received (Nehring *et al*, 1993). Not only do such projects provide a source of creative activity which can enhance self-esteem, they also provide the potential to break down the stigma attached to mental illness by demonstrating people's capacities to take on valued social roles. Users themselves have been active in developing and running such projects. The Clubhouse model, introduced into this country from the US, is based on reciprocal working relationships between members (users) and staff. Transitional Employment Schemes have been developed by Clubhouses such as Mosaic in Lambeth and users are very positive about the opportunities this offers for supporting gradual engagement in the world of work. A different model has been developed by users working under the umbrella of the Nottingham Advocacy Group (Davey, 1994). There, users have developed small scale employment based on principles of sustainable development, including a perma-culture project based in local allotments and a project to supply more efficient energy to local hostels.

Giving a voice to user views

The voices of mental health service users are being heard in a number of forums from which they have previously been excluded (Barnes, 1997). User self-organisation is supporting the expression of voice in user councils, in more strategic local planning forums and in national and international conferences and task groups. The key objectives of user groups relate to: advocacy; improving the quality and variety of mental health services; providing support to their members, and confronting stigmatising attitudes and practices outside mental health services. Fewer groups are directly involved in service provision than in the United States, although some have adopted this approach in preference to seeking to change the nature of services provided by statutory agencies. Some users have worked together to design and conduct their own research (Beeforth *et al,* 1994; Davis, 1992; Faulkner, 1997), whilst others are actively involved in training the professionals who will become their own and others' helpers.

In a variety of ways users are contributing to change in mental health services, and professionals are opening up to learn from the knowledge which comes from the experience of mental distress and of being on the receiving end of mental health services. Nevertheless, the day-to-day experience of using services is still too often one of difficulties of access and powerlessness once access has been gained, and barriers to participation are still placed by professionals who find the idea of power sharing threatening. We all need to develop new ways of learning from users' experiences to build more effective ways of supporting people with severe mental health problems.

References

South West Mind (n.d) *Avon Mental Health Measure*. Bristol: South West Mind.

Bailey, D. (1994) *Partnership in Practice: Developing a user led approach to the delivery of mental health services in primary care*. University of Birmingham: Department of Social Policy and Social Work.

Barnes, M. (1997) *Care, Communities and Citizens*. Harlow: Addison Wesley.

Barnes, M. & Shardlow, P. (1996) Identity Crisis? Mental Health User Groups and the 'Problem' of Identity. In: C. Barnes and G. Mercer (Eds) *Accounting for Illness and Disability: Exploring the Divide*. Leeds: The Disability Press.

Barnes, M. & Shardlow, P. (1997) From passive recipient to active citizen: participation in mental health user groups. *Journal of Mental Health* **6** 289–300.

Barnes, M. & Stephenson, P. (1996) Secure Provision – The Special Hospitals. In: R. Perkins, Z. Nadirshaw, J. Copperman & C. Andrews (Eds) *Women in Context: Good Practice in Mental Health Services for Women*. London: Good Practice in Mental Health.

Barnes, M. & Wistow, G. (1994) Learning to hear voices: listening to users of mental health services. *Journal of Mental Health* **3** 525–540.

Beeforth, M., Conlan, E., Field, V., Hoser, B. & Sayce, L. (1990) *Whose Service is it Anyway? Users' Views on Co-ordinating Community Care*. London: Research and Development for Psychiatry.

Beeforth, M., Conlan, E. & Graley, R. (1994) *Have We Got Views For You: User evaluation of case management*. London: Sainsbury Centre for Mental Health.

Bowl, R. & Barnes, M. (1990) Race, racism and mental health social work: Implications for local authority policy and training. *Research, Policy and Planning* **8** (2) 12–18.

Briere, J. (1984) *The Effects of Childhood Abuse on Later Psychological Functioning: Defining a Post Sexual Abuse Syndrome*. Paper presented at the 3rd National

Conference on Sexual Victimisation of Children, Washington DC, Children's Hospital Medical Centre.

Bryer, J. B., Nelson, B. A., Miller, J. B. & Krol, P. A. (1987) Childhood sexual and physical abuse as factors in adult psychiatric illness. *American Journal of Psychiatry* **144** (11) 1426–31.

Chamberlin, J. (1988) *On Our Own: Patient controlled alternatives to the mental health system.* London: Mind.

Copeland, J., Dewey, M., Wood, N., Searle, R., Davidson, I. & McWilliam, C. (1987) Range of mental illness amongst the elderly in the community: prevalence in Liverpool using the GMS-AGECAT package. *British Journal of Psychiatry* **150** 815–23.

Davey, B. (1994) *Empowerment through holistic development: a framework for egalitarianism in the ecological age.* Nottingham: Nottingham Advocacy Group/Ecoworks.

Davis, A. (1992) Who Needs User Research? Service Users as Research Subjects or Participants. In: M. Barnes and G. Wistow (Eds) *Researching User Involvement.* Leeds Nuffield Institute for Health.

Davis, A. & Betteridge, J. (1990) *Cracking Up – Social Security Benefits and Mental Health: Users' Experiences.* London: Mind.

Eaton, M. & Humphries, J. (1996) *Listening to Women in Special Hospitals.* University of Surrey: St Mary's University College.

Faulkner, A. (1997) *Knowing Our Own Minds.* London: Mental Health Foundation.

Fernando, S. (1991) *Mental Health, Race and Culture.* Basingstoke: Macmillan.

Harrison, L. (1993) Newcastle's Mental Health Services Consumer Group: A case study of user involvement. In. L. Gaster, L. Harrison, L. Martin, R. Means and P. Thistlethwaite (Eds) *Working Together for Better Community Care.* Bristol: School for Advanced Urban Studies.

Hart, L. (1995) *Phone at Nine Just to Say You're Alive.* London: Douglas Elliott Press.

Hemingway, C. (Ed) (1996) *Special Women? The experiences of women in the special hospital system.* Aldershot: Avebury.

HeppleWhite, R. (1988) *Introduction* at Common Concerns International Conference on User Involvement in Mental Health Services. Brighton: University of Sussex/East Sussex County Council/Brighton Health Authority/Mind.

Hutchings, S. (1989) Sectioning – A Last Resort. *Openmind* **39** 12–3.

Ignatieff, M. (1993) *Scar Tissue.* London: Chatto and Windus.
Lipsedge, M. (1994) Dangerous Stereotypes. *Journal of Forensic Psychiatry* **5** (1) 14–19.

Lorencz, B. (1991) Becoming Ordinary: Leaving the Psychiatric Hospital. In: J. M. Morse and J. L. Johnson (Eds) *The Illness Experience: Dimensions of Suffering.* Newbury Park: Sage.

Matthews, J. J. (1984) *Good and Mad Women.* Sydney: Allen and Unwin.
Millett, K. (1991) *The Loony Bin Trip.* London: Virago.

Moodley, P. & Thornicroft, G. (1988) Ethnic Group and Compulsory Detention. *Medicine, Science and the Law* **28** 324–8.

Murphy, E. (1982) Social origins of depression in old age. *British Journal of Psychiatry* **141** 135–142.

Neeter, A. (1993) NO to Community Supervision Orders – again. *Openmind* **62** 8–9.

Nehring, J., Hill, R. & Pole, L. (1993) *Work, Empowerment and Community.* London: Research and Development in Psychiatry.

Perkins, R. (1996) Serious Long Term Mental Health Problems. In: Perkins *et al*

Perring, C. (1992) The Experience and Perspectives of Patients and Care Staff on the Transition from Hospital to Community Care. In: S. Ramon (Ed) *Psychiatric Hospital Closure: Myths and realities.* London: Chapman and Hall.

Prior, P. M. (1995) Surviving psychiatric institutionalisation: a case study. *Sociology of Health and Illness* **17** (5) 651–67.

Read, J. & Baker, S. (1996) *Not Just Sticks and Stones: A survey of stigma, taboos and discrimination experienced by people with mental health problems.* London: Mind.

Ritchie, J., Morrissey, C. & Ward, K. (1988) *Keeping in Touch with the Talking: The community care needs of people with mental illness.* Birmingham: Community Care Special Action Project, Social and Community Planning Research.

Roger, A. & Pilgrim, D. (1991) Pulling down churches: accounting for the British mental health users' movement. *Sociology of Health and Illness* **13** (2) 129–48.

Rogers, A., Pilgrim, D. & Lacey, R. (1993) *Experiencing Psychiatry: Users' views of services.* Basingstoke: Macmillan.
Sayce, L. (1996) Sexual Abuse in Childhood. In: R. Perkins, Z. Nadirshaw, J. Copperman and C. Andrews (Eds) *Women in Context: Good Practice in Mental Health Services for Women.* London: Good Practice in Mental Health.

At the Core of Mental Health © Pavilion 2000

Smith, H (n.d) *Strategic Planning of Mental Health Services*. London: Centre for Mental Health Services Development, King's College.

Ussher, J. (1991) *Women's Madness: Misogyny or Mental Illness?* Hemel Hempstead: Harvester Wheatsheaf.

Wallcraft, J. (1996) Some Models of Asylum and Help in Times of Crisis. In: D. Tomlinson and J. Carter (Eds) *Asylum in the Community*. London: Routledge.

Warner, R. (1994) *Recovery from Schizophrenia: Psychiatry and Political Economy*. London: Routledge.

Wood, D. & Copperman, J. (1996) Sexual Harassment and Assault in Psychiatric Services. In: R. Perkins, Z. Nadirshaw, J. Copperman & C. Andrews (Eds) *Woman in Context: Good Practice in Mental Health Services for Women*. London: Good Practice in Mental Health.

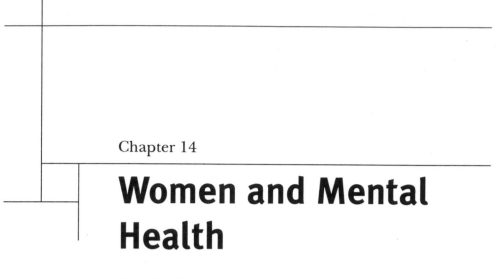

Chapter 14

Women and Mental Health

Ann Davis

Introduction

The majority of people who use mental health services in Britain are women. The evidence suggests that women are more vulnerable to emotional and mental distress and are more likely to receive diagnoses of mental illness than men. Women are prescribed more psychotropic drugs, more ECT and more psychosurgery than men (Catalan *et al*, 1988; Gabe, 1991). Research has shown that in comparison to men, women are also more frequently assessed by approved social workers (ASWs) for admission under the *Mental Health Act 1983* (Barnes *et al*, 1990) and receive more hospital treatment, psychotherapy and counselling in both the public and private mental health sectors (Abel *et al*, 1996; Allgulander, 1990; Busfield, 1995; Foster, 1995).

This chapter provides a brief overview of approaches to explaining this profile of women's emotional distress and illness. It goes on to look at the ways in which mental health services currently treat women. Finally, it considers ways in which practitioners and services can work with women to make a positive difference to their management of the mental distress and illness in their lives.

The focus on women in this chapter is not designed to ignore or devalue the distinctive ways in which men experience emotional distress and are treated for mental illness. There is much still to be discovered about the similarities as well as the differences in the origins and nature of the mental distress experienced by women and men. Explorations in this area need to be informed by gendered considerations of the roots of emotional distress as well as the ways it is expressed. Such considerations should actively influence the range of responses made by mental health professionals to women and men's mental health problems.

For those currently using, as well as working in, mental health services, a gendered view needs to incorporate considerations of the way in which gender relates to other major social divisions in society. In Busfield's words, **mental disorder is:**

> *'a gendered landscape in which some diagnoses are linked to women, some to men, and others do not have very marked gender associations – a landscape in which gender also intersects with other social characteristics such as age, marital status, social class and ethnicity':*
> (Busfield, 1995)

This chapter is part of this gendered landscape. However, in considering what women may have in common, it recognises that, in practice, it is vital to recognise the uniqueness of each woman. To quote Ussher:

> *'Each woman is different. Each woman's pain has its own history, its own roots – and its own solution...We must stop treating women as a homogeneous group, expecting one solution for all, one analysis for all. We do not need either to celebrate or deny difference, whether between women, or between women and men. We share a lot as women, but as individuals we cannot be subsumed under some category, some all encompassing label which predicts that our experiences will all be the same. Each women's experience is still unique to her.'*
> (Ussher, 1991)

Factors influencing women's mental health

The growing research and practice literature on women and mental health offers a great deal to those interested in understanding the mental health profile of women. In starting to unravel why women have a greater vulnerability to mental distress, three broad, interrelated accounts can be usefully identified. The first highlights biological explanations of women's mental ill health. The second argues that the social inequality and oppression experienced by women lies at the root of their mental distress. The third points to the ways in which the **gender-biased diagnostic classifications** used in the psychiatric services result in an over representation of women amongst those diagnosed as mentally distressed and ill.

Focusing on the biological

Research and user accounts of contact with medical professionals in the mental health care system suggest that the prevailing view of women presenting with emotional distress is that mental ill health is rooted in women's biological, biochemical, hormonal or genetic characteristics. As Foster has summarised it:

> '*Women's biology, or more specifically their raging hormones, are still regarded by many doctors as key determinants of women's excess vulnerability to mental ill health. Women are still perceived as the emotionally weaker sex by some doctors... most doctors still appear to believe that women suffering from more serious forms of depression, anxiety, phobias and baby blues are suffering from real, physically based illnesses and are not just reacting logically to intolerable circumstances.*'
> (Foster, 1995)

This response to emotional distress or variations in mood in part reflects the concerns of psychiatry to locate and sustain itself as a recognised part of medical science. Although it acknowledges that it is a less 'hard science' and more 'uncertain' branch than most, psychiatry remains rooted in a medico-biological framework (Rowe, 1991; Ussher, 1991; Foster, 1995). This has particular consequences for women, who find themselves, by virtue of their biology, *'deemed by the medical profession to be inherently more vulnerable to mental disturbances at virtually every stage of their adult life from menarche to menopause and beyond'*. And, as a result *'targeted as the main potential and actual consumers of a whole range of mental health care services'* (Foster, 1995).

The view that it is women's biological characteristics that make them more vulnerable to emotional and mental disturbance has a long established history (McNamara, 1996; Showalter, 1987; Ussher, 1991). It is a history that demonstrates the shifting (and socially constructed) nature of explanations of the profile of women's 'madness'. It is a history in which biological accounts have absorbed and influenced notions of gender as well as sexuality, race, culture, age and class. The resulting notions reflect judgements about inferiority as well as abnormality and pathologised difference (Fernando, 1995).

As commentators have noted, where the evidence for a biological contribution to mental ill health is at its strongest, it is for the most severe and enduring conditions, such as schizophrenia. Yet it is in this part of the spectrum that the distribution of mental ill health between men and women is most equal (Johnson & Buszewicz, 1996). Medical research has failed to establish a conclusive association between women's higher rates of mental health problems and their biology. Cochrane, amongst others, has argued this means that *'any kind of biological explanation must be placed firmly in a social context for it to be able to provide a useful explanation for differences in mental illness'* (Cochrane, 1983).

Despite the limitations of the biological account of women's vulnerability to mental ill health it continues to have a powerful influence on service responses to women's mental distress (Ussher,

1991; Cockerham, 1992). One of the defining features of biological accounts of vulnerability to mental ill health is that women are described as passive victims of biology; prey to organically, biochemically or hormonally-generated pathologies over which they have no control.

This view of women as hapless victims of their own biology underpins the perspectives that many psychiatrists and other mental health professionals bring to their understanding of women's mental distress as well as their relationships with women. It also impacts on the ways in which some women locate the origins and causes of their own mental distress and illness. This view is also reflected in the way some women talk about their emotional and mental distress to mental health workers – explaining their state of mind by reference to biological changes they are experiencing such as menstruation, pregnancy, childbirth and the menopause (Ussher, 1991).

While biological accounts of women's mental distress use the language of illness, symptom and cure, there is in fact no cure on offer. Emphasis is on future hopes rather than current certainties. Attention is focused on possible 'breakthroughs' in organic, biochemical and genetic research which will lead to 'wonder drugs' or other physical interventions. In the meantime, within the confines of its vision, the biological approach can only offer treatments which attempt to alleviate distress, disorientation and pain. Treatments which encompass medication, electrotherapy and occasionally surgery. Treatments which may offer respite to some, but not to others, as the growing literature from women who have been on the receiving end of services highlights.

> *'I have no doubt that ECT has the potential for abuse and has been abused; it has the potential to cause harm and has been harmful... I also know from my own experience and those related to me by others that it can be beneficial'.*
> (Perkins, 1996)

*'To give me tranquillisers for my distress is your answer
to my problem. All those tranquillisers can ever do for me
is subdue me, keep me quiet, make sure I don't behave
in a socially unacceptable manner. Tranquillisers do
not make the problems go away, they disempower me.
They take away my ability to think and speak clearly.
They rob me of my dignity, my self-respect, my ability to
communicate. They disempower me by depriving me of
my adult status. I become child-like, dependent, have no
control over my thoughts or words. Eventually I can no
longer remember how I became like this. I cannot
remember what worried me so, what frightened me. I am
powerless. I am scared. I am unable to remember who I
really am.'*
(Gifford, 1996)

Living with social inequality and oppression

This second account locates women's vulnerability to mental distress
and ill health in their responses to their day-to-day experiences of
inequality and oppression. It is women's reactions to their lack of
power in a male dominated society that is seen to be at the root of
their despair and distress. As Busfield notes:

*'...the different structural and material circumstances
of men and women and the differences in power and
status are highly pertinent to understanding the genesis
of men's and women's mental disorder'.*
(Busfield, 1996)

A focus on social inequality and oppression as a means of
understanding the origins of women's mental distress is rare amongst
mental health professionals and service providers (Williams &
Watson, 1996). This is a reflection of the individualising and
medically oriented training of such professionals. It also reflects the
traditionally narrow vision of policy makers and service
commissioners in developing mental health services. Yet, as the Audit

Commission acknowledges, the strongest indicator of the need for mental health services in a given geographical area is the measure of its social disadvantage and inequality (Audit Commission, 1994). Such measures have gendered characteristics. In the UK, women of all ages outnumber men in poor and socially disadvantaged groups (Glendinning & Millar, 1992).

An examination of women's daily lives from this perspective reveals the negative impact of social structure and process on mental wellbeing. Acknowledgement is given to the ways in which social forces impact differentially on the diverse range of women in contemporary Britain. Attention is paid in this account to characteristics such as age, race, ethnicity, sexuality and class as they intersect with gender in contributing to the patterning of women's mental health and illness.

To focus on the social in this way is not to ignore or devalue the personal. As many commentators have noted, social forces influence how women think of themselves, and value themselves (Barnes & Maples, 1992; Butler & Wintram, 1991; Fenton, 1993; Goodwin, 1997; GPMH, 1995; Holland, 1995; Pembroke, 1993; Williams & Watson, 1996). Women's sense of self and the control they have over their lives reflects their social roles and opportunities. As mothers, wives, daughters and carers women face specific difficulties that can trigger mental health problems. These difficulties reflect not only social inequalities but the associated economic disadvantages and lack of choice and opportunity (Bruce *et al*, 1991).

In their summary review of the risk factors that emerge when this perspective is used to consider the origins of women's mental distress, Williams and Watson (*ibid*) suggest that at least eight aspects of women's everyday life are critical to understanding their greater vulnerability to mental ill health:

- **Marriage**, which, is more detrimental to the mental wellbeing of women than men.

- **Childbirth and motherhood**, which can trigger depression for a significant number of women.

- **Caring responsibilities for children and adults** that carry high risk of mental distress and ill health because of the associated stress, isolation, low social value and lack of resources.

- **Poverty**, which is more widespread amongst women than men and impacts particularly on lone mothers, older women and women who are Black and members of minority ethnic groups.

- **Domestic violence**, which is estimated to affect women in 1 in 4 households.

- **Childhood sexual abuse**, which can substantially increase the likelihood of mental health problems.

- **Sexual violence against women**, which has been shown to increase the likelihood of mental distress in women.

- **Being female**, which, compared with being male, increases the risk of thoughts and feelings to be diagnosed as mental illness (Heller *et al*, 1996).

The ways in which such factors impact on women are complex but key themes have emerged from the work of researchers and practitioners. For example, in their seminal study of the social origins of depression in women, Brown and Harris explored why depression is more often diagnosed in women than men. In researching the circumstances associated with depression amongst a group of working class women living in London, they suggested that these women were more likely to experience depression if three or more 'predisposing factors' were present in their lives. These were having three children or more under the age of 14 living at home, being unemployed, losing their mothers in childhood or lacking an intimate confiding relationship (Brown & Harris, 1978).

Such findings are echoed in practitioner accounts of work with women and women's groups. Such work has identified fear, isolation and loneliness as playing a significant part in the lives of women vulnerable to mental distress and the diagnosis of mental illness (see for example, Butler & Wintram, 1991; Perkins *et al*, 1996).

This account of the roots of women's vulnerability to mental distress has a strong message for mental health practitioners. It calls for a radical re-orientation of their thinking and their practice. It promotes the view that it is vital for mental health workers to integrate consideration of the social, economic and political in their understanding of the distress they encounter amongst women. As Johnson and Buszewicz (1996) argue:

> *'Rather than seeing women as inherently vulnerable, clinicians need to understand the social roles and experiences that may be important in the genesis of distress'.*

However, those mental health workers who take this step and develop their social awareness of the origins of women's distress will need to think carefully about what this means about their expertise in working with women. They will need to think through the part they can play in identifying and addressing the gendered structures and processes which shape women's experiences. They will need to identify and develop skills which are relevant to working with women to change the circumstances and conditions in which they find themselves experiencing mental distress. In doing this they will have to begin to constructively counteract the observed tendency of mental health practitioners to have a *'narrowness of vision and an exclusion of any real concern with the structure of people's lives'* (Busfield, 1996).

Gender-biased diagnoses

This third account highlights the gendered nature of diagnostic procedures and processes. It takes as its starting point the socially contested nature of mental illness and disorder and notes the distinctly different ways in which women and men's mental distress is identified, understood and diagnosed.

Community-based surveys of psychoactive drug treatments in a number of countries in Western Europe and North America have found twice as many women as men are likely to be diagnosed and treated. Studies have also found that women experience higher rates of anxiety and affective disorders, while men tend to experience more personality disorders. Women tend to experience depression more often, particularly when they are married and even more so when they have children. Ninety per cent of people diagnosed with eating disorders are women (Dennerstein & Astbury, 1995; Nicolson, 1996).

Some commentators, in exploring these gendered diagnostic patterns, have emphasised the part that women play in this process (Barnes and Maple, 1992; Briscoe, 1982; Busfield, 1996). They note the tendency for women to talk about, as well as seek help for their emotional difficulties more often than men. This contact with GPs in which feelings are shared, appears to lead to more women being diagnosed as having depression and other common mental disorders than men. However, there are two parties to these interactions, and the responses of GPs as well as other mental health workers to women play a critical part in the diagnostic process.

Research has explored the gendered stereotypes of women and men's mental distress and illness held by those working in the mental health field. Some commentators argue that there is research evidence that suggests that the standards being applied to the assessment of women's distress increase the likelihood of them being diagnosed as mentally ill.

In their much quoted 1970 study, Broverman and her colleagues gave 79 psychiatrists, psychologists and social workers a questionnaire in which they were asked to choose between pairs of descriptions to indicate what in their view characterised a healthy mature adult, a healthy mature man and a healthy mature woman. The results showed great similarity between views held about healthy adults and healthy men. However, healthy mature woman were viewed somewhat differently. They were seen as more submissive, less independent, more easily influenced, more easily hurt, more emotional and less objective beings than men.

The conclusions reached in this study were that women are caught in a double bind. If they behave in ways that conform to mental health professionals' expectations of mature healthy women, they will fail to reach the standards set for mentally healthy adults, thus increasing their chances of being diagnosed as mentally ill. If they deviate from the stereotype of healthy women held by professionals, they are at risk as being labelled deviant and abnormal. Both stereotypes – conformity and non conformity – place women at risk of being defined as mentally ill or disordered.

Again, issues of age, sexuality, class, race and ethnicity need to be acknowledged as influencing this process, as women who have been on the receiving end of services have testified. In her contribution to an account of Black women's experiences in Britain in the 1980s, a woman who had spent time in prison observed:

> *'The prison system treats all women prisoners as if they are mad because they can't see how women would be in prison unless something was wrong with them. They've got this belief that Black women are violent or "savage", as they put it, and that therefore we are mad. When I was in prison in the ordinary block, I'd say that more than half of the Black girls were being given largactil.'*
> (Bryan *et al,* 1986)

Working for women's mental health

Each of these three accounts makes a contribution to understanding the profile of women's mental health. Taken together they suggest that it is important for practitioners, providers and service users to critically consider how the social, psychological and physiological interact to shape the uniqueness of each woman's life as well as her subjective understanding of her situation (Ashurst & Hall, 1991; Davis *et al,* 1985).

This means that mental health practitioners need to reflect on the ways in which social institutions and divisions in society reinforce particular forms of response to women's expression of distress and anger, rendering them objects of psychiatric treatment and intervention. For practitioners, as well as women experiencing mental distress, this can result in fruitful connections being made between women's lives and their mental health and wellbeing. Such connections need to be rooted in the agendas that women bring to services. They also need to address how practitioners and managers can change the traditional scope and focus of their interventions and services in order to fully engage with what is troubling the women that come to them.

Women and the mental health system

In considering how women are currently treated in the mental health system, two recent reviews of mental health services in the UK are helpful (Williams *et al*, 1993; GPMH, 1994). Both suggest that primary and mental health services are prone to:

- view women as passive, emotional and childlike and less capable than men

- misdiagnose women's distress

- fail to help women deal with the causes of their problems

- mistreat women's distress by using inappropriate medication, ECT and hospital admission

- be unsafe for women

- encourage women towards relatively dependent roles and domestic pursuits in which paid employment is viewed as unimportant

- set low programme expectations for women, which reinforce feelings of helplessness and hopelessness and provide less input for them compared with men

- use culturally and sexually specific measures of 'feminine' behaviour as an index of recovery.

These findings indicate that in the primary health care services, as well as in the specialist services, many women are not receiving a positively helpful response to the difficulties with which they are living and the despair and distress they are suffering.

It is GPs who diagnose and treat most women with mental distress. Yet little in their training prepares them for dealing with this area of their work. The predominantly biological and medicalising orientation used results in many women finding that their distress is ignored or trivialised. In the words of one of the women who contributed to Beliappa's survey of 98 Asian people's experiences of mental health problems:

> *'I am fit now, but for years I was suffering from aches and pains, sleeplessness and lack of appetite... I could see that all this was caused by stress. I had three miscarriages because of this... my experiences in my marriage led to physical ailments... they (doctors) would treat me for physical problems, gave me pain killers, but never bothered to find out what the problem was.'*
> (Beliappa, 1991)

When GPs recognise that the difficulties facing women are resulting in extreme mental distress it is rare for them to respond by providing opportunities to talk about things with someone else or to meet with others in similar circumstances. The dominant reaction is the prescription pad, used, as advertisements for psychotropic drugs graphically show, to keep women coping with the difficulties of poverty, poor housing, and caring for children and others. As one woman familiar with this response explained, it has its limitations.

> *'I've been on and off drugs – anti-depressants, 'tranx',* *for many years – since I was 17. I think they help* *initially, maybe for a week or so, but then I think I'm* *only living to take another tablet. It doesn't solve*

> *anything you still have to go back and face all the*
> *problems that were there before.'*
> (Corob, 1987)

Women who receive a psychiatric diagnosis or a referral to mental health agencies often find that their feelings of helplessness and dependency increase. As do their chances, especially if they are older, of receiving physical rather than talking treatments. Such responses and the feelings they trigger can increase the problems women already face in relation to powerlessness and violence in their domestic situations. With both hospital and community studies providing strong evidence of the links between women's experiences of abuse and mental distress, there is a risk that specialist services mistreat women by compounding rather than confronting the causes of their distress (Breggin, 1993; Hemingway, 1996; Rose *et al*, 1991).

As Pilgrim (1990) has argued, the lack of safety in mental health services, especially for women with serious long-term mental health problems, is alarming. Women are at higher risk than men of encountering sexual exploitation and violence in the hospital, residential, criminal justice and homelessness systems. The Mental Health Act Commission has recently identified safety for women as being 'a major issue' on psychiatric wards where staffing is low and 'violence considerable' as well as in Regional Secure Units *'where there may be few other female patients and a lack of female staff'* (MHAC, 1997).

Mistreatment and lack of safety within services for women is also a reflection of a failure to recognise and work with the diversity of women. Racial stereotypes, cultural assumptions and gendered ideas of normalisation are embedded in current services (Martin & Lyon, 1984; Perkins, 1996). Difference can be pathologised in ways which render women from minority ethnic groups either invisible or subject to excessive physical treatments. Such extremes of response are rooted in inaccurate assessment and understanding of need, shaped by lack of knowledge of religious, linguistic, ethnic and cultural differences. Women from minority ethnic communities report that it is difficult for them to discuss their problems and needs without the cultural preconceptions of mental health practitioners coming into play. In the experience of Dewan, who has Irish and Indian parentage and has lived with distress and depression for a great deal of her adult life:

> *'My mental health, race and culture are inextricably linked. This link has been ignored, denied, mocked, excluded, avoided, misunderstood, rejected by institutions and individuals – and also by me in many disorientated moments of my life'.*
> (Read & Reynolds, 1996)

Building better responses to women's distress

The picture, which has emerged so far in this chapter of women's experiences of mental ill health and the mental health services, suggests that strategies to improve women's mental wellbeing need to take account of mental health promotion as well as the provision of care, treatment and ongoing support. Such strategies need to be rooted in women's agendas as well as their survival skills.

The starting point for mental health promotion as well as crisis and support services is a consideration of how to respond to women in ways that do not compound the difficulties they face in their daily lives. This means that the collective problems as well as the diversity and uniqueness of women's lives must be recognised. As Johnstone has persuasively argued, mental health services have all too often exacerbated women's problems by pressuring them to conform to the very social roles that led to their mental distress (Johnstone, 1989). An awareness of this is critical to those aiming to build better responses to women's distress.

Services need to be equally accessible to women and men to ensure that women receive a share of resources in proportion to their needs. In creating this access, services have to take account of the barriers to seeking help which women using services have identified. These include the stigma attached to psychiatric services and the acquisition of diagnoses; the fear of losing custody of children; the fear of violence and harassment that service use might bring; the fear of the consequences of disclosing experience of abuse or sexual identity.

Responding to these concerns means that service development for women should aspire to provide as safe and confidential an environment as possible. Important too are service developments that prioritise issues central to women's lives rather than promoting the specialisms, power and status of professionals. The key here is to work in ways that are continuously informed by an understanding of the variation in living situations, relationships, employment experiences, ethnic origins, attitudes and values that characterise women's lives.

Acceptance and respectful concern for women is important. Making provision which encourages mutuality and peer support as well as being given at a pace which is jointly agreed. Recognition is needed of the way in which ageism operates in the mental health field The needs of older women need to be seen in context of their whole lives. Time must be given to listen to what women are saying about their pasts, presents and futures.

This is a way of responding to women's distress that necessarily challenges the traditional manner in which mental health training has neatly separated the personal from the social. This is because it explicitly acknowledges the need to reframe women's distress in community, specialist and primary health care settings.

In getting down to the detailed work of transforming practice and service provision to embrace these aspirations, practitioners and women using services could find the *Good Practices in Mental Health Project on Women and Mental Health* useful reference material (GPMH, 1994). This project developed a set of general principles and criteria for use by agencies striving to develop good mental health practice for women.

- There is a need to establish clear policies which make explicit reference to gender issues. Policies should be examined to consider whether they disadvantage women in any way. For example, by referring to 'diagnoses' such as personality disorder which are applied to women in very different ways from those in which they are applied to men.

- We need to enable women to make an input to service decision-making and to contribute to service monitoring and evaluation.

- It is necessary to provide support for those working with women with severe mental health problems to enable them to deal with the personal and professional stress generated.

- The project suggested that those working in and providing mental health services who wanted to develop good practice with women should:

  - promote self-esteem

  - provide care to each woman in her own right

  - provide space to talk through feelings and experiences in a non-threatening atmosphere

  - enable each woman to take control of her life

  - acknowledge that bad feelings are common to everyone

  - acknowledge the 'normality' of mental distress amongst women.

In addition services need to:

- be accessible without women having to leave children or have them taken into care

- provide the opportunity to meet with other women in similar circumstances

- provide access to sources of practical help as well as counselling, therapy and drug treatments

- enable each woman to receive help from a woman worker if that is her choice.

In thinking about how such services might be delivered, the project listed a wide range of UK programmes which aspire to provide good practice for women's mental health. Amongst them was the work of the White City Project. This project has provided a response to women's distress for almost two decades (Holland, 1995). Housed in a multi-racial inner city council estate in London, it provides a service for women with depression and anxiety based on a model of social action psychotherapy. It is an approach which promotes mental health through combining techniques drawn from sociological, psychological and therapeutic sources. Developed to work with both the social oppression and the personal psychic pain experienced by women living in socially disadvantaged circumstances, it aims to move women, through collective and individual experiences, from considering themselves as passive victims or patients to being active participants in their own and their neighbours' wellbeing. The project offers a service to women taking pills for 'nerves' on prescription from their GP. It goes on to offer them the alternative of psychotherapy, and moves women on to work in groups and to taking action to change the choices and opportunities in their individual and collective lives.

It is an approach which in Holland's words is *'disrespectful of existing professional boundaries'* (Holland, 1995), because it challenges the knowledge and vested interests of mental health professionals. It also promotes the idea that women should not only take more charge of their lives and circumstances, but also that in doing so they may become assertive and angry. This, it is argued, should not be suppressed but directed towards individual and community change. This is a message which needs to be heard by all practitioners and services considering making a positive difference to women's lives, health and mental wellbeing. Commitment to improving services for women's mental health is about working with women by working for change in mental health practice and services.

Summary

This chapter has stressed the need for mental health practitioners to work with women as individuals. Women who experience mental health problems are vulnerable to their mental distress being misunderstood by virtue of overemphasising biological explanations and paying scant attention to social inequality and oppression. Care must also be taken to guard against diagnoses based upon gender biased assumptions. Fruitful connections need to be made between women's lives and their mental health and wellbeing, including issues arising from race and cultural influences.

Services need to respond to women in ways that do not compound their difficulties. They need to be underpinned by clear policies to which women make a meaningful contribution to shape the mental health services of the future.

References

Abel, K., Buszewicz, M., Davidson, S., Johnson, S. & Staples, E.(Eds) (1996) *Planning Community Mental Health Services for Women: A Multi-Professional Handbook.* London: Routledge.

Allgulander, C., Nowck, J. & Rice, J.(1990) Psychopathology and treatment of 30, 344 twins in Sweden. I. The appropriateness of psychoactive treatment. *Acta Psychiatrica Scandinavica* **80** 325–334.

Ashurst, P. & Hall, Z. (Eds)(1991) *Understanding Women in Distress.* London: Routledge.

Audit Commission (1994) *Finding a Place: A review of mental health services for adults.* London: The Stationery Office.

Barnes, M., Bowl, R. & Fisher, M. (1990) *Sectioned: Social Services and the 1983 Mental Health Act.* London: Routledge.

Barnes, M. & Maples, N. (1992) *Women and Mental Health: Challenging the stereotypes.* Birmingham: Venture Press.

Beliappa, J. (1991) *Illness or Distress? Alternative models of mental health.* London: Confederation of Indian Organisations.

Breggin, P. (1993) *Toxic Psychiatry.* London: Fontana.

Briscoe, M. (1982) Sex differences in psychological wellbeing. *Psychological Medicine Supplement* **1**.

Broverman, D., Clarkson, F., Rosenkrantz, P., Vogel, S. & Broverman, I. (1970) Sex-role stereotype and clinical judgements of mental health. *Journal of Counselling and Clinical Psychology* **34** 1–7.

Brown, G. & Harris, T. (1978) *Social Origins of Depression: A study of psychiatric disorder in women*. London: Tavistock.

Bruce, M. L., Takeuchi, D. T. & Keaf, P. J.(1991) *Poverty and psychiatric status*. *Archives of General Psychiatry* **48** 470–4.

Bryan, B., Dadzie, S. & Scafe, S. (1986) *The Heart of the Race: Black women's lives in Britain*. London: Virago.

Busfield, J. (1996) *Men, Women and Madness: Understanding gender and mental disorder.* Basingstoke: Macmillan.

Butler, S. & Wintram, C. (1991) *Feminist Groupwork*. London: Sage.

Catalan, J., Gath, D. H. & Bond, A. (1988) General practice patients on long-term psychotropic drugs: a controlled investigation. *British Journal of Psychiatry* **152** 263–8.

Cochrane, R. (1983) *The Social Creation of Mental Illness*. London: Longman.

Cockerham, W. (1992) *Sociology of Mental Disorder.* London: Prentice Hall.

Corob, A. (1987) *Working with Depressed Women*. London: Gower.

Davis, A., Llewelyn, S. & Parry, G.(1985) Women and Mental Health: Towards an understanding. In: E. Brook and A. Davis (Eds) *Women, the Family and Social Work*. London: Tavistock.

Dennerstein, L. & Astbury, C. (1995) *Psychosocial and Mental Health Aspects of Women's Health*. Geneva: World Health Organisation.

Fenton, S. (1993) *The Sorrow in My Heart – the experiences of sixteen Asian women in Bristol*. London: CRE.

Fernando, S. (1995)(Ed) *Mental Health in a Multi-ethnic Society: A multidisciplinary handbook*. London: Routledge.

Foster, P. (1995) *Women and the Health Care Industry: An unhealthy relationship?* Buckingham: Open University Press.

Gabe, J. (Ed)(1991) *Understanding Tranquiliser Use*. London: Tavistock/Routledge.

Gifford, G. (1996) To Whom it May Concern... *Women and Mental Health Forum Newsletter* 1, May.

Glendinning, C. & Millar, J. (Eds)(1992) *Women and Poverty in Britain in the 1990s.* Hemel Hempstead: Harvester Wheatsheaf.

GPMH (1994) *Women and Mental Health: An information pack of mental health services for women in the United Kingdom.* London: GPMH.

Goodwin, S. (1997) *Comparative Mental Health Policy.* London: Sage.

Heller, T., Reynolds, J., Gomm, R., Muston, R. & Pattison, S. (Eds)(1996) *Mental Health Matters: A Reader.* Basingstoke: Macmillan.

Hemingway, C. (Ed)(1996) *Special Women: The experience of women in the special hospital system.* Aldershot: Avebury.

Holland, S. (1995) Interaction in Women's Mental Health and Neighbourhood Development. In: S. Fernando (Ed) *Mental Health in a Multi-ethnic Society: A multidisciplinary handbook.* London: Routledge.

Johnson, S. & Buszewucz, M. (1996) Women and Mental Health in the UK. In: K. Abel *et al* (Eds) *Planning Community Mental Health Services for women: A multiprofessional handbook.* London: Routledge.

Johnstone, L. (1989) *Users and Abusers of Psychiatry: A critical look at traditional psychiatric practice.* London: Routledge.

Martin, D. & Lyon, P. (1984) Lesbian Women and Mental Health Policy. In: L. E. Walker (Ed) *Women and Mental Health Policy.* London: Sage.

McNamara, J. (1996) Out of Order: Madness is a Feminist and Disability Issue. In: J. Morris (Ed) *Encounters with Strangers: Feminism and Disability.* London: Women's Press.

Mental Health Act Commission (1997) *Seventh Biennial Report 1995-97.* London: The Stationery Office.

Nicolson, P. (1989) Counselling women with post-natal depression. *Counselling Psychology Quarterly* 2 123–132.

Pembroke, L. R. (1993) *Eating Distress: Perspectives from Personal Experience.* Chesham: Survivors Speak Out.

Perkins, R. (1996) Women, Lesbians and Community Care. In: K. Abel *et al* (Eds)(1996) *Planning Community Mental Health Services for Women: A multi-professional handbook.* London: Routledge.

Perkins, R., Nadirshaw, Z., Copperman, J. & Andrews, C. (Eds) (1996) *Women in Context: Working papers on women, mental health and good practices.* London: GPMH.

Pilgrim, D. (1990) Competing Histories of Madness. In: R. P. Benthall (Ed) *Reconstructing Schizophrenia.* London: Routledge.

Read, J. & Reynolds, J. (Eds) (1996) *Speaking our Minds: An anthology.* Basingstoke: Macmillan.

Rogers, A. & Pilgrim, D. (1996) *Mental Health Policy in Britain: A critical introduction.* London: Macmillan.

Rose, S. M., Peabody, C. G. & Stratigeas, B. (1991) Undetected abuse among intensive case management clients. *Hospital and Community Psychiatry* **42** (5) 235–50.

Rowe, D. (1991) *Breaking the Bonds.* London: Fontana.

Showalter, E. (1987) *The Female Malady.* London: Virago.

Ussher, J. (1991) *Women's Madness: Misogyny or Mental Illness.* Hemel Hempstead: Harvester Wheatsheaf.

Williams, J., Watson, G., Smith, H., Copperman, J. & Brown, D. (1993) *Purchasing Effective Mental Health Services for Women: A framework for action.* Canterbury: University of Kent.

Williams, J. & Watson, G. (1996) Mental Health Services that Empower Women. In: T. Heller, J. Reynolds, R. Gomm, R. Muston and S. Pattison (Eds) *Mental Health Matters: A reader.* Buckingham: Open University Press.

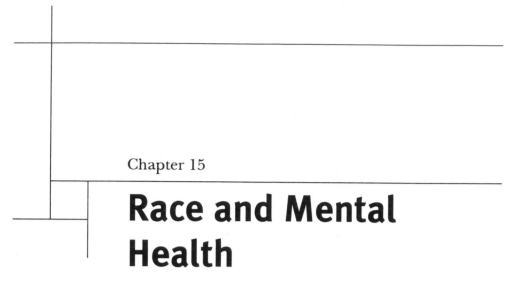

Chapter 15

Race and Mental Health

Peter Ferns

An historical perspective

Racism and psychiatry

The history of racism in psychiatry and psychology is as old as the disciplines themselves. Many of the basic concepts and theoretical approaches were formulated at a time when pseudo-scientific racism was being postulated as a justification for the exploitation and colonisation of Black people.

The effects of racism on psychiatry can be directly linked to the early stereotypes about Black people arising from pseudo-scientific racism. Bizarre mental 'diseases' such as 'drapetomania' were described which literally meant the uncontrollable urge for slaves to run away from 'home' ie the plantation (Cartwright, 1851). Generally, Black people were seen as:

- lacking civilisation (Tuke, 1858)

- degenerate primitives (Lewis, 1965)

- noble savages (Pritchard, 1835)

- childlike races (Evarts, 1913)

At the Core of Mental Health © Pavilion 2000

■ subhuman species (Hunt, 1863)

(Quoted in Fernando, 1991)

Many of these early stereotypes are still reflected in recent research studies (Fernando, 1988) and are evidenced in practice involving Black service users such as decisions about 'dangerousness' (Browne, 1997). For instance, African Caribbeans in Britain have been described as having suffered 'cultural stripping' leaving their family life weak and unstable (Pryce, 1979). Conversely, Asian families have been seen as too stable and rigid – almost too strong a culture (Lawrence, 1982).

Mental 'illness' has always had a social construction and as such is open to the influences of racism in society. One fairly spectacular illustration of the social construction of mental 'illness' was the declassification of homosexuality as an 'illness' by the American Psychiatric Association in 1973. Political, ideological and social forces always impact on the diagnostic process by influencing the judgement of behaviour and its underpinning beliefs and assumptions. Clinical practice is based upon theories and models of practice which are covertly value-laden as well as social customs and practices which are directly culturally defined.

The Western Scientific Tradition

The basic scientific methodology underpinning psychiatry and psychology derives from a Western tradition of science and more precisely, a 'reductionist' approach, which in Western psychiatry not only divides the mind from the body and spirit but also compartmentalises the mind into cognition (intellect and thinking) and affect (emotions and feelings). The 'reductionist' approach increases the danger of objectifying people and their feelings as collections of facts or bits of data that can be sifted independently of each other and brought together to provide a rational solution to mental distress. The messy reality of human experiences can get lost in a blizzard of half-truths and conjectures which are then ordered using scientific methodologies to provide a comfortingly tidy resolution to a painful problem being presented to mental health services.

Many Black and ethnic minority service users find the 'reductionist' approach unhelpful and irrelevant to their experiences of mental distress. The unity of mind/body/spirit is a lived experience for many African and Asian service users. Feelings, emotions and behaviours are inextricably linked with the individual's wider social, physical and spiritual existence. Mental distress may well involve a disturbance of several of these interlinked fields of existence and can only be treated by addressing the problems presented in an holistic way.

The legacy of racism today

The legacy of racism in the past is still with us today. It may not be as overt or easily identifiable, but its very covert nature makes it even more insidious and difficult to eradicate. Society currently carries the scars of this legacy in the form of structural inequalities which have built up over a very long period of time both nationally and internationally. It is reflected not only in the operation of institutions and structural processes within nations but also in relations between countries in terms of world-trade, economic barriers and tariffs, and 'Third World debt'.

The result of structural inequalities in society are reduced life opportunities for Black people in, for example, employment, health, education and housing. The flip-side of this situation is the continued privilege accorded to the White majority who, whether conscious of it or not, have benefited from the reduction in competition for jobs, health, housing and education. White people in positions of power and authority have not had to deal with the issue of racial discrimination in any meaningful way due to the imbalance of power between Black and White people in society. Influential people can maintain their position and status in society without having to develop skills and knowledge in responding to the needs and interests of Black people in their communities. The issue of racism then becomes an unpleasant reality that powerful people would rather forget or ignore as it raises uncomfortable questions about competence and fairness regarding their own position. The standard response has been to engage in a process of denial and apathy, providing all the fuel that institutional racism requires. People do not have to be actively racist to discriminate in organisations, they merely have to follow the rules and regulations which conveniently discriminate for them. Denial and apathy are the greatest challenges in racism today as in an organisational environment this results in 'lazy' thinking taking over, and stereotypes becoming more influential in practice as ignorance and incompetence are rewarded equally with good practice. The reinforcement of racist stereotypes often leads to the introduction of other stereotypes about women, disabled people, lesbians and gay men. The result is an increase in covert and intractable racism within the organisation and, at best, a growth in structural inequality; at worst, a justification of it. Overall, the outcome is a self-reinforcing cycle of institutional racism.

Research findings

Diagnosis of 'mental illness'

There have been consistent patterns of higher rates of diagnosed 'severe mental illness' over the last two decades for African Caribbean people compared to White people. Figures vary from between 3 to 6 times, up to 18 times higher (McGovern & Cope, 1987; Harrison *et al*, 1988). Evidence of levels of 'mental illness' amongst Asian people is less consistent. Cochrane (1977) suggested that rates for Indian and Pakistani people were lower than for English and Caribbean people. Whereas, Dean *et al* (1981) showed higher rates of admission for Indian men compared to Whites. Hitch (1981) showed higher admissions for Pakistani women and lower rates for Indian women compared to White British women. Some research shows that schizophrenia is 1.5 times more prevalent in Asian people compared to White people (Dean *et al*, 1981).

On the whole, evidence shows that the rates of diagnosis of schizophrenia are lower for Asians compared to African Caribbeans. Young Asians have a higher compulsory admission rates compared to other Asians and there are higher rates of informal admissions for young Asian women (Bowl & Barnes, 1992). Nazroo (1997) found that 'mental illness' was more prevalent amongst Asians who were born here or who migrated at a very early age and who were fluent in English compared to other Asians.

Explanations of lower rates of 'mental illness' amongst Asian people include the reduction of risk due to family and community support (Beliappa, 1991). However, other research has contradicted this explanation finding that family support does not protect people from the risk of 'mental illness' (Butt & Mirza, 1997). Another explanation put forward by several researchers has been that symptoms have not always been recognised (Littlewood & Lipsedge, 1989; Furnham & Sheikh, 1993). Soni Raleigh (1995) has suggested that unwillingness and difficulties in approaching services along with language barriers and the lack of culturally appropriate services may be more likely reasons.

Compulsory detention

There has also been higher usage of Compulsory Orders against African Caribbean people, especially young men. One study shows that the greatest disparity between African Caribbeans and Whites was in the 16–29 age range, with migrant African Caribbeans having an admission rate 17 times that of their White counterparts for Part II (civil sections) of the *Mental Health Act 1983,* and 25 times the rate for Part III (forensic sections) (McGovern & Cope, 1989).

According to another study, African Caribbean people were more likely to be compulsorily detained than White people after an assessment for an emergency admission (Section 4 of *Mental Health Act 1983*) and none in the study were persuaded to enter the hospital voluntarily. They were generally less likely to be offered alternatives to hospital and there were similarities in outcomes found between White people and people of Asian origin (Bowl & Barnes, 1992).

Explanations for the over-representation of Black people amongst those who are compulsorily detained have included genetic or inherent factors for this group, the reactions of Black people to White racism and cultural dissonance between Black patients and White practitioners (Browne, 1997). Biological factors and other inherent factors for African Caribbean people are not borne out by other studies in the Caribbean that do not show higher rates of diagnosed schizophrenia compared to White Europeans. Other explanations have been put forward are to do with cultural and Eurocentric bias in the diagnostic process, racism and stereotyping (Shashidharan, 1989; Fernando, 1997). A study by Nazroo found that rates of psychosis among people of Caribbean origin were much less when measured in the home by people of the same ethnic background compared to the assessments of made by White psychiatrists in hospitals (Nazroo, 1997).

Links with the Criminal Justice System

Cope's (1989) study of source of referrals for two secure units found that 91% of African Caribbeans were referred by prisons compared to 54% of White referrals. It was also found that African and Caribbean patients who were compulsorily detained were four times more likely than White patients to be transferred to high security units (Bolton, 1984). Judgements about 'dangerousness' involving Black people are often influenced by racial stereotypes and Black people are more likely to have 'required' physical restraint prior to or upon admission – 16%, compared to 2% for White patients (Browne, 1997).

A study found that Black women (18%) were much more likely to be detained by the police on a Section 136 of the *Mental Health Act* compared to White women (2%). Overall, Black people were much more likely to be held under a Section 136 compared to White people (24%, compared to 15%) (Browne, 1997).

Treatment

Over-medication of Black people has been found by several studies. A typical study in East London by Littlewood and Cross, found that Caribbean, African and Asian patients were more likely than Whites to be receiving major tranquillisers, intra-muscular medication and electro-convulsive therapy without a diagnosis of depression (quoted by Grimley & Bhat, 1989; see also Browne, 1997). One study found that many more White people had experienced talking therapy at some time in their lives compared to African Caribbean people; 75% compared to 45% (Wilson & Francis, 1997).

Low take-up of services has also been well-documented in various studies (Beliappa, 1991; Baylies *et al*, 1993) but it is important to note that when appropriate services are available to Black people they do use them and benefit (Wilson & Francis, 1997).

Summary

It appears from the research evidence that Black people are experiencing a poorer quality service compared to White people. There are greater risks of being misdiagnosed and they are more likely to experience over-medication with fewer options for psychological treatments such as talking therapies. Many Black people are entering the psychiatric system through compulsory detention or through the Criminal Justice System. This may be linked with the lack of preventative services and the likelihood of coming to mental health services in times of crisis. There is a clear pattern of under-reaction to serious areas of need arising from mental distress which leads to crisis intervention when severe damage triggers an emergency. Alternatively, there is evidence of over-reaction to minor problems which often becomes punitive in nature and actually precipitates a crisis where one could have been avoided with a less heavy-handed approach. The overall outcome is that Black people tend to be concentrated in the more formal and secure end of the mental health system rather than the informal and preventative end. It also suggests that the basic rights of Black service users are more vulnerable compared to other patients and in need of greater safeguarding within the system. Through all the negative data about the experiences of Black people in the psychiatric system, it is important for practitioners to remember that Black people still want and need good mental health services. Francis and Wilson (1997) found that Black service users:

> '...*appear to be concerned to carry on a meaningful dialogue with mental health professionals, to exercise their rights as people and as patients, and to express their views in order to help bring about a system of care and treatment more responsive to their particular needs.*'

Understanding discriminatory barriers

One of the major challenges facing mental health services in the future is overcoming the consequences of discriminatory experiences of Black people in the past. Unless mental health services can begin to engage Black people who need them in a positive and proactive way, there will not be sufficient opportunities to build up a critical mass of beneficial experiences of services for Black communities. Negative expectations of Black people and mental health practitioners all too often result in self-fulfilling prophecies of poor and discriminatory service (Westwood *et al*, 1989). In order to address this familiar 'litany' of institutional racism inherent to the whole mental health system, it is important to identify precisely the barriers to services in order to focus an effective planning process needed to overcome them.

Engaging Black and ethnic minority people in mental health services

Most communities have negative views about mental distress and stigma is usually attached to the use of psychiatric services. The effects of this stigma can be devastating in some communities where social status, marriage prospects, personal economic future and the 'saving of public face' are essential for the achievement of socially valued roles. Mental health services must be more aware of the negative social impacts of mental distress and work actively to counteract them.

Through recent survey work with Black people in mental health services, it has emerged that the fear of stigma and shame can directly lead to the avoidance of using services at an earlier stage of mental distress and serious damage to the fabric of the family and the community may occur before a person uses services as a 'last resort'.

The lack of preventative services compounds the feeling of dread many Black and ethnic minority people feel when they or their families realise that they need skilled assistance. The issue of mental distress has often never been discussed and there are many myths and negative fantasies about its effects. Services have to take on a more educative role in relation to Black and ethnic minority communities to inform people of the realities of mental distress, the treatments available and support for people and their families. Preventative services which are part of everyday community services or linked to specific community cultural and religious groups would be an invaluable source of education and support and engage people at an early stage in their mental distress.

The problems of misdiagnosis and over-medication are well-documented, as mentioned earlier. Black and ethnic minority service users have been very clear that they wish to be offered alternatives to purely physical forms of treatment (Wilson & Francis, 1997). Over-medication and over-reliance on physical treatments such as ECT are often born out of the practitioner's lack of understanding of the cultural explanations and meanings of the person's experience of distress or fear arising from racial stereotyping.

Lack of understanding and fear results in practitioners resorting to the 'quick fix', which is often cheaper and quicker in the short-term from the practitioner's viewpoint, but it means storing up longer-term and more intractable problems for services in the future. Black and ethnic minority service users have suffered the 'quick fix' for too long and have sustained a great deal of physical, social and spiritual damage from this superficial and ineffectual approach.

During the process of engagement and relationship-building with service users, practitioners must stop and question a reliance on physical treatments – particularly with Black and ethnic minority people – and explore alternative therapies which are less intrusive, with less potential for damage and which are more culturally appropriate. A good discipline to safeguard the rights of service users is to ensure that they participate in the decision-making and implementation process around any treatment programmes – engagement will be optimised if people are actively encouraged to have a say in the process of how they are to get better.

Mental health services have frequently been experienced by Black and ethnic minority communities as being more geared to social control rather than genuine concern for the wellbeing of people who need assistance due to their mental distress. Evidence for this fear is clear in the stronger links between psychiatry and the Criminal Justice System that often exists for Black and ethnic minority people compared to White service users (Fernando *et al*, 1998).

Recent audits of race equality practice undertaken by the author in a few mental health services have thrown up a number of issues. Firstly, that services must begin to demonstrate that they can provide genuine assistance to Black and ethnic minority people in mental distress in the least restrictive way possible, in line with the principles underpinning the *1983 Mental Health Act*. The use of compulsory orders with Black and ethnic minority people must be clearly justified and not littered with vague fears about not taking medication, broad assumptions about future behaviour or anxieties due to the lack of appropriate support services in the community.

Whilst the mistakes of the past cannot be undone, what is most important for Black and ethnic minority service users is that professionals learn from their mistakes. There needs to be an acknowledgement of institutional racism in services and an earnest commitment by practitioners to eradicate it and promote an holistic approach to service provision. Black and White practitioners must build trust with Black and ethnic minority service users by adopting a social model approach to mental health and openly working with the tensions and contradictions of the current psychiatric system which exist for Black and ethnic minority people (Sashidharan, 1994). Openness and genuine commitment from practitioners will build trust and confidence. The majority of Black service users in recent consultations by the author have expressed a strong desire to be treated in a human way by mental health professionals, and that humanity can only be expressed through a more equal relationship with all service users, based on mutual trust and respect.

Limitations in current service provision

Black and ethnic minority service users are often faced with a narrower range of options than White service users, due to the lack of culturally appropriate services (Webb-Johnson, 1991). Religious and cultural needs for food and personal care are not taken seriously enough by service providers. The fundamental basis of providing therapeutic help is to ensure that basic physical needs are met before tackling issues of coping, getting better, personal development and self-actualisation. Practitioners need to develop a range of treatment options and packages of assistance which are culturally appropriate and relevant to Black and ethnic minority people. A new partnership has to be forged between mental health professionals, traditional healers and other community resources to maintain the wellbeing of Black and ethnic minority people who are vulnerable to mental distress.

Based on fieldwork in over 20 local authorities undertaken by the author for the Department of Health, it was often the case that Black and ethnic minority service users had to travel longer distances to access appropriate services. The 'block' nature of many services militates against meeting the specific individual cultural and religious needs of Black and ethnic minority people and services are planned according to the level of demand measured in the numbers of people requiring a particular form of service. Small and scattered ethnic minority communities are unlikely to reach the threshold at which the planning process for culture-specific services is triggered. The result is that some independent sector services are commissioned which are targeted in terms of need but cover a broad geographic area as their catchment. Even when there are substantial numbers of Black and ethnic minority people in an area, it was not unusual to find poorly located services for those particular communities.

Service development plans must reflect the whole community's needs, taking into account those in most need, and culturally specific services must be located in an accessible way for Black and ethnic minority communities. Mainstream services must also be developed in parallel with culturally-specific services to ensure that all services are appropriate for an ethnically diverse community. In this way, a range of choices can be offered to Black and ethnic minority people which would be on a par with other groups of service users.

Examples have been found by the author where 'residential' and 'therapeutic' environments have been provided for Black people and where staff have been unable to even communicate with a person from a non-English speaking background. Therapeutic and other forms of assistance cannot be offered to mental health service users unless there is clear communication with them. Services must have easy access to a range of interpreter services, particularly for mental health assessments of non-English speaking people.

Community interpreters should be trained in working in the mental health field and have some basic knowledge of mental health legislation and the rights of service users. The role of community psychiatric nurses, doctors, approved social workers and others should be explained to interpreters in training and they should be given an opportunity to clarify their own role in relation to all of these other practitioners. Black and ethnic minority practitioners and family members should not be expected to provide an informal interpreting service unless practitioners have this written into their job descriptions with appropriate remuneration for their additional skills. It would be preferable to recruit more first language practitioners and develop policies to achieve this in areas where there are large populations of Black and ethnic minority communities should be of highest priority.

There have been several initiatives to inform Black and ethnic minority communities about local mental health services but these have often been in the form of written documents translated into the main local languages. Studies have shown a poor level of knowledge about existing services amongst Black and ethnic minority communities (Soni Raleigh, 1995) as well as other barriers of poor experiences in the past and the lack of trust mentioned earlier. There needs to be a more creative usage of different formats and the media available in an area such as video, radio, Black press and the Internet. The use of stories and plays has also been very successful in work with Black elders.

Mental distress increases threats to self-identity for any service user and for Black and ethnic minority people additional threats of racial and cultural stereotyping increase their vulnerability (Fernando *et al*, 1998). Practitioners must guard against stereotyping creeping into their practice, especially in relation to assessments of needs and risks, decision-making and the recording of data about people. If stereotyping is not addressed, it tends to result in a self-fulfilling prophecy where people are exposed to environments and service settings which are based on oppressive assumptions about them, and these environments then elicit the expected responses due to the behaviours which are consequently shaped by them.

The effects of stereotyping on individuals can be extremely damaging, particularly where it leads to the internalisation of oppression resulting in low self-esteem, negative racial and cultural identity and a lack of motivation to take action or accept change in one's life (Stephen, 1996). It is easy in such a situation for people to enter a state of 'learned helplessness' and some Black and ethnic minority service users may even reject assistance from anyone who may be influential in maintaining their racial and cultural identity, especially Black practitioners. Recent findings from consultancy by the author have indicated that some Black and ethnic minority service users may eventually become 'rootless' and isolated within their own communities, often presenting difficult and complex problems for families, friends and services trying to help them.

All practitioners must actively challenge racial and cultural stereotypes wherever they find them. They should also ensure that Black and ethnic minority service users have access to positive role models of other Black and ethnic minority people who have survived the psychiatric system and are now contributing their skills and talents in the community. Self-help and self-advocacy groups are a useful source of such role models. Black and ethnic minority service users are often in need of facilitation around their self-advocacy and assertiveness skills, so training and development opportunities should be built into assistance and treatment programmes. 'Learned helplessness' can be overcome through a focus on achievable goals set with the service user, which take into account their cultural context, and which addresses their interests and concerns. It is important for practitioners to celebrate improvement and progress and ensure that adequate community supports are in place on a continuous basis. The remainder of the chapter suggests how progress may be made towards an holistic approach to service provision.

Outlining an holistic approach to service provision

The patterns of racial discrimination in services highlighted by research and the practical barriers summarised above help us to clarify the shape of holistic service provision for Black and ethnic minority people. Holistic service provision is defined in the following way:

> '*A holistic model takes into account a wide range of social, economic, political and psychological factors influencing Black people's lives. Assessment of individual need would be based on all of these factors and would seek to identify discriminatory barriers in order to remove them. A holistic approach more clearly acknowledges the effects of social stress in Black people's lives and the variety of ways in which individuals cope with this. The model is based on an understanding of personal and institutional discrimination. It seeks to identify and work with the strengths of Black families and others who are vulnerable to oppression and work with them in an empowering way. Cultural diversity is valued, and culturally appropriate services are central to a holistic model. To achieve this agencies, must work together to provide a comprehensive and coherent network of services.*'
>
> (Dutt & Ferns, 1999)

The diagram overleaf represents an holistic model which was discussed in a recent Department of Health publication.

Holistic assessment

For Black and ethnic minority people, assessment is one of the most important 'drivers' of change and development in services; unless needs are identified and assessed accurately in the first place, there will be no pressure in the system to change, or reliable data on which

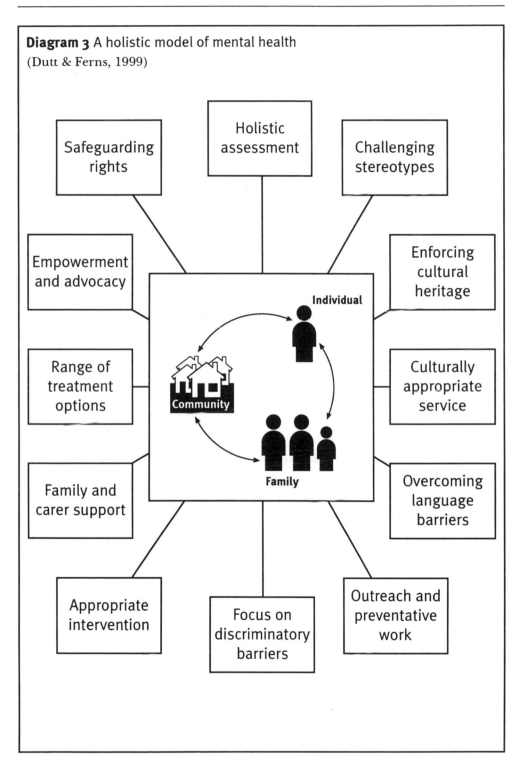

Diagram 3 A holistic model of mental health
(Dutt & Ferns, 1999)

Safeguarding rights

Holistic assessment

Challenging stereotypes

Empowerment and advocacy

Enforcing cultural heritage

Range of treatment options

Individual

Culturally appropriate service

Community

Family

Family and carer support

Overcoming language barriers

Appropriate intervention

Focus on discriminatory barriers

Outreach and preventative work

to base the future development of services. Assessment of needs has to take a broader and more holistic view of personal needs. The mental health service user movement maintain that an over-emphasis of medical diagnosis merely leads to a pathologising approach where the individual person is seen as the 'problem' to be tackled by services instead of addressing the discriminatory barriers and the mental distress, feelings or behaviours that are troubling the person. The mental distress of Black and ethnic minority people has to be seen in the context of their social circumstances in an institutionally racist society. In a social model approach, the wider socio-economic context can never be divorced from the sources of stress and mental distress which exist in their lives due to the all-pervasive quality of racism in society. Medical diagnosis tells us little about actual support needs for community living, as one individual with a similar medical condition or diagnosis to another may have very different personal and support needs from someone else.

There are a variety of possible formats for holistic assessments but any assessment format should incorporate an examination of individual factors which represent a mind/body/spirit unity as well as an individual's social and physical environment. Assessment questions should cover the following issues:

- the sense of purpose and deeper meaning in a person's life

- the sense of wellbeing and positive racial and cultural identity of the person

- their physical health

- the relationships and valued social roles in the person's community

- the provision of adequate material and financial requirements for the person's chosen lifestyle.

Challenging stereotypes and discriminatory barriers

The existence of racial stereotypes in mental health work has been discussed earlier; the danger of pathologising any mental health service user is great. The additional dimension of institutional racism makes the Black mental health service user more vulnerable to a process of blame. An holistic approach would entail the avoidance of making assumptions about people based on any categorisation or ascribed characteristics of the individual due to their membership of a particular social group. Stereotypes would be exposed and challenged through a process of reflective practice, informed questioning of traditional practices and constructive challenge between peers. An holistic approach would also involve and emphasise dealing with the social processes of discrimination and devaluation addressing these issues through assessment and planning to meet individual needs.

Reinforcing cultural heritage

Poor assessment and planning with Black and ethnic minority service users is often due to cultural misunderstanding and lack of appreciation of the importance of cultural heritage on the part of practitioners (Fernando, 1991). Cultural heritage and spirituality must be maintained and developed through mental health services as it can often be a valuable source of personal growth and development. It may form a route through to recovery and healing for Black and ethnic minority people who are experiencing trauma or mental distress in their lives. Understanding and supporting the chosen lifestyle of Black and ethnic minority people within their specific cultural and religious context is essential for improving the quality of their lives and this goal must be the bottom line for all mental health services.

Culturally appropriate services

All mental health work takes place in a social and cultural context. The service user and practitioner often represent two different cultural contexts coming together and often for different purposes. The social interaction between them takes place at several different levels simultaneously, both macro and micro. At the macro level, societal and political factors, as well as cultural differences, influence the diagnostic and treatment process. There are repercussions on clinical observations, the use of psychological theories and the choice of a social or medical model in the process. At the micro level, the service user and practitioner bring with them a whole set of their own cultural assumptions, beliefs and mythologies, including their prejudices and stereotypes of each other. The complexity of this micro level is often masked by the use of the simple phrase 'common sense'. Often, it may not be 'common' to both parties at all, moreover it can easily make very little 'sense' if seen from different cultural perspectives. Practitioners must be self-aware, not only of their own prejudices or stereotypes (for we all have them), but also of regulating their cultural assumptions, which may not be shared by a Black and ethnic minority service user. Culture is complex and is not an easy concept to understand – practitioners must make conscious efforts to get to grips with this aspect of their professional practice if they wish to engage in reflective practice (Fernando, 1991).

The conceptualisation and expression of emotions and mental distress itself is shaped by cultural influences.

> '*Complicated personal, cultural and social meaning complexes may fashion the way in which emotion is expressed through behaviour; and the socio-cultural context in which an emotion is felt and expressed may effect the outcome. Not only that, but emotions may be suppressed, distorted or exaggerated for psychological, social or cultural reasons; and some feelings, or the way they are expressed, may be designated as "illness".'*
> (Fernando, 1991)

The basic approach to the measurement of health itself varies from one culture to another. In Chinese culture, it may be dependent on the balance between 'yin' and 'yang', the two complementary poles of all-pervasive life energies. It is common in Indian culture to view good health as being dependent on the degree of harmony between the person and his or her social group. African views of health are more social than biological and dependent on social and religious behaviour or maintaining moral principles in everyday living. In Tibetan psychiatry, there are no general treatments but diagnosis is based on specific causes of illness for a particular person. There are often subtle, interwoven factors taken into consideration and the individual's behaviour, regardless of their confused mental state, is imbued with meaning. Hence, mental 'illness' can result from leading a life that runs counter to one's natural disposition, or from 'poisons' which may be spiritual, physical or environmental in nature, or from ghosts or other invisible forces.

Culturally appropriate services incorporate culturally appropriate treatment options which address a mind/body/spirit unity that exists in many ethnic minority cultures. The use of spiritual approaches, talking therapies and other non-physical treatments should also be promoted through a holistic approach.

Transcultural mental health work cannot by definition be monocultural. The understanding and employment of different cultural perspectives must be inherent to the practice of transcultural mental health work. Practitioners must not only be aware of their own cultural 'style' but they must also reflect other people's cultural styles in their practice, most importantly the cultural 'style' of the Black and ethnic minority service user. One model being developed seeks to examine different dimensions of culture which are common to everyone. In a recent publication (Dutt & Ferns, 1999), three dimensions of cultural style were put forward as a starting point in the process of increasing the cultural flexibility of practitioners and reflect the cultural preferences of Black and ethnic minority service users in mental health work. The three dimensions chosen were: understanding mental distress, the response to mental distress and the approach to intervention and treatment.

The first dimension involves understanding mental distress on a continuum of increased self-awareness and a contemplative style to one of analysis of factual detail involving a problem-solving style. In the second dimension, the continuum ranges from acceptance of one's situation and nature, leading to striving for more harmony and balance of energies in one's situation. Here, there are attempts to get in touch with the causes of distress. The other end of this continuum is a control-oriented approach where efforts are made to deal directly with the effects of distress, regardless of its causes, in line with a Western approach of controlling and eradicating unwanted symptoms of illness. The third dimension involves a range of promoting the harmony of the social group over and above the individual as opposed to primary concern for the personal rights and autonomy of the individual. These dimensions of cultural style are a useful first step for practitioners to begin to explore a range of alternative styles to intervention in situations involving Black and ethnic minority service users. There are no wrong and right ways of dealing with each situation but it does encourage practitioners to become more flexible in their approach to practice.

The development of culturally specific services and the adaptation and improvement of mainstream services is central to an holistic approach. Feeling welcome, experiencing unconditional concern for one's wellbeing, and feeling 'at home' in service settings is an important part of recovery from mental distress. Many Black and ethnic minority people in the psychiatric system never experience these feelings in current services. They are always the stranger on the edge of a crowd of devalued mental health service users – the 'most isolated' amongst a group of the 'most rejected'. Feeling comfortable in therapeutic settings for Black and ethnic minority service users is a real challenge for mental health services in the current system. Culturally appropriate services is one way forward in achieving this outcome.

Outreach and preventative work

The stigma attached to mental distress mentioned earlier can only be broken down through better mental health education programmes and good communication channels between services and Black and ethnic minority communities. A proactive approach to dealing with psychological stress will reduce the current crisis-oriented stance taken by services with Black and ethnic minority communities. Positive action should be taken, in developing viable community support services, reinforcing informal networks and working in partnership with Black-led organisations and community groups, to establish a network of preventative services for Black and ethnic minority communities.

Preventative work can take place on various levels and a model developed in the child protection field (Hardiker *et al*, 1995) has been adapted here, as it provides a useful template for the development of appropriate preventative mental health services for Black and ethnic minority people.

Level 1 – Community development

This level of preventative work focuses on education, information and empowerment work in Black and ethnic minority communities. The main aim of this level is to create more 'inclusive' communities which do not attach stigma to mental distress and are more tolerant of a range of behaviours from people experiencing mental distress. Through strengthening existing supportive natural networks in Black and ethnic minority communities, it is possible to increase the capacity of communities to work more positively to meet the needs of mental health service users. Work at this level should also address the wider social conditions which increase people's vulnerability to psychological stress and health problems. This would include poverty, unemployment, homelessness and poor housing as well as other related issues such as policing, availability of general health services and environmental health.

Level 2 – Strengthening individual support networks

This level involves supporting personal relationships of Black and ethnic minority people with emerging problems of mental distress, especially their family relationships. Practitioners would have to understand the cultural religious context in which the family is operating to intervene in a culturally appropriate manner. If intervention is not forthcoming at this level it is likely that these problems will become more severe and require more intrusive interventions. Emphasis at this level is put on short-term and focused interventions which do not create longer-term dependency on services. The nature of these interventions may be more of a generalised therapeutic nature with greater usage of non-statutory, community-based or user-led services. The main aim of this level of work would be to prevent entry into more formalised and longer-term psychiatric services.

Level 3 – Focused therapeutic intervention

At this level, individuals and their families are at risk of experiencing serious problems which may involve abuse or neglect of the individual or may present dangers for the family or others. Effective risk assessment and crisis intervention may be required at this level but to maintain a preventative stance it would be necessary to engage in this action in an empowering and non-discriminatory way. This may appear to be contradictory to some people, but the setting of clear boundaries and the application of external controls when a person is fearful of being out of control can be an extremely empowering process on the road to gaining autonomy in one's life. Timely intervention is thus paramount so that unnecessary harm is prevented to Black and ethnic minority people and their families, but punitive and over-reactive measures are avoided. A cautionary note has been sounded by several inquiries into the care and treatment of Black and ethnic minority mental health service users, where it has been highlighted that practitioners must not enter a state of inaction due to the fear of being accused of being racist – avoidance and inaction are just as discriminatory as punitive over-reaction. More use of specialised therapeutic and remedial services may be required at this level in addition to similar community-based resources at Level 2. The main aim of this level of preventative work should be to return the person to their chosen lifestyle and enable the family to operate in a healthy manner within its particular cultural context.

Black and ethnic minority families have to be fully involved in the process of treatment where this is desired by service users. If there are conflicts, mental health services should be working hard to mediate and resolve these difficulties. In many ethnic minority cultures, the role of the individual in the family and the maintenance of good family relationships is a fundamental part of good mental health. Black and ethnic minority families require better information and a range of culturally appropriate support services to ensure accessible and reliable back-up for their efforts to assist their family members in distress.

Level 4 – Consistent support and personal development

The most important aspect of work at this level is the consistent and facilitative quality of support offered to individuals who may have well-established mental health problems with regular periods of mental distress. The aims of practitioners would be to create contingency plans for periods of distress in order to avoid future crises and counteract the effects of institutionalisation and other damaging effects arising from using psychiatric services over a long period of time. The importance of maintaining and strengthening racial and cultural identity should not be underestimated as people are most vulnerable to internalised oppression at this level.

Black and ethnic minority service users have tended to be dealt with at Levels 3 and 4 at a point when they are already in crisis and damage has been sustained to family and personal relationships. Preventative services at Levels 1 and 2 need to be developed for Black and ethnic minority communities to create a better range of culturally appropriate services that begin to redress the power imbalance.

Redressing the power imbalance

Internalised oppression can be tackled effectively through empowerment and actions to increase self-confidence, self-esteem and reinforce racial and cultural identity. Empowerment is a process which can be facilitated by practitioners; it is not about conferring power onto service users as this recreates an unequal power relationship between service user and practitioner. Black and ethnic-minority service users may require facilitation and assistance to gain access to legitimate means of power over their own lives. Practitioners must use their professional power to enable Black and ethnic-minority service users to have greater autonomy in their lives which may initially require work to improve self-identity, particularly racial and cultural identity. Once Black and ethnic minority people feel confident and positive about who they are, they would be in a position to express their needs and wishes more clearly. Assertiveness and skills around self-advocacy are especially important for people who have been institutionalised in the psychiatric system over a period of time. Contact with Black and ethnic minority role models of other service users who have successfully recovered or coped with their mental distress and self-advocacy groups involving Black and ethnic minority people would be most effective. There would always be a need for independent advocacy services, if only as a transitional measure for those who need or prefer more direct assistance with advocacy at points in their recovery.

The use of compulsory detention with Black and ethnic minority people must always be carefully considered in light of the research in this area, bearing in mind the problems of under-reaction and over-reaction. Black and ethnic minority service users and their families must have access to complaints procedures and other mechanisms for redress if they feel that they have been unfairly treated. Such procedures should be framed within general anti-discrimination policies so that procedures are sensitive to the needs and circumstances of Black and ethnic minority people who may experience additional barriers to using complaints procedures compared to others.

Complaints procedures tend to be reactive, and a more proactive approach would be to ensure that quality assurance systems are based on the views and expectations of Black and ethnic minority service users and their families. Accurate monitoring mechanisms and enforcement of any findings are essential to avoid tokenism in this area. Black and ethnic minority service users should be directly involved in the process of monitoring and making judgements about service quality. Quality criteria must be explicitly tied to improvements in the quality of life for Black and ethnic minority service users as well as anti-discriminatory practice in services.

Conclusion

Finally, it is worth emphasising a couple of points for practitioners who may still feel a little distant from issues of race and culture in their work. Take some time to reflect on your own cultural heritage and identity. How important is it for you? How does it influence your behaviour and lifestyle today? What about your racial identity? What feelings does it leave you with being described as Black or White? How do all the issues above influence your practice? Race and culture are powerful influences on the shaping and delivery of mental health services. For many Black and ethnic minority people on the receiving end of these services this is a self-evident truth that does not require much persuasion.

Are we as mental health practitioners really in touch with our service users if we cannot see this reality for Black and ethnic minority people users? It may be an old-fashioned word but a sense of humility in approaching mental health work by practitioners is required more than ever today in an increasingly demanding and complex field of work. We must be prepared to learn from service users as well as use our expertise and skill in an empowering way. We must never lose sight of the basic humanity that binds us tightly with service users, whatever their cultural background, and we must respond to people in distress with the same commitment as if they were our relatives or friends.

A poem by Odiri

My life is a river
A river in which I gather
In the centre
Flowing down stream positively
Banks broadening
Soil enriching
My water clearing
Letting through light
Breeding colours
Changing tone
Slowing sweetly in my wealth of
Collected journeys
Carrying all of myself with me
Water of creek and stream
Brook and sea
My rivers flowing
Maketh me

One truth is worth remembering: cultural diversity is a strength in our society to be celebrated, not a problem to be feared. If practitioners try and live this truth, the nature of mental health services will be irrevocably changed. This truth cannot be summed up any better than by the following poem by a Nigerian story-teller whom I have had the privilege of working with in various consultation events with Black and ethnic minority mental health service-users. What has been highlighted in this chapter is no more than good practice in the context of a multi-ethnic society. It is not 'special' or different practice applied to a small group of Black and ethnic minority service-users, it should be integral to practice that goes on in any mental health service. Discrimination reduces the quality of service for all and racial discrimination against people in mental distress demeans us all. Black and ethnic minority communities need and deserve high quality mental health services. If we do not address this need urgently we are consigning the next generation of young people in these communities to further damage by mental health services, rather than support and assistance in achieving good mental health. Mental health practitioners who are committed to improving their services for Black and ethnic minority people are in a unique position to make a significant contribution to the future of our society through promoting social justice and equality for all in their everyday practice.

References

Baylies, C., *et al* (1993) *The Nature of Care in a Multi-racial Community: Summary report of an investigation of the support for Black and ethnic minority persons after discharge from psychiatric hospitals in Bradford and Leeds.* University of Leeds.

Beliappa, J. (1991) *Illness or Distress? – Alternative Models of Mental Health.* Confederation of Indian Organisations.

Bolton, P. (1984) Management of compulsorily admitted patients to a high security unit. *International Journal of Social Psychiatry* **30** 77–84.

Bowl, R. & Barnes, H. (1992) *Monitoring the Mental Health Act 1983: Approved Social Worker Assessments, Race and Racism — Local Authority Policy and Practice.* London: CCETSW North Curriculum Development Project.

Browne, D. (1997) *Black People and 'Sectioning': The Black Experience of Detention under the Civil Sections of the Mental Health Act.* PLACE?: Little Rock Publishing.

Butt, J. & Mirza, K. (1997) *Social Care and Black Communities – A Review of Recent Research.* London: The Stationery Office.

Cartwright, S. A. (1851) Report on the diseases and physical peculiarities of the Negro race. *New Orleans Medical and Social Journal* May, 691–715.

Cochrane, R. (1977) Mental illness in immigrants to England and Wales – an analysis of mental hospital admissions 1971. *Social Psychiatry* **12** 23–25.

Cope, R. (1989) The compulsory detention of Afro-Caribbeans under the Mental Health Act. *New Community* **15** (3) 343–356.

Dean, G., Walsh, D., Downing, H & Shelley, E. (1981) First admissions of native-born and immigrants to psychiatric hospitals in South-East England, 1976. *British Journal of Psychiatry* **139** 506–512.

Dutt, R. & Ferns, P. (1999) *Letting Through Light – a training pack on Black people and mental health.* London: Department of Health & REU.

Evarts, A. B. (1913) Dementia Precox in the colored race. *Psychoanalytic Review* **14** 388–403.

Fernando, S., Ndegwa, D. & Wilson, M. (1998) *Forensic Psychiatry, Race and Culture.* London: Routledge.

Fernando, S. (1991) *Mental Health, Race and Culture.* London: Macmillan.

Fernando, S. (1988) *Race and Culture in Psychiatry.* London: Croom Helm.

Fryer, P. (1984) *Staying Power: The History of Black People in Britain.* London: Pluto Press.

Furnham, A. & Sheikh, S. (1993) Gender, generational and support correlates of mental health in Asian immigrants. *International Journal of Psychiatry.*

Grimley, M. & Bhat, A. (1989) Mental Health. In: A. Bhat, R. Carr-Hill and S. Ohri (Eds) *Britain's Black Population.* London: Gower.

Hardiker, P., Exton, K. & Barker, M. (1995) *The Prevention of Child Abuse – A framework for analysing services.* London: NSPCC.

Harrison, G., Owens, D., Holton, A., Neilson, D. & Boot, D. (1988) A prospective study of severe mental disorder in Afro-Caribbean patients. *Psychological Medicine* **18** 643–657.

Hitch, P. (1981) Immigration and mental health: local research and social explanations. *New Community* **9**

Hunt, J. (1863) *On the Negro's Place in Nature.* London: Trubner.

Lawrence, E. (1982) In the Abundance of Water the Fool is Thirsty: Sociology and black 'pathology'. In: Centre for Contemporary Cultural Studies (Ed) *The Empire Strikes Back: Race and Racism in 70s Britain.* London: Hutchinson.

Lewis, A. (1965) Chairman's Opening Remarks. In: A. V. S. De Rueck and R. Porter (Eds) *Transcultural Psychiatry.* London: Churchill.

Littlewood, R. & Lipsedge (1982) *Aliens and Alienists: Ethnic Minorities and Psychiatry.* London: Penguin.

Littlewood, R. & Cross, S. (1980) Ethnic Minorities and Psychiatric Services. *Sociology of Health and Illness* **2** 195–201

McGovern, D. & Cope, R. (1987) The compulsory detention of males of different ethnic groups with special reference to offender patients. *British Journal of Psychiatry* **149** 265–273.

Nazroo, J. Y. (1997) *The Fourth National Survey of Ethnic Minorities – Ethnicity and Mental Health.* Findings from a National Community Survey, Policy Studies Institute.

Pritchard, J. C. (1835) *A Treatise on Insanity and Other Disorders Affecting the Mind.* London: Sherwood, Gilbert and Piper.

Pryce, K. (1979) *Endless Pressure.* Harmondsworth: Penguin.

Shashidharan, S. (1994) The need for community-based alternatives to institutional therapy. *Share Newsletter* **7** Jan, 3–5.

Shashidaran, S. (1989) Schizophrenia or just Black? *Community Care* **783** 14–15.

Soni Raleigh, V. (1995) *Mental Health in Black and Minority Ethnic People: The fundamental facts.* London: Mental Health Foundation.

Stephen, S. (1996) The need for the re-education of the Black community. *Journal of Black Therapy* **1** (1) 41–4.

Schweitzer, P. (1997) *A Place to Stay.* London: Age Exchange.
Tuke, D. H. (1858) Does civilisation favour the generation of mental disease? *Journal of Mental Science* **4** 94–110.

Webb-Johnson, A. (1991) *A Cry for Change: An Asian perspective on developing quality mental health.* London: Confederation of Indian Organisations.

Westwood, S., Couloute, J., Desai, S., Matthew, P. & Piper, A. (1989) *Sadness in My Heart – A research report.* University of Leicester: Leicester Black Mental Health Group.

Wilson, M. & Francis, J. (1997) *Raised Voices: African Caribbean and African Users' Views and Experiences of Mental Health Services in England and Wales.* London: Mind.

Concluding Comments

Di Bailey

As stated in the **Introduction** this core text aims to provide mental health practitioners with a starting point in respect of the underpinning knowledge necessary to inform competent practice. From the foregoing chapters a number of important interconnected themes emerge from the constituent parts of the book that span the domains of individual practice and service delivery.

With regards to the signs and symptoms of presenting mental distress, the chapters reveal a move away from a traditional medical approach to understanding symptomatology to one that looks towards the goals of recovery (Davies) rehabilitation and resolution (Stokes). Whilst treatment with medication may be one element of an attempt to achieve these goals, medication levels need to be appropriate and well managed, invariably accompanied by approaches that target the social and psychological components of an individual's mental distress (Kingdon). All this is a co-ordinated response to a holistic assessment that is based around the needs of individuals and their families and facilitates targeted intervention at the earliest opportunity to address the needs identified.

Such an approach on an individual level can only be achieved through effective working between the component parts of the health and social

At the Core of Mental Health © Pavilion 2000

care system particularly across the interface of primary and secondary care (Armstrong) and more generic mental health and specialist services such as those provided in the forensic domain (Houlders). More effective integrated services are needed, particularly for people with interrelated needs such as those who have mental health problems and also use substances (Bailey). Important ingredients to effective care delivery include good communication and information sharing, teamworking and follow-up through discharge and care planning. What is needed is a co-ordinated, multi-professional, interagency approach that takes a longer term view of improving services for people with mental health problems, as supported by the *National Service Framework*. This must work together with an increasing emphasis on the education and training of all staff involved in providing mental health care in both primary and more specialist settings.

In essence, the 'bricks and mortar' with which to build this integrated framework have been identified largely through Government policy and a growing evidence base about those approaches to mental distress that are deemed to deliver effective outcomes.

The Care Programme Approach provides the vehicle for encapsulating an individual's needs as part of a systematic care plan that is centred upon a clearly stated aim and a number of measurable objectives. Whilst the focus of care planning should be on achieving the goals of recovery, rehabilitation and resolution identified in **Part One**, additional positive by-products of this approach, if done properly, are improved information-sharing within the multidisciplinary team (Bailey) which supports an approach to risk assessment that is constructive and not defensive (Moore). Also it provides a foundation from which to launch an approach targeted at early intervention that involves team members in intensive and regular symptom monitoring together with a framework of intensive support, counselling and rapid access to services, if needed. The Care Planning process must form the basis of a collaborative partnership between the individual, their family and social networks.

The establishment of a collaborative partnership supports mental health practitioners together with users of mental health services to challenge the 'cure model' in psychiatry (Radford) and the resistance to recovery-oriented community-based practice that is still evident in the practice of many psychiatrists. The collaborative approach also opens up opportunities for practitioners to learn first-hand from users about the kinds of strategies they employ to manage their distress. This promotes the inclusion of complimentary therapies within an overall approach to optimise coping strategies. Thus practitioners may find themselves involved in facilitating personal empowerment of users to access therapies that may be more in tune with cultural needs and belief systems (Mitchell) and provide an alternative source of pleasure and relaxation to enable users to manage stress at times of crisis.

Whilst listening and learning from users of services is the cornerstone to effective practice at an individual level there is a need to develop such collaboration further. Collectively, user groups should be in a position to influence the way services are designed and delivered in order to improve the quality and variety of services that also confront stigmatising attitudes and practices (Barnes). This is particularly important in the current climate of social inclusion and in the light of historical developments in mainstream psychiatry that have continually identified the marginalisation of certain groups such as women and Black people.

In respect of anti-discriminatory practice, both women and Black people are vulnerable to the misunderstanding of their mental distress and being treated as homogenous groups rather than individuals (Davis). Good anti-discriminatory practice is no more than good practice in the context of a multi-ethnic society and is not special or different when applied only to marginalised groups (Ferns).

By focusing on the quest for services and individual practice that are anti-discriminatory, socially inclusive and built upon the foundations of mental health as opposed to illness, recovery, rehabilitation and resolution, we optimise the chances of improving the mental wellbeing of future generations and eradicating the stigma and social isolation that surrounds and compounds mental distress. By restoring 'humanity' in the way mental health services and practices are organised and delivered, we invite individuals to use their own strengths as human beings to cope with mental distress if and when necessary in ways that are supported and not undermined by the professionals' response.

Also Available from Pavilion

A Stakeholder's Approach to Innovation in Mental Health Services: A reader for the 21st century

Edited by Professor Shulamit Ramon

A collection of reports on the experience of, and suggestions for, setting up innovative services in mental health

This book brings together the real and varied experiences of professionals and service users, working together to develop new and imaginative services from concept to policy and practice. It looks at the need and opportunities for innovation, as well as identifying the barriers to it – physical, social, political and bureaucratic – and offers suggestions and advice on how to avoid such barriers.

This book is a must for all those working in the field of mental health looking for inspiration and practical help in challenging poor services and in setting up new ones.

Format: handbook (300pp)

Price: £29.95

Code: 60P   **ISBN** 1 84196 019 5

Looking to the Future

Edited by Thurstine Basset

This book was written to accompany the training materials developed for the Certificate in Community Mental Health Care. It contains a range of papers, each giving an up-to-date overview of a key area of mental health, exploring central issues and debates and outlining key research findings. Written by a variety of professionals, carers, and family members, the book is illustrated throughout with photographs and poems.

Apart from its direct relevance to the Certificate, it also provides underpinning knowledge for S/NVQ Level 2 in Care.

Format: handbook (220pp)

Price: £14.95

Code: 67D   **ISBN** 1 84196 031 4

Assertive Outreach in Practice

A development tool for team members, leaders and project managers

Deborah Davidson for the Institute of Applied Health and Social Policy

The aims of assertive outreach are to enable women and men with profound and enduring mental health problems to live reasonably stable lives – lives of quality – in the community, and thereby reduce the dreadful upheaval and turbulence of episodic mental illness with the knock-ons of hospitalisation and homelessness.

The assertive outreach team must deliver a service which contains the client, in the sense that it delivers a dependable and accessible, regular service. Also, by being open to the client's messages of distress, workers have the opportunity to process their thoughts and feelings in order to engage in therapeutic work.

This video training pack looks at the day-to-day challenges and practical necessities of working together in an efficient and positive way. It is split into three sections:

- weekly planning
- the daily handover
- long-term benefits and staff support.

The 40-minute experiential video is supported by group training materials.

Format: 40 minute video with supporting training materials

Price: £95

Code: 84P

Young Minds: Looking after the mental health of looked after children

This bright, accessible training pack provides research, training and resource material for all those working with, and caring for, children and young people in public care.

The pack aims to develop an understanding of the mental health needs specific to this very vulnerable and diverse group, and to help professionals and carers to recognise and support those children at risk of developing mental health problems, or who are already experiencing mental distress.

Of particular interest to: all those professionals working for looked after children and young people in the statutory, voluntary and independent sectors, including: foster carers; residential childcare staff; social workers; leaving care teams; health visitors; school nurses; paediatricians; teachers; education social workers; education welfare officers and pupil referral units.

Format: bound materials including trainer's notes, OHP and handout masters

Price: £75

Code: 68P   **ISBN** 1 841960 44 6

Whose Reality is it Anyway?

Putting social constructionist philosophy into everyday therapeutic practice
Isabelle Ekdawi, Sue Gibbons, Elizabeth Bennett and Gillian Hughes
How we make sense of the world depends on our past experience, current context and social interactions with others. The social constructionist approach to therapy aims to view a person in their total social, cultural and experiential context in order to find a way through present mental health problems. A group of clinical psychologists from Newham Community NHS Trust have put together this video-accompanied training pack presenting practical guidance to introducing a social constructionist philosophy into everyday therapeutic practice. The text explains the basis of 'social constructionism' and provides a step-by-step guide to how to use it as a key to good mental health.

Topics include:

* The social construction of reality
* Systematic techniques
* Use of language in therapy
* 'Reflecting teams'
* Ethical dilemmas
* Addressing racism

The resource employs both visual and written resource material to develop an understanding of the benefits of applying social constructionist theory in a clinical practice setting.

Format: boxed materials including video (35 mins) plus trainer's notes (80pp) incorporating illustrations, exercises and OHP masters.

Price: £125 + VAT (Total: £146.88)

Code: 62P   **ISBN** 1 84196 022 5